Introduction to Healthcare for Chinese-speaking Interpreters and Translators

Introduction to Healthcare for Chinese-speaking Interpreters and Translators

Ineke H.M. Crezee
Auckland University of Technology

Eva N.S. Ng
The University of Hong Kong

John Benjamins Publishing Company
Amsterdam / Philadelphia

The paper used in this publication meets the minimum requirements of the American National Standard for Information Sciences – Permanence of Paper for Printed Library Materials, ANSI z39.48-1984.

DOI 10.1075/z.202

Cataloging-in-Publication Data available from Library of Congress:
LCCN 2016017987 (PRINT) / 2016022097 (E-BOOK)

ISBN 978 90 272 1235 1   (HB) / ISBN 978 90 272 1236 8 (PB)
ISBN 978 90 272 6684 2 (E-BOOK)

John Benjamins Publishing Co. · https://benjamins.com

Table of contents

Part III. Healthcare specialties

Table of illustrations

List of tables

Authors' notes

This book is based on the previous, more internationally oriented (2013) version and is intended mainly for interpreters working between the English and Chinese languages. English-Chinese glossaries have been added to chapters and terminology has been localized to align with usage in Hong Kong, Taiwan and Mainland China. The chapter on medical terminology touches on traditional Chinese medical terms, which are very easy to understand for native speakers of Chinese. This chapter will explain the Latin and Greek roots which make up the majority of medical terms in English, since even native speakers of English may find these difficult to understand.

First and foremost, this book is meant to be a guide for all those who are working or wishing to work as interpreters or translators in healthcare settings but who have not had any formal training as health professionals. Healthcare interpreter trainers may also find this book useful as a course text for programs aimed at preparing interpreters for work in the healthcare setting. There is no point in simply learning medical terminology lists or surfing the internet without a good basic understanding of health and healthcare. The workings of the body are very complicated but will be explained only in very broad terms in relevant chapters, so as to enable the interpreter to have a good general understanding of what doctors and other health professionals are talking about when they explain a patient's condition to the patient or the patient's family. This publication is intended to give healthcare interpreters who do not have a professional healthcare background some very basic insights into the health system, as well as anatomy, physiology and common disorders. The field of medicine is ever evolving: researchers keep unpeeling more and more layers of previously unknown details, however the aim of this book is, first and foremost, to enable healthcare interpreters to do their job with a better knowledge of the subject area. Secondly, the book aims to provide interpreters with a good basis for ongoing self- and professional development. For this reason, language has been kept fairly plain throughout the book and information has been restricted to main points, to avoid losing readers in a jungle of details.

The blueprint for this book was based on feedback from students in one of the lead author's healthcare interpreting courses. Students said they wanted a three-part book that would firstly give a brief introduction to health interpreting, followed by an overview of various settings and finishing with a number of chapters dedicated to medical specialties. They wanted the overview of the various settings to incorporate questions commonly asked by health professionals. Students requested that the final part of the book be organized by medical specialty. Students asked that each chapter in the final part be named by specialty (e.g. Orthopedics) and organized so as to optimize preparation for assignments. Accordingly, each chapter in Part III of this book will start with an overview of anatomy and physiology of a particular body system. This will be followed by a brief look at the Latin and Greek roots which are the building blocks of much of the terminology to do with particular body systems. Healthcare interpreters will be able to go to relevant chapters prior to an interpreting assignment to re-familiarize themselves with anatomy, physiology, Latin and Greek roots and most common conditions, tests and treatment options.

This work will be equally useful to medical translators, since both interpreters and translators need to be thoroughly familiar with a setting in order to 'interpret' it. Translators working on medical reports will be able to find commonly used abbreviations. Translators who have been asked to translate health information material into community languages will be able to gain a good basic overview of related background information. Court interpreters, who often have to interpret evidence of medical doctors testifying as expert witnesses or to sight-translate medical reports in court cases such as wounding or murder, will find this book extremely useful as well.

This book will not discuss general aspects of interpreting or translation in great detail. Interested readers are referred to the excellent publications by Scimone & Ginori (1995); Pöchhacker & Shlesinger (2007); Gile (1995); Gentile, Ozolins and Vasalikakos (1996), and Hale (2004, 2007) for thorough studies on the main issues in community and legal interpreting and the need for pre-service training (Hale 2007). Pöchhacker & Shlesinger (2007) address discourse in healthcare interpreting, while issues in healthcare interpreting settings across countries are discussed in Valero-Garcés & Martin (2008).

Care has been taken to provide information which may prove useful to interpreters working between the English and Chinese languages in a range of countries. Those interpreting for new immigrants or refugees are referred to the excellent work on specific health risks in different regions of the world by Walker & Barnett (2007) and on traditional cultural values and cross-cultural communication by Jackson (2006), Camplin-Welch (2007) and particularly Holmes (2013).

The authors are under no illusion that this book will be so comprehensive as to cover the entire range of areas interpreters may come across when working in healthcare settings. With the continuing developments in the fields of technology, biophysics, biochemistry and integrative medicine, healthcare delivery will see the introduction of ever changing procedures, tests, and approaches to treatment. There is no doubt that publications like the current one will need to be updated fairly regularly to keep abreast of new procedures and changes in the use of terminology.

The authors also wish to stress that the present publication contains some anecdotal evidence relating to ethical conflicts in healthcare settings. Such anecdotes were commonly shared by experienced interpreters who wished to remain anonymous.

US spelling has been followed throughout. This means that words originating from the Greek words containing 'αι', which are spelled with 'ae' in the UK tradition, have been spelled with 'ɛ' instead. Where possible alternative spellings have been included in the index because these may come up in reference works.

The authors have attempted to avoid jargon. As an example, the term diagnostic studies has been used throughout rather than the word workup, and, similarly, the term 'blood tests' has been used rather than blood work.

The authors welcome any suggestions or comments!

Ineke Crezee and Eva Ng
Affiliations: Auckland University of Technology, Faculty of Culture and Society, Auckland, New Zealand.
The University of Hong Kong, Faculty of Arts, Hong Kong.

Notes relating to the format of English-Chinese glossaries

English words and phrases appear in alphabetical order in the glossary for each chapter. English words, phrases and explanatory notes are written in standard, non-italicized format, e.g.: nurse; Chinese translations appear in both traditional and simplified characters. All Chinese translations have been checked by three different reviewers. Where readers have other suggestions, the authors would welcome their feedback.

Disclaimer

Nothing in this book should be construed as personal advice or diagnosis and must not be used in this manner. The information provided about conditions is general in nature. This information does not cover all possible uses, actions, precautions, side-effects, or interactions of medicines, or medical procedures. The information in this book should not be considered as complete and does not cover all diseases, ailments, physical conditions, or their treatment. Any decision regarding treatment and medication for medical conditions should be made with the advice and consultation of a qualified healthcare professional.

Acknowledgments

I wish to thank Dr Ineke Crezee for inviting me to co-author this book with her. I was thrilled to be asked and to accept her invitation, because I have always had a huge interest in interpreter education and I believed this book to be a major contribution, not simply to the field of healthcare interpreting, but also to legal interpreting, as interpreters in legal settings often have to interpret medical evidence or sight-translate medical reports in court. I am indebted to Ineke for the opportunity to embark on this exciting project. As a former staff court interpreter and now an interpreter educator and researcher, I believe this practical book, completed with the wide range of medical terms and their Chinese translations, will prove an indispensable toolkit, not just for healthcare interpreters, but also to legal interpreters working between English and Chinese in their day to day work. During the process of this new endeavor, I have learned a lot from Ineke, who has long been an expert in the education of healthcare interpreting. It has been a great experience working with her as she is such a wonderful person, always inspiring and reassuring. All I see in her is nothing but positive energy, which I believe is what has enabled her to cope with her super hectic schedule of teaching and research activities.

I would also like to join Ineke in thanking all the scholars and friends (named below) for their contributions to this book, which could not have come into existence without their kind assistance and support.

Eva Ng, February 2016

First and foremost, I need to thank experienced interpreter and translator educator Dr Eva Ng for agreeing to work on this book with me. Eva gave the book her full attention, somehow finding the time alongside her many research and teaching activities: She edited chapters, liaised with reviewers and found the most excellent Steven Wing Kit Chan willing to dedicate a lot of his time to working on proofing the book and the glossaries, adding references and ensuring a polished product overall.

Peter Zen, who was born in Hong Kong, (college) educated in Canada and who spent many years living in Mainland China, put this wonderfully international background and meticulous attention to detail to good use when researching and translating all terms for the glossaries.

A huge thanks must also go to Dana Lui, Nurse Specialist – Neonatal Advanced Practice and NAATI accredited Mandarin and Cantonese-speaking interpreter and translator, for freely giving many hours of her time in extensively reviewing the glossaries. There is no doubt that Chinese-speaking interpreters and translators will find these glossaries extremely helpful.

I also owe a huge debt of gratitude to my friend Leigh (Li Chin) Hsu for all her invaluable help with the very first iteration of this book.

We also wish to give thanks to Professor Jing Chen and Dr Ester Leung for their invaluable feedback on the book.

This publication is dedicated to my parents, Han and Nelie, my husband Paul and my brother Hans. I am indebted to Dana Lui, Maureen Kearney and Linda Hand, for their valuable contributions! I also owe a debt of gratitude to Sandra Hale, who wrote the foreword to the international version of this book. Sandra Hale, Jemina Napier and the late Miriam Shlesinger, all practicing interpreters and interpreter educators, have been ongoing sources of inspiration to me.

Jenny Liang, graduate of the Auckland University of Technology degree in Graphic Design did an outstanding job in creating wonderfully clear illustrations for this book.

Many thanks to Isja Conen, Patricia Leplae, and John Benjamins Publishing Company, for their ongoing support!

Ineke H. M. Crezee, February 2016

Foreword

As interpreting and translation educators and practitioners, we are privileged to meet interesting people from different professional, educational and ethnic backgrounds with a wealth of knowledge about language and culture and about life in general. The people we interpret for and the students we teach are usually our inspiration to do better. We learn from them and they learn from us. As practitioners, we are constantly confronted with new topics, new settings, new language and new challenges. The interdisciplinarity of our work leads to constant gaps in our knowledge and skills, and as educators we feel the responsibility to do something about filling those gaps. One way is to conduct research to find answers, another is to disseminate our newly acquired knowledge in the form of teaching resources. This book is an example of the latter. Written by a healthcare professional, practicing interpreter and educator, *Introduction to Healthcare for Interpreters and Translators* is an easily accessible, practical guide for students and practicing healthcare interpreters. Ineke Crezee's motivation for writing this useful resource came from her own students, who specifically asked for a book of this kind.

Interpreters do not work in isolation. They work in specific settings with their own cultures, organizational practices, institutional goals, participant roles, and context-specific discourses. In order for interpreters to be able to interpret accurately, they must first understand the context in which they are working, the content they are to interpret, the discourse strategies used by the different participants and the discipline-specific terminology. This book aims to provide guidance on many of those context-specific issues. It describes different health settings, hospital procedures and healthcare interactions; explains the roles of primary care providers, nursing, medical and other hospital staff; provides easy-to-understand descriptions of anatomy and the different biological systems, complemented with figures and pictures; presents samples and explanations of typical illnesses and conditions, diagnoses, tests, medical procedures, treatments and medications; and descriptions of common equipment used in hospitals. The book also provides a section on the language and discourse of health and medicine, firstly by presenting an overview of its Greek and Latin origins, followed by glossaries of terms with clear definitions and lists of typical medical and other health related questions.

The book complements the content pertaining to the healthcare context and setting with anecdotes from practicing interpreters and practical advice from the authors as educators. Continuous reference to the work of interpreters and their ethical obligations is made throughout in a didactic way to make relevant links to the work of interpreters and at times translators.

Practicing interpreters and interpreting students will be able to achieve the authors' goal of increasing their knowledge of the medical field and apply it to the improvement of their practice by using this book as a practical guide. *Introduction to Healthcare for Interpreters and Translators* is a welcome addition to the training resources available.

Sandra Hale
Professor of Interpreting and Translation
School of Humanities and Languages
University of New South Wales
Australia

Foreword to this edition

Knowledge of the world and situation is a basic component of an interpreter's knowledge base. The better the accumulation of the knowledge and familiarity with all the elements of the communicative situation are, the more effective her/his integration into the communication community will be. *Introduction to Healthcare for Chinese-speaking Interpreters and Translators* serves both as a good textbook and a handy reference book for healthcare interpreters as well as an informative guide to healthcare settings, healthcare interpreting and healthcare specialties, which readers can use in long-term knowledge buildup and advance task preparation.

The book is a good example of disseminating general and systematic subject-specific knowledge which interpreters need in order to understand adequately the context and the discourse. More significantly, as the major target readership are Chinese-speaking interpreters and translators, the book, the first of its kind, boasts ample information on Chinese medicine and medical terminologies and the differences between Chinese and Western healthcare cultures. Interpreters and translators working between the English and Chinese languages will find them most relevant, practical and instructive.

What is worth special mentioning is the English-Chinese glossaries. Words are to a language what bricks are to a building. What an interpreter has to get right from the very first is what is in a word and what is in a word in the other language. The English-Chinese glossaries in *Introduction to Healthcare for Chinese-speaking Interpreters and Translators* serve well as comprehensive and accurate resources of medical jargon for both practicing interpreters and interpreter trainers and trainees, especially those who lack formal medical training. The glossaries, organized into 21 sections and added on to the end of relevant chapters, represent nearly all the subjects in the medical system. Chinese and English readers across the globe will find them extremely useful as they provide accurate renditions from English to both traditional Chinese and modern Chinese, presented side by side and perfectly grasp all the nuances of expressions. The glossaries are a coherent addition to the text proper and valuable assets to the readers.

What is equally impressive is the user-friendly blueprint and the plain language used to explain the complicated subject matter, which I believe, will make the book well-received.

Jing Chen
Professor of Interpreting
College of Foreign Languages and Cultures
Xiamen University
China

PART I

Interpreting

Chapter 1

Introduction

1. How to use this book

This book contains 28 chapters, divided into three separate parts. Part I provides a brief introduction to healthcare interpreting, while Part II provides an overview of a range of healthcare settings. Part III offers a brief overview of the main body systems, conditions and disorders, diagnostic tests and treatments, organized around the body as a framework. Some items may of necessity be mentioned under different headings, however it is hoped that this will strengthen understanding. Each chapter will be completed by a summary of the main points, to assist learning and understanding. Healthcare interpreter educators may want to use this book as a course text, while healthcare interpreters may want to use the book as a reference, checking briefly on anatomy, terminology and most commonly encountered conditions before leaving to interpret in a certain setting.

As mentioned under the authors' notes, this work will be equally useful to medical translators, since they too need to be thoroughly familiar with healthcare settings and terminology in order to successfully carry out translation assignments (Gonzalez-Davies 1998). Sections of this book will concentrate on healthcare interpreters and issues they may face in practice, including the pressures which result from being in the setting, at close quarters to both healthcare professionals and patients. Translators will not usually find themselves in the actual setting, but will still need to possess a good basic knowledge of healthcare and medical terminology to carry out their assignments. Translators will find these described in Parts II and III of this book, while cultural issues with particular relevance to those working between health professionals and patients across traditional Chinese and 'Western' medical cultures will be described in Chapter 3.

This chapter and the next will focus mainly on the development of the interpreting profession and the demand for healthcare interpreters. The wide range of studies in the area of health interpreting will be touched upon only very briefly, the reader being referred to other publications for further reading. The chapter will also touch on teaching healthcare interpreting, since healthcare interpreter educators may wish to use the book as a course text.

2. Development of the interpreting profession

Before discussing specific aspects associated with healthcare interpreting, some thought needs to be given to the development of the interpreting profession in general. Interpreting is probably one of the oldest professions in the world, the presence of interpreters being mentioned in the Bible when Joseph talks to his brothers through an interpreter (Genesis 29–50). Interpreters are also mentioned by Roman and Greek historians including Cicero, Plutarch and Herodotus (Hermann 2002; Mair 2011).

In contrast to translation theory, which has been discussed in detail by a considerable number of authors from the classical period to the current time, interpreting studies have only claimed the attention of theorists, linguists and educators much more recently. We might surmise from this that perhaps the services of interpreters have long been taken for granted and not been given much thought. It might also be assumed that, for a long time, interpreters were merely viewed as bilingual individuals who were incidentally called upon to use their linguistic skills on certain occasions (e.g. commercial or military). Such examples include Tupaia, the Tahitian, who, while engaged as a pilot and navigator, also acted as an interpreter for Captain Cook when visiting New Zealand. For centuries too, the demand for interpreters may not have been that obvious, as the residents of many countries sought to use one 'common language' (or *lingua franca*) for the purpose of communicating with speakers of other languages. In this way, Latin was long used as the *lingua franca* by scientists and statesmen from a wide range of European countries. The Renaissance and the advent of nationalist movements in many European countries were reflected in the resurgence of a feeling of national identity and a renewed interest in and emphasis on national languages. The influence of Latin (and Greek) in medical terminology remained, however, and as a result, those engaged in healthcare interpreting between English and other languages need to acquire a good knowledge of Latin and Greek roots, affixes and suffixes.

3. The demand for interpreters around the world

From the early part of the 20th century, there has been an increasing demand for interpreters worldwide. After the First World War, interpreters were employed during lengthy international negotiations over the terms of the Treaty of Versailles. After World War II, interpreters were needed for proceedings such as the Nuremberg War Crime Trials, which were attended by participants from a wide range of countries. In more recent times, civil wars, unrest and fighting in various hot spots around the world have led to an increase in the number of refugees settling in new countries, while globalization has led to international trade and the establishment of organizations such as the European Common Market, the United Nations and World Health Organization.

These changes have brought with them an ever growing demand and need for interpreters and translators.

Immigrants, in particular, bring great diversity to countries like the United States (US), the United Kingdom (UK), Canada, Australia and New Zealand (NZ). Gill, Shankar, Quirke and Freemantle (2009) suggest that linguistic diversity is such that in the UK interpreting services need to meet the needs of almost 300 different community languages, excluding dialects. Gill et al. estimate that interpreting services might be needed during some 2,520,885 general practice consultations per year.

In the US, 25% of the population speaks a language other than English at home (US Census Bureau 2011), with approximately 47 million people speaking a language other than English (Swabey & Nicodemus 2011) and more than 24 million residents speaking English "less than very well" (US Census Bureau, 2011). The first US telephone interpreting service was offered in 1981, with many others following. Today courts and hospitals in the US make extensive use of face-to-face, telephone and video interpreters. Phelan (2001) offers a good overview of the services and range of training programs offered. Roat & Crezee (2015) cover the history of health interpreting in the US and beyond.

In Australia in the 1970s, the influx of immigrants from a wide variety of cultural, ethnic, religious and linguistic backgrounds led to an increased and ongoing demand for interpreters who were able to work in various community contexts, including health, legal and public service. An accreditation system was set up for the identification of different skill levels and for the accreditation of individual translators and interpreters who were able to work at these differing levels. The National Accreditation Authority for Translators and Interpreters (NAATI) was set up (Chesher 1997), which remains involved in training, accreditation and certification of translators and interpreters to this day. Bontempo, Goswell, Levitzke-Gray, Napier & Warby (in press) report an exciting step forward in recognizing, legitimizing and professionalizing the work of Deaf Interpreters (DIs) in Australia, with the accreditation of the first DI by NAATI.

Hale (2007, 2012) argues that interpreters need specialized pre-service training to work in special settings such as the legal and medical contexts. The authors wholeheartedly agree, and would argue that, likewise, there is no doubt that healthcare interpreters need specialized training to enable them to work in health-related settings.

In the late 1980s, NZ faced controversy surrounding a large cervical cancer research project involving many women who did not have English as their first language (Coney 1988). The subsequent findings of the committee of inquiry concluded that trained interpreters should be used in interactions with patients from non-English speaking backgrounds (NESB). Subsequently, the need to use trained interpreters where practicable was included in the Health and Disability Act 1996. New Zealand society has since become increasingly multilingual and multicultural (Crezee 2009a, 2009b), with services reportedly providing services in up to 190 different community languages.

4. Health interpreting studies

Today, the need for interpreters is acknowledged around the world, with interpreting being increasingly recognized as a profession in its own right. This has led to widespread discussion of the ethics and standards of the profession, a debate which is reflected in the literature.

Since the 1980s there has been an increasing number of studies associated with interpreting in public service settings, in particular those related to health and justice. Hale (2007) provides an excellent summary of such studies. Of special interest to healthcare interpreting studies is 'the loss of crucial information in the medical encounter mediated by unprofessional interpreters' (Hale 2007, p. 200). This is also discussed in studies by Vasquez & Javier (1991) and Cambridge (1999). There is no doubt that the use of untrained interpreters can have a considerable impact on the communication between health professionals and patients. The various codes of ethics developed for interpreters (see Hale 2007, for an overview) therefore tend to focus not only on ethical conduct during the interpreting session, but also on the need for ongoing professional development and education, and the necessity to decline interpreting assignments which the interpreter should reasonably know to be beyond his or her area of competence. Many studies have therefore focused on issues relating to the interpreter's role and the interpreter's impact on interactions between healthcare professionals and patients (Athorp & Downing 1996; Wädensjö 1998; Cambridge 1999; Bolden 2000; Meyer, Apfelbaum, Pöchhacker F. & Bischoff 2003; Flores, Barton Laws & Mayo (2003); Flores 2005, 2006; Tellechea Sanchez 2005) and on ethical dilemmas (Kaufert & Putsch 1997; Angelelli 2004; Mason 2004; Hale 2005; Clifford 2005; Rudvin 2004, 2007). In New Zealand, Gray, Stubbe & Hilders (2012) developed a toolkit for the use of interpreters in general practice. In Australia, Napier, Major and Johnston have developed a medical terminology sign bank for signed language (AUSLAN interpreters). See also Major, Napier, Ferrara & Johnston (2012), Napier, Major & Ferrara (2011) and Johnston & Napier (2010). Other areas related to health interpreting (education) and translation have been explored by Lai, Heydon & Mulayim (in press); Crezee, Jülich & Hayward (2013); Ferner & Liu 2009; Fischbach 1998; Hale & Napier 2013; Holt, Crezee & Rasalingam 2003; Meyer 2001; Napier 2010, 2011; O'Neill 1998; Pöchhacker 2004; Roat 1999a, 1999b, 2000; Roberts-Smith, Frey & Bessel-Browne 1990; Roy 2000, 2002; Stewart 1995.

Researchers such as Bontempo and Napier are carrying out important work on signed language interpreter education, including the academization of interpreter education (Bontempo 2013a) and work focused on identifiying cognitive abilities and personality traits that might be predictive of interpreter ability and competence (Bontempo 2013b; Bontempo & Napier 2011). Slatyer (2014) has done important work on designing a language neutral interpreter education curriculum for student interpreters with languages of limited diffusion.

Several researchers have commented on the lack of empirical studies as to what goes on in interpreter-mediated health encounters (Angelelli 2008; Chen 2003; Swabey & Nicodemus 2011). This is most likely due to the fact that such studies would include a complex process involving ethics approval and consent from all those involved in such encounters: health professionals, interpreters and patients. Thus studies aimed at protecting a patient's right to effective communication (and protection from potential breaches of the interpreters' code of ethics) often appear to fall at the first hurdle, namely that of obtaining the approval of ethics committees who are equally intent on protecting patient rights. This apparent paradox still looks to be some way from being resolved. This is primarily due to the fact that arguably only large scale studies into interpreter-mediated encounters would yield the statistically significant findings needed to gain real insights into healthcare interpreting practice. However, large scale studies are typically less likely to gain ethics approval than small scale studies, where the latter might allow the researcher more control over variables. In the case of clinical studies, ethics approval is usually obtained because the perceived benefits are seen to outweigh possible objections. Quality interpreting research may be said to be comparable to clinical studies in terms of their importance for patient outcomes.

5. Teaching healthcare interpreting

One challenge may involve training interpreters in languages that the teachers may not be familiar with, because of the ongoing demand in an ever-changing range of community languages (Crezee & Sachtleben 2012; Slatyer 2014). A second challenge is to teach healthcare interpreting in such a way that students feel empowered and ready to develop further in practice, as lifelong learners. Health is a huge and complex area: the more layers you unpeel, the more are revealed underneath. The challenge is to give aspiring student healthcare interpreters enough information to empower them, setting them off on a path of effective lifelong development, without confusing and undermining them.

Learning starts with a good textbook. Student feedback on what they wanted in a course book has resulted in the book before you now. The challenges of preparing students for interpreting in healthcare comprise:

- reducing the virtual Mount Everest of Latin, Greek and complex science to a seemingly surmountable molehill;
- allowing students to practice interpreting while also getting immediate feedback on their performance, as that is effective and powerful (something the lead author learnt from a friend who trains football referees);
- familiarizing and preparing students for the ethical dilemmas they will face in practice.

The authors would advise educators to keep thinking of how they can make the learning experience better still, not being afraid to draw on personal experiences as a health professional and/or interpreter in telling helpful anecdotes. Miming, drawing cartoons and telling stories are very powerful teaching methods and consolidate the 'drier' points of learning.

The authors believe that healthcare interpreting needs to be taught following a situated learning model (Gonzalez Davies 2004) where learning is partly co-constructed, especially in team and pair work. Teaching should center on:

– theoretical knowledge of healthcare settings and terminology,
– theoretical and practical knowledge of the professional code of conduct, and
– semi-authentic simulated opportunities for interpreting practice, also using video clips.

In some cases, the teacher may be both a practicing healthcare interpreter and health professional. In other cases, the teaching team may consist of an experienced interpreter plus an experienced healthcare professional.

Care should be taken to choose a healthcare professional who has the ability and skill to explain the necessary information clearly, without overwhelming the students with too much detail, as this will merely lead to confusion. The knowledge base provided should prepare student interpreters for the knowledge required to accurately and comfortably interpret between healthcare professionals and patients.

Sessions should involve a presentation, interspersed with video clips showing patients in hospitals during related doctor-patient interviews and/or undergoing certain procedures.

Watching video clips will serve to give student interpreters the feeling of being 'right there' in the hospital room. This simulated presence in the healthcare setting may help give student interpreters the feeling that they are being induced into the community of practice of practicing healthcare interpreters (Lave 1990, 1991, 1996; Lave & Wenger 1991). Once they are practicing interpreters, they will repeat this experience in real life, and this will consolidate their knowledge of healthcare settings, allowing them to develop as healthcare interpreters.

Medical equipment such as real angiography catheters, nebulizer masks, stents, inhalers, peak flow meters should be passed around the class. It is much easier to interpret the word "catheter" when you have held a real one in your hands. Such *realia* can be obtained from healthcare settings, e.g. when a pack has been opened by accident and the catheter can no longer be used as it is no longer sterile. Induction into the professional code of conduct and into interpreting practice should be led by an experienced healthcare interpreter. Interpreting practice may involve students working in pairs or in triads, reading out scripts in English and in languages other than English

(LOTE). In this way, student A can act as the health professional, reading out the script for that role in English. Student B can act as the patient, doing a sight translation from English into the LOTE while Student C does not have a script, but has to interpret what he or she hears. This practice enables *immediate feedback* from Students A and B on word choice and interpreting competence.

In the authors' experience, students find this type of practice thoroughly enjoyable and effective (Crezee & Sachtleben 2012).The lead author and her colleagues utilize Blackboard Collaborate Voice Authoring® technology in the computer lab, where students record their responses to pre-recorded interpreting dialogues. This technology also allows student interpreters to get their language buddies or family members at home or anywhere in the world to listen to their interpreting practice and give them language-specific feedback.

Other valuable practice may take the form of field trips. As an example the lead author took her student interpreters off campus to practice interpreting with speech language therapists (SLTs)*, some of whom spoke the same LOTE as the students. Students and SLTs spent hours practicing interpreter-mediated real life scenarios, with some playing the role of interfering parents, incompetent interpreters, four-year old children with speech problems, or stroke victims. The students were there for three hours and when it was time to stop, nobody wanted to stop. It was a great deal of fun, and not hard to organize (Crezee 2015).

Post-graduate students who were already qualified SLTs

Summary of main points

This chapter has identified three possible categories of readership for this book:

- healthcare interpreters
- medical translators
- healthcare interpreter educators

This chapter has touched on the development of the interpreting profession and the increasing demand for healthcare interpreters. It has also briefly touched on the range of publications in the area of health interpreting as well as on the challenges involved in healthcare interpreter education.

Chapter 2

Interpreting in healthcare settings

This chapter will touch on some of the challenges faced by professionals interpreting in healthcare settings and will move from there to an overview of what skills, abilities and knowledge healthcare interpreters need to possess. It will also provide a brief look at the status of health interpreting in Hong Kong, Taiwan and Mainland China. Healthcare interpreter training should address all these areas to allow (student) interpreters to develop the knowledge and capabilities required.

1. Interpreting in healthcare settings

There is a great demand for trained and competent interpreters in healthcare settings. Unfortunately, all too often, providers may feel tempted to utilize the services of the so-called ad hoc interpreters. Alternatively, they may ask anyone who happens to speak the patient's language, be this a visitor, a medical assistant or the housekeeping staff, to act as interpreter. This may happen because staff is in a hurry, for instance because the patient has to go to the operating room for a lifesaving operation, and there is no time to lose. In most cases, however, the real reason for not using a trained interpreter may be that staff, who are often monolingual, have a poor understanding of what is involved in interpreting (e.g. linguistic skills, cultural knowledge, interpreting techniques, understanding of the code of ethics), or of the risks of using untrained interpreters in healthcare settings. Sometimes the cost and delay involved in bringing in a trained healthcare interpreter also come into play.

Most countries have a healthcare interpreting system in place, which may involve *on site* (face-to-face) interpreting, telephone interpreting or video remote interpreting (VRI). Many Asian countries however do not have such healthcare interpreting systems in place. In some Asian countries, healthcare interpreting is still in the early stages of development.

In Hong Kong, for example, the need for healthcare interpreting was not recognized until 2008 when the Race Discrimination Ordinance (Cap 602, Laws of Hong Kong) was passed to promote racial equality and ensure equal access to key public services including healthcare services for all members of the public regardless of their race and ethnic origins. Since then ethnic minorities who do not speak Cantonese or English have been able to request interpreting services. Such services, which are provided by a service contractor, are restricted to public hospitals and clinics and were initially provided in only twelve languages, namely, Urdu, Hindi, Punjabi, Nepali, Bahasa Indonesia, Vietnamese, Thai, Korean, Bengali, Japanese, Tagalog and German (Constitutional and Mainland Affairs Bureau 2009). The range of languages offered now also includes Hong Kong Sign Language, French, Sinhala, Spanish, Arabic, Malay, Portuguese and, Taiwanese (Food and Health Bureau, Department of Health & Hospital Authority 2015). In recent years, the government has expanded the sources of the service by seeking help from the Hong Kong Christian Service's Centre for Harmony and Enhancement of Ethnic Minority Residents (CHEER) and from part-time interpreters from the Judiciary of Hong Kong, who provide interpretation services in more than 50 different languages and Chinese dialects. As in many other healthcare settings, the service is provided onsite or over the phone (ibid.). For scheduled appointments, patients are encouraged to give advance notice of their need for an interpreter, or to bring friends and relatives to interpret for them (Equal Opportunities Commission 2008). Utilizing the services of such untrained 'interpreters' in healthcare settings may lead to information being censored, omitted or misinterpreted, which may put the patient's health and wellbeing at risk. It is essential that professional and reliable services are provided to patients in need to avoid medical errors (Hong Kong Human Rights Commission Society for Community Organization Asylum Seekers' and Refugees' Voice 2008).

There is a lot of medical translation in Taiwan, however medical interpreting is still at an early stage of development. Community interpreting (which by definition includes medical interpreting) used to be provided by volunteers due the lack of government funding (Chen 2011). It was not until 2006 that the Department of Health of Taipei City Government established a database of foreign language interpreters for new immigrants through the Pearl S. Buck Foundation of Taipei. The interpreters recruited under the progam provided services at the 12 regional healthcare centers in Taipei city and the Taipei City Hospital (Yang, Ye & Sha 2010).

Following the ratification of the International Covenant on Civil and Political Rights and the International Covenant on Economic, Social and Cultural Rights in 2009, many governmental departments have put in place measures for the provision of community interpreting services in recent years (Chen 2011). For example, in April 2009, the National Immigration Agency of the Ministry of Interior established a translation service database, which incorporated translators and interpreters trained in various governmental bodies including the public health sector (Yang et al., 2010). As of 2014, the database has a total of 1,467 interpreters in 18 languages providing services for government agencies and NGOs (National Immigration 2015).

In Mainland China, the need for medical interpreting was not recognized until recently when some of the larger Chinese cities, such as Beijing, Shanghai and Guangzhou, have become more internationalized, however such services remain underdeveloped to date (He 2006, 2010; You 2014; Yang 2010; Zhan & Yan 2013).

There are hardly any professionally trained medical interpreters and very little research has been done on medical interpreting (He 2010; Su 2009; Zhan & Yan 2013). With no legislation to guarantee ethnic minorities' equal access to healthcare services, hospitals are left to their own devices when encountering patients who do not speak Chinese. Some hospitals seek help from staff members who possess some bilingual skills. Often patients have to bring along friends or relatives or hire university students to act as ad hoc interpreters. Most of these ad hoc interpreters however do not possess the required knowledge or terminology to equip themselves for the challenge of medical interpreting, and many are not able to effectively bridge the communication gap. A survey conducted by Zhan and Yan (2013) reveals that most foreign language speaking patients were not satisfied with the interpreting services provided in healthcare settings. One American interviewee even cited an example of a university student he had hired to interpret for him at hospital rendering a "suppository" as a "pill", which resulted in his misuse of the medicine though his life was fortunately not put at risk. Most of the healthcare workers interviewed also expressed their dissatisfaction with the quality of interpreting as the interpreters failed to comprehend and express references to the patient's condition (ibid.), which may lead to an incorrect diagnosis, the consequences of which can be matter of life and death.

2. Different healthcare systems

Most countries have healthcare systems offering healthcare at the primary and secondary care level. Differences between countries' healthcare systems are mainly due to differences in historical development and funding. The healthcare systems in former Commonwealth countries (like Canada, Australia and New Zealand) tend to be quite similar to that which operates in the UK, being mainly publicly funded. The healthcare system in the US, in contrast, is still primarily funded and operated by private entities, though the scene is rapidly changing in the wake of the Affordable Care Act of 2010 (Roat & Crezee, 2015; ibid.).

In the early days of most healthcare systems, patients were only seen when they were ill, with little or no emphasis placed on disease prevention. More recently, healthcare emphasis has moved to include illness prevention. Preventive care involves education, screening and preventive measures. These may include such things as breast cancer and cervical cancer screening programs and diabetes educators. Chapter 4 offers some information on medical terminology in Chinese and English, with the latter section focusing on some of the Latin and Greek 'building blocks' of medical terms, while Chapters 5 through to 8 will provide information on both primary and hospital care settings.

So let us have a look at what is involved in healthcare interpreting and what qualities a good healthcare interpreter needs to possess.

3. Accuracy

Accuracy has been a problematic concept in interpreting and translation over the centuries (Venuti 2000; Pöchhacker & Shlesinger 2002) and the discussion is still evolving. Hale (1996, 2004, 2007) has provided an excellent overview of the discussion, which includes the very important pragmatic aspects of communication. Hale states that the interpreter's very difficult role is to understand the intention of the utterance and portray it as faithfully as possible in the other language (Hale 2008, p. 115). Morris (1999, as cited in Hale 2008) with reference to court interpreting, asserts that interpreting involves "gaining an understanding of the intentions of the original-language speaker and attempting to convey the illocutionary force of the original utterance," adding that this "understanding will be to some extent a personal, i.e. a subjective one." Hale agrees that while it may not be possible to ever be sure about the intention behind other people's utterances, it is possible for the interpreter to be faithful to their own understanding of the original utterance' as that is the best they can be expected to do (Hale 2008, p. 115).

In most cases, healthcare interpreters will be involved in situations where *information needs to be exchanged*. See also Wadensjö (1998, 2002), Meyer (2000, 2003) and Tebble (1998, 2004) for just some of the discussion on the discourse analysis of such interviews). Such exchanges may include:

– the healthcare professional trying to elicit information from the patient or client by asking questions, e.g. when taking a patient's history or when trying to assess the patient's condition after surgery or other forms of treatment.

– the healthcare professional giving the patient instructions which are essential for preventing complications and for managing the patient's condition, e.g. the healthcare professional may tell the patient what to watch out for after a head injury, or may instruct a patient with diabetes about lifestyle changes, which are essential to prevent further complications.

– the healthcare professional giving information about a procedure for which he requires the patient's informed consent. In this situation, the patient may be asking for further information in relation to the proposed benefits of the procedure, as well as its side-effects, risks and any possible alternatives.

– the patient may also ask for information, e.g. about the disorder, the disease process, further treatment options and medications.

– alternatively, the interpreter may be needed in a *counseling* situation. Here, the interview between the client and the health professional or counselor will revolve not so much around an exchange of information, as around an expression of feelings and emotions on the part of the client, and an understanding of these on the part of the professional.

It is clear that, in order to interpret accurately, a healthcare interpreter needs a good knowledge and understanding of the anatomy and physiology of the main body systems, common diseases and/or disorders, diagnoses and treatment methods, including pre-operative instructions. Interpreters should be familiar with informed consent procedures, and with commonly used healthcare terminology, including their Latin and Greek roots, prefixes and suffixes. Healthcare interpreters also need to be familiar with idiomatic language. In some countries, health professionals like to use idiomatic expressions in order to make the patient feel at ease, not realizing that non-native speakers may not have learned such expressions (Crezee & Grant 2013; Crezee & Grant, in press). Similarly, patients may use everyday expressions to describe their symptoms and interpreters need to understand these in order to interpret them accurately. Chinese speaking interpreters need to be familiar with a wide range of expressions used in different Chinese-speaking countries or provinces, or ask for clarification whenever they encounter any unfamiliar expressions. Crezee & Grant (in press) point out that the use of idiomatic language may pose a real challenge to (student) interpreters.

If the interpreter does not interpret information accurately, the consequences may be disastrous. One of the authors was told about a New-Zealand-based interpreter who had rendered the words 'major surgery' as 'a small operation'. The family had signed the consent form, believing the procedure to be a minor one. When the child ended up in the intensive care after surgery, they expressed shock and a feeling of distrust towards the doctor who had given them this 'false' information.

Accuracy is similarly important in history taking. Most of the studies reviewed by Stewart (1995) demonstrated a correlation between effective physician-patient communication and improved patient health outcomes. Healthcare professionals are very much aware of the fact that people who cannot express the history of their complaints are at risk of not having their underlying disorders fully diagnosed. An incorrect diagnosis may lead to either an inappropriate course of treatment or to the patient being discharged in error. This may lead to frequent re-admissions or deterioration in the patient's condition.

Immigrants or visitors from other countries who do not speak English (well enough) may not be able to express exactly how they came to be in the condition they are in, or what their family history or social background is; in other words, they may be unable to give the healthcare professionals the exact information needed in order to reach the correct diagnosis and to institute the most appropriate treatment. Therefore the importance of a trained interpreter who is very familiar with health terminology, anatomy and physiology cannot be underestimated. Interpreters who do not know the difference between heartburn, heart failure, a heart attack or cardiac arrest, cannot interpret such terms accurately and this may cause significant problems for patients and health professionals. See Chapters 18 and 26 for more information on the differences between these conditions.

To summarize: In order to interpret accurately and appropriately, healthcare interpreters need to have a very wide knowledge base. They need to be familiar with the healthcare system in their current country of residence and in the patient's country of origin. This familiarity should include at least the following:

i.   Organization and procedures in the healthcare system of the patient's country of origin, today and in the past, and organization and procedures in the healthcare system of the host country.
     Sometimes healthcare interpreters may find it difficult to keep abreast of new developments in the healthcare system, or of the current situation in other countries. Sometimes it is the patient who simply does not understand the organization of the healthcare system, even if it is interpreted into the healthcare terminology currently used in their country of origin.

ii. The professionals involved in the healthcare systems – both biomedical and traditional – of the patient's country of origin and various professionals involved in the healthcare system of the host country.

iii. Appointment and referral system in the patient's country of origin, and appointment and referral system in the host country.
     One might presume that all countries have a system whereby the patient sees his or her primary care physician first and is then referred on to a specialist. In practice, however, there are enormous differences in appointment and referral systems, also dependent on the way in which the healthcare system is funded. In some countries, patients do not have a primary care physician but are allowed to self-refer to the specialist they think they need to see. This may lead to unrealistic expectations of any other healthcare system in which they may find themselves.

iv. Informed consent forms and their implications as legal documents.
     The 'informed consent' or 'agreement to treatment' form is a legal document. It protects both the patient and the healthcare professional. The patient cannot undergo any procedure without having been fully informed of the reasons why the procedure is necessary, the expected outcomes, the risks and benefits, possible side-effects, any alternatives and the qualifications and experience of the person(s) performing the procedure. The informed consent procedure protects the professional in that, if things do not work out as expected during the procedure, the professional can state that the patient was aware of the possible risks before they agreed to the procedure.

v.   Common pre- and post-operative procedures and instructions.
     The interpreter must have a sound understanding of common pre-operative procedures and instructions in order to be able to interpret these accurately. 'Nothing by mouth after midnight' means just that: *no food, no drink, no smoking.*

It is extremely useful if the interpreter has a good understanding of what is involved in common pre-operative tests such as an EKG or chest X-Ray. This is particularly true for languages which do not have a direct equivalent for words such as *gastroscopy* or even *vertebrae*. Some interpreters always find themselves having to paraphrase words, as, traditionally, their languages do not have words for vertebrae, bipolar disorder, laparotomy or pre-medication. Similarly, those interpreting into signed languages may find themselves developing a new sign for a term they have not previously encountered. The need to paraphrase medical terms requires a very good understanding of the concepts involved.

4.   Understanding common responses to bad news

Interpreters should also be aware that patients may resort to different coping strategies when they are admitted to the hospital or when they are coping with bad news. The hospital environment has an uncanny way of stripping patients of their normal social status and turning them into a 'case' in pajamas. Some patients feel threatened and may resort to some kind of coping strategy. As a result, some patients may get abusive, in what seems an attempt to regain some sort of control over others, if only by annoying them. In other cases, patients and relatives may get abusive and sometimes even aggressive towards staff, because they are genuinely worried about themselves or their loved ones and want to ensure that the health professionals try their very best to help them.

Dr Elizabeth Kübler-Ross (1969; Kübler-Ross & Kessler 2008), a world famous physician, spent hours listening to people who were trying to come to terms with their impending deaths. She described the following **five stages of grief**:

> **Denial** – 'No! It's not true!' 'You must have mixed up the test results! It must be somebody else!'
> **Anger** – 'Why me?' 'It's not fair! I have always lived such a healthy life!' 'I am too young to die!'
> **Bargaining** – 'What if I give up smoking now?' 'What if I try this new wonder diet?' 'What if I see a faith healer?' 'What if I go to church every week from now on...' and so on.
> **Depression** – the patient may become withdrawn and refuse to speak.
> **Acceptance/Introspection** – patients may accept that they are going to die, but may only wish to speak to those closest to them; many patients will choose to whom they want to talk or say good-bye.

It is important to realize, however, that not everybody ends up accepting their loss. Occasionally people keep returning to earlier phases, such as anger and denial. In addition, the word 'loss' should not be used solely to refer to 'life and death' situations. Loss may mean the loss of fertility, losing a limb, or moving to a different unit.

Another situation which may pose problems for the doctor and/or interpreter later on is where the patient goes into denial upon being told that he has cancer and that this must be operated on straight-away. Let us say that a woman is told that she has breast cancer. The specialist explains the situation to her and says that surgery is the best option. The woman gives her consent for surgery, with the interpreter interpreting exactly all the woman's questions and all the explanations given by the doctor. After surgery, the woman is horrified to find that one breast has been removed and maintains that she was never told that she had breast cancer.

The phenomenon of denial of bad news may serve to emphasize, once again, the importance of full and accurate interpretation. Only in doing so will the interpreter ensure that no accusations of 'inaccurate rendition of the message' will ensue. Health professionals involved may realize that the woman's statements are probably due to denial, this being one of the most common responses to 'bad news'.

Health professionals learn about the five stages of grief during their training, and **so should interpreters**. Interpreters should be aware of the reasons why patients may respond to certain information in a certain manner and should use this understanding to help them remain 'cool, calm and collected'.

Obviously interpreters should not admonish patients who get angry with a health practitioner when confronted with bad news. They should not take it personally when the patient denies that he has ever been told about the cancer in his prostate. They should not try and get the depressed person to talk.

It is important that interpreters understand and respect people's individual responses to loss. It is also important that they acknowledge that the professional also understands the various stages of grieving, and that they leave it to the professional to deal with the situation.

5. Culture broker

Interpreting is not a matter of language alone (Hale 1996, 2004, 2007; Rudvin 2007). The patient's cultural background also needs to be understood and taken into account. In some cultures it may be inappropriate for a woman to discuss gynecological problems such as spotting or vaginal blood loss after intercourse, with a male interpreter present. Given that such blood loss may be an indication of cancer, the woman's unwillingness to discuss such symptoms may have serious consequences. *Patient preferences as to the interpreter's gender should be respected.* Similarly, in some cultures, it may not be acceptable for patients to question the doctor, while in others it may be usual practice for patients to be extremely assertive. In some countries, again, the words 'We cannot do anything further' may equate to a demand for payment of additional fees. Even if the interpreter interprets such words accurately, a culture-specific misunderstanding may arise, and the interpreter may need to act as a culture broker and resolve the resulting communication breakdown.

We usually assume our own cultural beliefs to be 'right' and we may therefore also assume that everyone else will (or should) share these beliefs.

Most people almost automatically fall back on their traditional cultural beliefs when their health is failing. It seems natural for humans to return to what they know best when they find themselves in a situation which they perceive to be threatening. Patients from particular ethnic communities may call in faith healers when told that they have a terminal illness. Some patients may insist on a traditional diet in accordance with the principles of *yin* and *yang* when faced with a particular disorder at a particular time of year.

Healthcare interpreters need to be aware of their own cultural backgrounds and of cultural beliefs held in the patients' community in relation to health, diet, 'patient' behavior and attitudes towards illness and disease (Helman 1991). This will enable them to brief healthcare professionals on a range of cultural attitudes in relation to health and to also recognize the differences and similarities between those beliefs and beliefs often held by people in the host country.

Cultural differences may also affect non-verbal behavior (e.g. eye-contact, facial expressions, physical distance, touching, gestures, posture), the use of politeness formulas; tone of voice; loudness of delivery; rhythm, and a whole range of other para-linguistic factors. These will be discussed in more detail in Chapter 3.

6.   Interpreter codes of ethics

In the US, the National Council on Interpreting in Health Care (NCIHC, 2004, 2005), a multidisciplinary body advocating for improved language access in healthcare, has suggested ethical guidelines with input from many stakeholders. Guidelines have also been formulated by the HIN (2007) in Canada, and by the IMIA/MMIA (1996) in the US. Weblinks to the websites of these professional bodies may be found in the reference section. When comparing the various codes, the similarities are immediately apparent. It is essential that healthcare interpreters adhere to such ethical guidelines, as they are often present in situations which may in themselves be potentially embarrassing and difficult for the clients. See Hale (2007) for a discussion of various aspects of ethical guidelines for Chinese-speaking Interpreters.

Professional healthcare interpreters understand the need for complete confidentiality. They do not go around telling others within their community that Miss X has had a termination of pregnancy, that Mr. Y is considering having a vasectomy, or that Mrs. Z has bowel cancer.

The interpreters' attitude has to be one where their minds 'go blank' as soon as they leave the room where the interpreting assignment has taken place. Interpreters who maintain strict confidentiality enjoy all-round respect and trust.

Unfortunately, untrained, non-professional interpreters may not feel bound by the Interpreters' Code of Ethics and may not feel obliged to keep things 'in confidence'.

Healthcare practitioners employing untrained interpreters need to be aware of the fact that the untrained interpreter may leave out information. Such interpreters may distort what is being said simply because they do not understand the medical condition and/or medical terminology, carrying on regardless and incorrectly interpreting information, because they do not want to lose face. In addition, untrained interpreters may censor the information given to the patient by the health professional, because the interpreter does not want the patient to know what is wrong with him/her. In some cultures, too, it is taboo to mention words such as cancer. Many of the author's former interpreting students recount having come under pressure from family members who would ask them not to interpret words like cancer, because the family did not want their (elderly) relatives to be given this bad news. One interpreting student once told the author that she would be inclined to interpret the words 'lung cancer' as 'chest infection' because of a cultural taboo on cancer in her home country.

Professional interpreters, however, are bound by their code of ethics to interpret what the patient is told. Professional interpreters should either disclose a conflict of interest or turn down an assignment in a given situation where they would not be able to remain completely unbiased or impartial, for whatever reason. So, by engaging professional interpreters, health professionals can be assured that the interpreter will be accurate and impartial. There is no such guarantee with ad hoc interpreters or other untrained 'language aides'.

In brief, health professionals should not use untrained interpreters because untrained interpreters may be ignorant of, or may not feel bound by a professional code of ethics. This means that they may (amongst other things):

- not maintain accuracy (see Chapter 2), leave out things they do not understand, change information or add information *they* feel should have been included;
- not maintain strict confidentiality;
- not maintain impartiality: they may be tempted to take sides with either party (the client or the professional) and 'interpret' what they want the other party to hear, rather than what was really said;
- not disclose any possible conflict of interest (including any personal connections with the patient);
- offer advice to the client, which may include giving the client the answers to a test the client is taking (e.g. when they are interpreting for someone who is taking their driver's license test!);

- not be able to provide the healthcare practitioner with cultural background information, as they may not be aware of, or able to elucidate, differences between their own culture and that of the host country;
- not be able to brief the professional on the 'triangle of communication' and the need to use the 'first person singular';
- not be able to use the correct interpreting technique or to explain to both client and professional about the various interpreting techniques which can be used.

7. Duty of care

Occasionally difficult situations may arise where the interpreter is 'torn between' the ethical conduct guidelines, specifically the duty to maintain complete confidentiality, and another obligation called 'duty of care'. Duty of care means that interpreters must speak out if they are aware of situations which could endanger the patient's life, but situations which they know the health professionals are not aware of. It will be obvious that interpreters may find it difficult to reconcile the concept of duty of care with ethical guidelines relating to confidentiality and impartiality. In general, the author's personal feeling is that the interpreter needs to weigh up whether there is in fact a serious risk to the patient's life if the interpreter does not speak up. Issues relating to duty of care and how this can be reconciled with the various interpreters' codes of conduct deserve much wider and more in-depth discussion. As stated, Hale (2007) offers an excellent discussion of various codes of conduct. In some situations, it may be an excellent idea to employ highly skilled bilingual Patient Navigators (Crezee 2014), rather than interpreters. Such Navigators can play more of an advocacy role.

8. Triangle of communication

Trained healthcare interpreters are able to explain to both patient and professional the best seating arrangements. They know that the main flow of conversation and communication should be between the professional and the client. They are also able to instruct the professional and the client as to the different interpreting modes, such as simultaneous or consecutive interpreting. Once all parties in the three-way communication are aware of the 'ground rules', the interpreter will do his or her job almost imperceptibly, thus enabling a natural flow of conversation and exchange of information between the professional and the client.

Untrained interpreters may unconsciously 'side' with either the client or the professional. As a result, either the client or the professional may feel uncomfortable and excluded.

In addition, *untrained* interpreters do not use the 'first person' when they are interpreting, which interpreting theorists agree is the best approach (Scimone & Ginori 1995; Tebble 1998; Hale 2004, 2007). Bot (2005, 2007) has observed that interpreters may on occasion use the third person singular possibly to distance or protect themselves from what they are interpreting. Untrained interpreters may therefore say things like: 'He says his name was Samuel Smith and he says he is glad he saw him before he went back to his house'. This method of 'interpreting' leads to a lot of confusion – with nobody quite sure who 'he', 'his' and 'him' refer to. Confusion is, of course, the opposite of accuracy.

Trained interpreters interpret accurately what the professional or the client has said, no matter how strange it may seem to them to say things like, "I am 84 and I have 3 sons and 21 grandchildren" or "I can hear voices coming out of the handlebars of my bicycle."

9. Note-taking

Trained interpreters are able to take notes which enable them to interpret what has been said completely and accurately. They will include dates, numbers, names, names of conditions, lab results, and so on in their notes. Often our short-term memory cannot cope with details such as numbers and dates, and note-taking skills are an essential tool in storing and retrieving important information such as the dates of the client's 'last menstrual period', blood-pressure readings, and instructions relating to the taking of medication.

In addition to being competent note-takers, trained interpreters will tell the client or the professional if they could not hear part of what was said, or if they are not familiar with the terminology used. As a result, the trained interpreter can maintain a high degree of accuracy and completeness. Those interested in techniques, memory training and note-taking should read the short introduction by Ginori & Scimone (1995) on these issues. They may also follow some of the note-taking practices used by doctors and nurses when it comes to commonly-used abbreviations such as IV abs (intravenous antibiotics), Hy, written as Hx, for history, on P/E (on physical examination), Ty, short for Therapy and written as Tx, for treatment, Ry (short for Recipe) and written as Rx for prescription, and SOB (shortness of breath). This book includes commonly used abbreviations wherever appropriate.

10. Terminology

It is essential that healthcare interpreters possess not only an excellent knowledge of everyday expressions and idioms but also specific knowledge of terminology.

A knowledge of everyday expressions is important because health professionals often 'switch' to everyday language in an attempt to make themselves more readily understood. The effect may be more confusing, however, if the interpreter is not familiar with everyday idioms such as "Are you keeping regular?" and "Are you feeling a bit under the weather?" An obstetrician was once heard to refer to *mastitis* (breast infection) as 'arthritis of the breast'. Since arthritis refers to an inflammation of a joint, this is very confusing.

It is also essential that the interpreter has a very good knowledge of healthcare terminology. The lead author has regularly encountered healthcare professionals who maintain that the interpreter does not need to know 'too much' about healthcare. On the contrary, the basic rule is that *you simply cannot interpret what you do not understand*. Healthcare interpreters should make every effort to gain a good basic understanding of healthcare terminology and to keep building on their knowledge base. They need to be familiar with existing resources. In most countries, health services put out excellent resource material, and with the advent of the internet, much information is easily accessible. However, once again, without a good basic knowledge of healthcare terminology, it may be difficult to fully utilize such material. This book offers lists of commonly-used medical terminology and English-Chinese glossaries in relevant chapters.

Summary of main points

This chapter has touched on some of the many challenges faced by professionals interpreting in healthcare settings. It has also provided an overview of the skills, abilities and knowledge that competent healthcare interpreters need to possess.

This chapter has also reviewed the provision of healthcare interpreting in Hong Kong, Taiwan and Mainland China.

Chapter 3

A word about culture

Special thanks to Amy Hewgill for her input on this Chapter.

1. Culture

What is culture? Anthropologists and other writers have produced a wide range of definitions of culture. In 1871, anthropologist E. B. Tylor defined culture as, "That complex whole which includes knowledge, belief, art, morals, law, custom and other capabilities and habits acquired by man as a member of society" (1871, p. 1). Keesing (1981, p. 518) defines culture as "systems of shared ideas, systems of concepts and rules and meanings that underlie and are expressed in the way that humans live." Helman (1990, p. 2) argues that culture consists of

> "a set of guidelines (both explicit and implicit) which individuals inherit as members of a particular society, and which tells them how to view the world, how to experience it emotionally, and how to behave in it in relation to other people, to supernatural forces or gods, and to the natural environment. It also provides them with a way of transmitting these guidelines to the next generation – by the use of symbols, language, art and ritual".

This chapter will limit itself to two important aspects of culture in relation to the work of the healthcare interpreter:

– aspects of communication that may be influenced by cultural beliefs
– cultural beliefs in relation to health, i.e. attitudes towards sickness and health, behavior, diet, etc.

2. Cultural influence on spoken communication

People with a certain cultural set of 'communication rules' may misunderstand the communication attempts of speakers who regard as normal an entirely different set of 'communication rules'. This applies to users of different spoken languages as well as to users of signed languages. Sign language interpreters need to be very familiar with Deaf culture (cf. Meador & Zazove 2005).

Culture influences communication in a large number of ways, including content, manner of delivery and pragmatics, (van Dijk 1977; Candlin 2003; Candlin & Gotti 2004a; Candlin & Gotti 2004b; Hale 1996, 2004, 2007; Hofstede 2003; Sarangi 2004; Scollon & Scollon 2001; Bowe & Martin 2007; Dysart-Gale 2007; Tate & Turner 2003).

Cultural impact on message content may pertain to levels of explicitness and implicitness, levels of directness, acceptability of topics, and the taboo nature of certain topics (usually topics relating to sex or death). Different cultures differ for example in the way people either give or respond to compliments. In most Western cultures people would most likely respond by saying "thank you". Chinese people on the other hand may feel too embarrassed to accept a compliment, as to them, acknowledging a compliment would go against social expectations and their cultural heritage of humility, a virtue they hold in high regard. Therefore the traditional response to praise or compliments may be a polite denial with words to the effect of "not really" or "I don't deserve the praise".

Nonverbal and paralinguistic aspects of communication are important components of the meaning of the verbal message as they help express attitudes, feelings and emotions. Nonverbal communication however differs from one culture to another and misinterpretation of such forms of communication is unfortunately commonplace. For example, when American troops in Iraq were greeted by small children giving them a thumbs-up sign, they took that as a sign of friendliness, not knowing that in Iraq the "thumbs-up" sign was traditionally a symbol of insult, equivalent to the American middle-finger salute (Woodward 2006, p. 290; Samovar et al. 2013, p. 267).

Nonverbal aspects of communication include, but are not restricted to, posture, physical proximity, gaze, eye-contact, facial expression, gestures and even style of dressing (Grice 1975; Searle 1969, 1975).

Eye contact – in some cultures, women should not look a man in the eye when talking to him as they can find themselves being misunderstood.

Physical closeness – physical closeness is closely linked with the concept of personal space. According to Hall (1990, p. 11), people have around them an invisible bubble that "expands and contracts depending on a numbers things", and cultural background being one of such things. Generally speaking, cultures which value individualism such as the United Kingdom or the United States (Samovar, Porter, McDaniel & Roy 2013) demand more personal space than collective cultures, where people are more interdependent (Samovar et al. 2013). Chinese culture is characterized as a collective culture, where group action or group wellbeing is valued over individual wishes (Lee & Ballard 2011; Samovar et al. 2013). It is thus not uncommon for two women (or even two men) to walk arm in arm or hand in hand even though they are not in a homosexual relationship. People from Western cultures may feel ill at ease when witnessing such companionable closeness. Therefore, English speakers may feel uncomfortable when a Chinese speaker moves very close to them when engaged in conversation and may move back to gain more physical space for themselves. The Chinese speaker in turn may feel offended when the other person distances him or herself in such a way.

Physical contact – in some cultures, it is acceptable to touch the person you are talking to. In other cultures, it is definitely not okay and may be misinterpreted completely. In China, it is now common for people to shake hands when they first meet, but not to hug or kiss each other as is the case in many Western cultures.

Facial expressions – sometimes facial expressions, such as smiles, can be totally misinterpreted by speakers from other cultures. A Laotian interpreter once recounted how he had interpreted for two refugees at a refugee camp in Thailand. As they recounted their harrowing journey, they kept smiling. Afterwards the UNHCR official told him he was shocked by their account, but could not believe they had smiled right through, and was therefore wondering whether they were telling the truth. The interpreter told him that in the refugees' culture it would have been very impolite to impose anger or sadness on the person to whom they were talking. By smiling, they tried to ensure that the other person would not be negatively affected by their story. Needless to say, most native speakers of English would interpret a smile as a sign of happiness, not of anger, shyness or sadness. Chinese, Japanese and Korean people, may use a smile to express politeness, confusion, embarrassment or even apology (Lee & Ballard 2011).

Nodding – nodding in most Western cultures indicates agreement but in Asian cultures including China and Japan, this may only indicates acknowledgment (Lee & Ballard 2011). The movement of the head in nodding may also vary from culture to culture. For example, in the US and many other Western cultures, vertical head movement denotes "yes" and horizontal head movement (or head shaking) indicates "no". In Bulgaria however, the reverse is true (Andonova & Taylor 2012).

Hand gestures – hand gestures are culturally embedded and may be interpreted differently in different cultures. For example, pointing at someone in the Chinese culture can be taken as a sign of rudeness while in the United States it does not usually carry negative connotations (Samovar et al. 2013). Beckoning people in the Northern European way, with the fingers pointing upwards, not downwards, may be perceived as very rude. In many cultures, including China and Korea, people hold their fingers downwards when beckoning people and upward only when beckoning animals.

Cultural attitudes also dictate paralinguistic aspects of communication, including volume or loudness, tone, pitch, speech rhythms, speed of delivery, pausing before responding, sentence stress, intonation and flow. Volume or loudness is but one aspect of the way in which a spoken message is delivered. Different cultures harbor different ideas on 'loudness'. In some cultures such as Japan and Thailand, speaking in a very low voice is a way of expressing respect towards the person you are addressing. For the Japanese, "a gentle and soft voice reflects good manners and helps maintain social harmony" (Samovar et al. 2013, p. 291). In other cultures, this might be interpreted as a sign of shyness, and may even be received with irritation. Among the Chinese, people speaking different regional dialects vary in the loudness of their speech. For example, people speaking Hakka or some southern Min dialects such as Chiuchow and Hoklo (which is the native tongue of one of the authors of this book) tend to speak in a louder voice than Mandarin or Cantonese speakers. When the way in which a message is uttered is interpreted in a way completely opposite to what was intended, so that illocutionary intent is lost, communication breakdown may result.

Other aspects of speech which may be misinterpreted might include the natural speech rhythms or speed of delivery. The natural speech rhythms which occur in some languages may be received by speakers of other languages as monotonous or akin to whining. The speed with which a message is delivered may also be misinterpreted by speakers of other languages. Recipients might think, "They speak too fast – they must be very nervous or upset," when that rate of delivery may be totally normal for users of that language.

For the speakers of some languages, pausing before responding is a sign that the question is taken seriously and given some thought. To speakers from other cultures, however, these long pauses may convey hesitation and be a sign that the speaker does not know what to say. It may even have a prejudicial effect on the speaker's credibility, for instance in refugee status hearings or during examination in the courtroom.

Stress-timed languages, such as English, emphasize the key words through stress, however this may be interpreted as rude by speakers in some other cultures. Similarly, speakers of certain languages habitually use a very loud voice, which may be perceived as either rude or aggressive by people not familiar with that language.

In short, paralinguistic features may play a considerable role in the way a spoken message is interpreted by the listener, especially if the listener does not share the speaker's cultural background.

3.   Implications for interpreting

Like translation, interpreting is by no means a word-for-word or sense-for-sense matching game, but a process in which cultural considerations of all sorts come into play. Since language and culture are intertwined, accuracy in interpreting "cannot be achieved at the basic word level" and that "words in interaction only take on meaning according context, situation, participants and culture (Hale 2014, p. 322). Before embarking on an interpreting job, interpreters need to ask themselves some of the following questions:

- How may speakers from this cultural background express respect in the way they deliver a spoken message, in their facial expressions, body posture and so on?
- How may these native speakers express anger?
- Are there any gestures, body postures or facial expressions used by speakers from this cultural background which may be misinterpreted by health professionals from a different background and vice versa?

Being aware of these differences will help interpreters become aware of the pitfalls of cross-cultural communication. Interpreters should always bear in mind that their own interpretation of such pitfalls may also be subjective and that every speaker is a unique individual. Hale (2014, p. 323) argues that people are both individuals and members of different groups or cultures and therefore have their own individual traits while sharing some traits with members of the cultures to which they belong. It may not be always easy for interpreters to separate the two. Care must thus be taken when approaching perceived instances of potential cross-cultural miscommunication. The more interpreters know about the background of the speakers including not only the cultural groups they belong to, but also their life experiences and beliefs, the better equipped they will be to eliminate any possible miscommunication or to attain pragmatic equivalence.

4.   Culture and health

With regards to health, Helman (1990) describes in some detail how members of different societies use different cultural definitions of anatomy and physiology. Cultural beliefs with regard to anatomy govern beliefs not only to do with desirable body size and how to clothe and decorate the body, but also with the body's inner structure and with how the body functions. Cultural beliefs include concepts of balance and imbalance. The belief system of *yin* and *yang* is quite well known, with *yin* representing that which is 'dark, moist, watery and female', and *yang* representing that which is 'hot, fiery, and male' (Helman 1990, p. 20). It is believed that *yin* and *yang* are two contrary yet complementary forces that interact to form a dynamic system. The concepts of *yin* and *yang* are the foundation of traditional Chinese medicine, which holds that disease or sickness is caused by the imbalance of the *yin* and *yang* energies around our human bodies (Low & Ang 2010).

The World Health Organization (WHO) provides a good definition of health, defining it as a state of complete physical, mental and social well-being and not merely the absence of disease or infirmity (WHO 1948). Cultural beliefs also influence our attitudes towards important areas of our lives, such as marriage and relationships, family relationships, child-rearing practices, education and, very importantly, health.

Even people who immigrated to another country many years ago, and who feel that they have assimilated to their new country in many areas of their lives, may return to their original cultural attitudes when faced with ill health.

Chinese women may want to use traditional Chinese herbs in before, during and after childbirth, when in fact Western health professionals would caution against the use of some of those herbs.

South East Asian mothers giving birth in hospital, may be told to have a shower straight after birth, in the interests of hygiene and to prevent perinatal infection. In practice, however, many of these women refuse, as they remember what their mothers and grandmothers told them about the dangers of catching a cold or getting wind (what is called *fung1*[1] in Cantonese or *fēng*[2] in Mandarin) into their bones by stepping under the shower. In particular, Chinese women after childbirth are told not to wash their hair to stop wind from getting into their heads through the scalp, or else they can expect to have frequent headaches for the rest of their life. If a woman insists on cleansing her body, she is strongly advised to use boiled gingery water as ginger is believed to be hot (*yang*) in nature and helps dispel cold or wind (*yin*). The Chinese also believe that a woman's body after childbirth is most vulnerable to ailments, so it is important for her to observe a postnatal confinement, which usually lasts a month from the birth of the child. During this month of confinement, the mother should avoid going out, as she may then 'catch wind'. The banquet at the end of this first month celebrates both the conclusion of the confinement and the fact that the baby has survived its first month of life – a vestige of earlier times when infant mortality was high.

The extent to which immigrants continue to adhere to their own traditional practices and beliefs in the area of health, depends on a lot of different factors: length of time spent in their new country, age, educational background and so on. In this way, a Chinese woman doctor may well shower after childbirth, as her traditional beliefs have been replaced by the medical knowledge she has gained in the course of training.

In some Chinese hospitals, parents may only be allowed to visit their premature babies once in a while, while in Western hospitals parents may be allowed to be at their child's bedside at all times.

We have decided to share with readers the story of a New Zealand couple called Amy and Greg who were faced with an urgent hospital admission in Mainland China, in July 2013, when they were travelling through Shanghai on their way to New Zealand. Amy was 26 weeks pregnant, when suddenly her membranes broke just 12 hours before they were due to fly out, and Amy found herself giving birth to her daughter Lily in a Chinese hospital without access to interpreters. Amy and Greg were asked to

---

1.   Cantonese Romanisation is based on *Jyutping*.

2.   Mandarin Romanisation is based on *Hanyu* pinyin.

prepay for care, something that is unheard of in New Zealand, where health professionals will always provide care first and present an invoice later. Because Lily was born prematurely, she had to stay in the Neonatal Intensive Care Unit (NICU) for several weeks. Amy recalls:

"As a new mother in China I had very few rights but many responsibilities. I had to deliver all of the breast milk that I could express (using a breast pump) to the hospital two to three times a week. In addition, I had to supply my daughter with any of the medical things she might require from the pharmacy, yet I did not know what they were or where to find them. I had to extend our visitor visas to emergency stay medical visas and get documents from the hospital to prove that we had a child there. All of this and more was on my shoulders and yet I could barely say "hello" and "thank you" in Chinese.

Misunderstandings happened daily throughout my stay. It took me one week of delivering my breast milk to the hospital before I finally understood that they were throwing my milk away. In fact, it was only five weeks later that I finally understood what should have taken the nurses ten seconds to tell me: "Put your breast milk is sterile bags in quantities of 10–20 ml each. You can buy them at this pharmacy located in X, and this is what they are called in Chinese." This is just one of very many of these miscommunications.

In New Zealand, as in most western countries, the family is allowed to see the patient (especially if it is a child) throughout their stay. In the case of a NICU, the parents can stay 24 hours a day, 7 days a week if they choose. Furthermore, parents have full access to any medical records and can get copies of any relevant hospital documents. Also, in New Zealand, an interpreter would be provided for you by the hospital if you ask for one. Lastly, in New Zealand and some other countries all of this would be provided for free to residents and citizens.

As the mother of a patient, I had expectations which were vastly different from those of Chinese parents, and which did not fit our new reality.

While the Chinese hospital was reasonably well equipped and staffed by good doctors and nurses, firstly, we were not allowed to see our daughter. Secondly, we were not allowed to have any of her medical records or documents that we were required to sign (so we could get them translated); In other words, I was asked to sign documents without understanding the content. Thirdly, an interpreter was never offered, and lastly, nothing was provided for free. If a mother was not allowed to see her child in hospital in New Zealand there would be an outcry in the media. In fact, it would be front-page news (and in our case it was).

What we needed most in our first few days was a bi-cultural/bi-lingual mediator to help us bridge the gaps. We also needed an advocate who knew the medical system. In my many exchanges with the doctors through 'interpreters' I found that the latter interpreted consecutively without notes, and some things appeared to be lost in translation. As an example, doctors would give long explanations, followed by the 'interpreter' asking the doctor a few questions, receiving responses from the doctor, but not telling me what was happening. Following this, I would receive what appeared to be a significantly shortened version of their conversation, so much so that it sometimes felt like a cruel joke. I felt incredibly powerless and vulnerable being entirely dependent on someone else to relay the message to me. I also felt I had missed some vital information. In hindsight, I think simultaneous interpreting would have been better for me but I did not feel comfortable asking for that. As a result I felt that the interpreter was acting as a "helper" by asking questions on my behalf without consulting me, something I felt was patronizing to me as the client. I think that there needs to be a pre-briefing session between the interpreter and the client as to how the interpreting will be done (consecutive or simultaneous) so expectations are met."

Amy is now a qualified New Zealand Sign Language (NZSL) Interpreter, having completed her Bachelor Degree in NZSL Interpreting at Auckland University of Technology, while Lily is a healthy, active and thriving toddler who keeps her parents very busy. Amy says the experience has made her more aware of the interpreter's role. She says: "As an interpreter you must be aware of cultural differences and expectations in both of your languages." Amy and Greg's experience is interesting because it highlights the importance of healthcare interpreters being aware not only of medical terminology, but also of different cultural expectations based on differing healthcare systems.

Similarly, in some cultures, the doctor may routinely ask the woman if she would like her husband to be present at the interview. In some cases, the woman may in fact want to tell the doctor that she does not want a particular procedure or form of birth control, or she may want to disclose other painful issues, however it may be impossible for her to say so when her husband is present. In such situations, it may be better to first ask the woman to come in and ask her through the interpreter whether she wants her husband to be present or not when the husband is not in the room.

So what are some of these traditional beliefs regarding health, and how can they constitute a problem for the healthcare interpreter?

5.   Cultural beliefs pertaining to health and their implications for the interpreter

Our attitudes towards health issues may be deeply influenced by cultural beliefs, which we have had passed down from our mothers and their mothers before them.

An interpreter needs to be aware of both traditional ideas around health and illness held by clients and of approaches advocated in the healthcare system in which they are working. This way, the interpreter can provide cultural background information if a complete breakdown of communication threatens. See also Rudvin (2004,

2007) and Dysart-Gale (2007) for a discussion of how interpreters negotiate cultural and linguistic aspects of the interpreting process in relation to their professional roles. The culture of the hospital system in countries like the US and Canada is largely bio-medical in nature. This means that spirits and malicious spells are not seen as a cause of illness. In addition, it means that natural remedies are not considered useful unless scientific research has proven otherwise. Those who have been educated within the healthcare system of the aforementioned countries usually have the same confidence in scientific evidence and may have little patience with patients who have faith in tra-ditional healers and unproven herbal remedies. This can lead to a fair amount of cul-tural misunderstanding with patients and hospital staff possibly getting upset at the 'obviously incorrect' beliefs of the other party.

As mentioned above, the traditional Chinese medicine is based on the concepts of *yin* and *yang* and on the belief that illness is caused by the imbalance of *yin* and *yang* in the body, i.e, having excessive *yin* and deficient *yang* or vice versa. Thus, a patient with a mouth ulcer (canker sore) is most likely to be diagnosed by a Chinese doctor practicing traditional Chinese medicine to be suffering from "heat-syndrome" (literally "hot air", usually believed to have been caused by the consumption of deep-fried food), thus resulting in excessive *yang* in the body and deficiency in *yin*, whereas a Western doctor may simply suggest a viral infection as the cause. Some Chinese patients may be seen nodding (as a sign of acknowledgement as mentioned above) when listening to the advice of a Western doctor, but may simply follow their own remedies for dealing with what they believe to be a health issues resulting from an imbalance between *yin* and *yang*.

5.1   Sickness and disease (or medical condition)

What is sickness? Obviously, we should be able to define sickness as the absence of health. Yet, what may be defined as a sickness by one person or one culture, may not be seen as such by another person at all. In a culture where the common cold is extremely common, people suffering a cold are not considered to be sick. If they take sick leave just because they have a cold, this will be frowned upon.

For many people, having a medical condition does not equate with being sick. Something the medical professional might diagnose as a disease or disorder, may not be seen in the same light by the patient at all. Often the patient will not consider him-self to be ill if he does not feel 'ill'. Such patients may only return to the doctor when the disease is in such an advanced stage that it has become incurable or has resulted in serious complications.

Diabetes is one example of different cultural attitudes towards sickness and dis-ease. Some patients may have been diagnosed with diabetes and been told to take their medications, change their life-styles and more specifically their diets, but they feel well and may then stop adhering to the prescribed treatment plan. They may stop taking their medication, since they feel it is not working, as they still have diabetes. They may only return to hospital when they 'feel sick'. By that stage they may have end-stage renal failure or necrosis.

5.2   Patient behavior

How a patient is supposed to behave differs from culture to culture. In some cultures, you have to lie in bed, and are not allowed to do anything for yourself. This type of behavior may be greeted with annoyance by caregivers from other cultural backgrounds, who have been taught to grin and bear it and to 'carry on' regardless.

Many hospital staff will encourage inpatients to mobilize and do things for themselves, as this has been proven to reduce the risk of many complications such as bedsores, contractures, chest infections and thrombosis. This approach reflects 'medico-scientific' ideas and may be greeted with dismay by patients who have always been taught that sick people should stay in bed and not exert themselves.

The cultural misunderstanding which results can easily lead to non-compliance. A patient who has been told that he has diabetes and needs to exercise, may well disregard his doctor's admonitions and spend most of his time lying in bed or sitting in a chair, because that sort of behavior befits an 'ill' person.

5.3   Cultural attitudes towards pain

Pain behavior can be another obstacle to effective communication. Patients from some cultures express the fact that they are in pain by yelling, shouting and moaning, whereas people from other cultural backgrounds may have learned to grit their teeth and 'suffer in silence'. The latter might well view the former as 'moaners' and treat them with disdain.

5.4   Causes of sickness

Medical professionals tend to look for scientific causes for illness and disease. Research is undertaken to find out the causes of those illnesses whose origins remain unknown. The underlying principles of treatment will also be based on scientific evidence. Patients may come from cultures where illnesses are believed to be caused by evil spirits. Sometimes, people believe that an adversary has put a spell on them. It seems logical to them that the only treatment in that case is to 'undo' the spell or to invoke other spirits to counter the attack on their health. The lead author remembers doctors and nurses being very much taken aback when a patient with melanoma was taken out of hospital by his family, be taken to a faith healer from his ethnic community.

Similarly, some people in Indochina may still practice 'mother roasting' to help dry up the woman's vaginal discharge after childbirth. One interpreter recounted how fire-fighters were called in to a suspected house-fire, with smoke coming out of the window of an apartment. When they entered the apartment, they found a woman lying on a bed. Under the bed were a few smoldering coals, put there to help dry up the woman's discharge after childbirth.

Many of these beliefs apply to the behavior of pregnant women. Some pregnant Cook Islands women have been known to refuse to wear the ID bracelet (or anything circular around their bodies, including rings and belts) for fear it may cause their babies to be born with their cords around their necks.

5.5   Diets in sickness and health

Many deep-rooted cultural beliefs come to the fore when it comes to what we choose to eat in sickness and health (Helman 1990).

It is no coincidence that many visitors can be seen carrying in pots and pans when visiting relatives in hospital. Chinese patients often prefer rice gruel above all else. It is well-documented that Southeast Asian patients often follow the philosophy of *yin* and *yang* (Adams & Osgood 1973). To them, sickness is the result of ill-balance and the diet needs to be chosen in such a way that this balance is restored. Interestingly, Southeast Asian patients may follow a different diet if they catch a cold in winter than if they catch a cold in summer. The only food they can eat all year round is rice, as rice is neutral and will therefore not cause any imbalances.

The belief in special diets for certain conditions and special remedies for certain ailments can be so strong that patients will adhere to these above all else. Sometimes the effect can be detrimental or interfere with medically prescribed treatments. For example, Chinese people believe that ginseng can invigorate the primordial Qi of the human body. Thus Chinese women during labor may chew on ginseng to give themselves more Qi, without being aware that this may actually increase the risk of postnatal hemorrhage. After childbirth or heavy periods, Chinese women are traditionally given a special strengthening soup, containing special herbs such as ginger, longan, red dates, Chinese angelica root (*dang gui*) and codonopsis pilosula (poor men's ginseng) which are said to make the body strong again. In some studies, ginseng has been linked to decreased anticoagulant effect (Albers et al., 2004; Ramsay, et al., 2005). According to other studies, the ginger and sesame oil in the food traditionally eaten by new mothers pass into the breast milk and may make their baby's jaundice worse, as the ginger specifically is thought to interfere with the breakdown of *bilirubin* in the baby's body. Anecdotal evidence suggests that some obstetricians simply tell these mothers to just stop breast-feeding, saying that the breast milk will make the baby's jaundice worse, without explaining that the reason lies in the ethnically varied food. Pregnant and breastfeeding women are advised to check with their health professionals before taking any natural herbs, to ensure these do not inadvertently pose a risk to their health.

5.6   Taboos

All cultures have taboos, many of which relate to sex or illness and death. This may explain why foul language often concerns sex or illness and death. In hospitals, taboos are understandably more to do with serious and potentially fatal health conditions than with sex. In the Chinese culture (Cantonese-speaking community), it is a taboo for a visitor to bring a patient a melon (gwaa1), which is homophonous to a Cantonese slang for "death". Likewise, the number "4" (sei3 in Cantonese and sì in Mandarin), which sounds similar to the more formal word "death" in both Cantonese (sei2) and Mandarin (sǐ) is avoided or even omitted in the numbering of the floors of high-rise buildings and even of wards and beds, especially in private hospitals.

5.7   The role of the interpreter as a culture broker

It is sometimes said that the interpreter's role is also to act as a culture broker when there is a threat of complete) communication breakdown which has its roots in cross-cultural misunderstandings (NCIHC, 2004: 18–19). As we have seen, cultural attitudes may affect communication between people from different cultural backgrounds in a variety of ways.

Patients may not comply with the doctor's instructions if these go against their own cultural beliefs. New mothers from Southeast Asian countries may not have the prescribed shower after birth if they believe it can give them *fung1* (wind). They may feel quite taken aback, and may not want to say 'no' directly, as it would be impolite to do this to a person in a position of authority, such as a medical doctor.

People who are sad may indicate that they have a pain in their heart. They may be sent off for cardiac tests and come through these with flying colors. Holmes (2013) gives examples of cross-cultural communication problems between US health professionals and migrants from Latin America in his moving book on migrant workers in the US horticultural industry.

It is the interpreter's role to be conscious of situations where different cultural attitudes towards sickness and health may potentially lead to communication breakdown and non-compliance. Interpreters need to be familiar with commonly held beliefs within a patient's cultural group. They also need to be aware of the hospital culture in the country they are working in, and of the scientific approach followed by the health professionals.

Interpreters should be aware of all these, without stereotyping. Some anesthetists may be fully convinced of the benefits of acupuncture and even practice it themselves. Some new immigrants may have trained as doctors in their home countries and share the scientific approach to health and illness. Every patient is shaped by his or her own life experiences, personal upbringing and family background, professional development and time spent in the new country of residence.

Ideally, interpreters should have the opportunity to discuss different cultural backgrounds during the pre-briefing session with the professional, or alternatively, during the de-briefing session following the interpreting assignment. Unfortunately, briefing and debriefing often do not take place in practice, although mental health professionals appear more willing to spend time with interpreters before or after assignments. Once the health professionals become aware of the impact of cultural beliefs in relation to sickness and health, they may start to value the interpreter's cultural knowledge more (Crezee 2003).

Finally, unaddressed differences in cultural beliefs may cause severe communication breakdown during interpreting assignments. The nature of cultural attitudes is such that we all think our own are the norm and should be or are shared by everyone else. For this reason, people are often not aware that the other party in the interview may approach health issues in an entirely different way. According to anecdotal evidence, a woman in an Australian hospital was told that she had an incurable illness and that nothing more could be done. In her country this meant that the doctor would 'pull out all the stops' as long as the patient paid a higher fee. When her husband pulled out his wallet, the doctor got upset and said: "No, you don't understand. Money doesn't enter into it. There is nothing more I can do." The man then pulled out more banknotes while both he and the doctor got increasingly upset. Had an interpreter been present, they might have been able to prevent this breakdown in communication by explaining cultural differences to both parties. When interpreters do this, they should put up their hand and ask for permission to provide some cultural background information. They need to state that this will be a subjective statement and that each individual is unique, before proceeding to make a general statement. They will need to repeat any cultural background information provided in both languages. This way both the patient and the professional will know what was said and will be able to express their agreement or disagreement if need be.

As patients' cultural beliefs will presumably influence how they describe their health problems and the way in which they communicate their symptoms to health professionals, it is believed that an improved communication between patients and health professionals will lead to improved therapeutic outcomes.

Interested readers are advised to read Samovar et al. (2013), Andonova & Taylor, (2012), Hall & Hall, (1990), Battle (2002), Angelelli (2004), Tellechea Sánchez (2005); Hale (2005, 2007, 2014); Rudvin (2004, 2007); Pym, Shlesinger and Jettmarová (2006); Bowe and Martin (2007); Dysart-Gale (2007); Lee, Lansbury and Sullivan (2005); Lim, Mortensen, Feng, Ryu and Cui (2012) and other authors for some of the extensive debate on cross-cultural communication involving interpreters in health settings.

Summary of main points

This chapter has touched on some of the impacts culture may have on interpreter-mediated cross-cultural communication in healthcare settings, including:

– cultural aspects of communication
– cultural beliefs relating to health and illness, in particular, how the concept of *yin* and *yang* may affect Chinese people in their approach to health problems, the diet chosen, and any medication or remedies they wish to use.

Chapter 4

Medical terminology

1. Introduction

(Student) interpreters preparing to work in healthcare settings using English as one of their working languages, will in fact need to acquire some basic knowledge of two additional languages: Latin and Greek. There are a number of excellent books available on medical terminology (Walker, Wood & Nicol, 2013; Chabner, 2011, Thierer & Breitbard, 2006), however, no book on healthcare interpreting would be complete without a brief section on medical terminology.

This chapter will provide a very brief introduction to the historical background of why these two languages are still reflected in healthcare terminology in English today, followed by an overview of basic Latin and Greek roots, suffixes and affixes. Each chapter in Part Three will start with a brief list of Latin and Greek roots used in a particular field of medicine. For this reason, the current chapter will restrict itself to a general overview only. Since this book is intended for Chinese-speaking interpreters and translators, the authors have included a short section on the history of Chinese medical terminology.

2. History of medical terminology in the western world

Medical traditions developed in various civilizations around the world, including Mesopotamia (ca. 3500 BC), Egypt (ca. 3000 BC), India (ca. 2500 BC) and China (ca. 1600 BC) (Pourahmad, 2010). It is likely that there was some contact between the various civilizations resulting in the sharing of certain health-related beliefs. Translations of health related writings have played a major role in the spread of health-related beliefs to other cultures as documented by McMorrow (1998), Van Hoof (1998a), Segura (1998) and many others.

Ancient Greek doctors were very skilled at diagnosing as evidenced by the continued use of Greek words denoting certain medical conditions: the term *diabetes mellitus* (literally: sweet-honey passing through) is but one example. The Ancient Romans liked to employ Greek doctors and many of these, including a famous physician known as Claudius Galen, travelled to and worked in Rome. In the 1st century BC, a Roman nobleman called Cornelius Celsus (53BC-7AD) recorded all that was then known about Greek and Roman medicine in a huge encyclopedia called *De Medicina* (about medicine).

The invasion of Spain by the Moors (718AD) also introduced into Spain what Segura (1998) calls 'a treasure cove of medical and scientific knowledge' from other countries, including Greece. The establishment of the Toledo School of Translators by Archbishop Raimundus (1125–1152) brought about the translation and dissemination of a wealth of scientific works, including medical writings (Segura, 1998). In the Middle Ages, a small group of doctors formed an influential medical school in Salerno (Italy), revisiting the teachings of Greek physicians such as Hippocrates and Galen. Medical schools all over Europe followed suit and Latin and Greek terminology is used by medical scientists to this day.

Even though Latin (L) and Greek (Gk) are distinct languages, roots from either language will be presented in this chapter without indicating their linguistic origins.

Overall, terms of Greek origins can often be recognized because they may include the English spelling conventions for the following Greek letters: χ (ch) as in *brachy* (short); θ (th) as in *pathology* (study of illness); φ (ph) as in *angiography* (blood vessel imaging), ψ (ps) as in *psychology* (study of the mind) and υ (y) as in *hysterectomy* (removal of the womb) and αι (ae) as in gynaecologist.

3.   Chinese medicine and medical terminology

Wiseman's (2000) very interesting doctoral thesis is a wonderful source of information on the history and development of Chinese medicine, as well as the nature of the often descriptive metaphors used to describe body parts, and mental and physical conditions and functions. Wiseman traces the history of Chinese medicine from the first and second centuries BC onwards (2000: 112 ff.), describing the main philosophical influences on its development. He also describes the five elements in medicine (wood, fire, earth, metal and water) and explains how these are used to not only classify internal organs, but also other parts of the body, as well as bodily substances, and both physical and mental functions (2000: 116).

Some traditional Chinese medical terms reflect political, cultural and historical aspects of the eras in which they originated, going beyond the purely biomedical meaning. In their very interesting paper outlining considerations in the translation of Chinese medicine, Pritzker, Hui and Zhang (2014: 15) note that it is sometimes a good idea to include dual translations such as "windfire eye/acute conjunctivitis" in order to facilitate a link between a traditional condition in Chinese medicine with a biomedical diagnosis." Pritzker, Hui and Zhang (2014: 8) point out that Chinese medical texts have a high level of 'interreferentiality': in other words, they are linked to other texts, social, cultural and historical contexts, not just to the human body.

Wiseman (2000:161) notes that Chinese medicine has always drawn on the linguistic resources of the Chinese language, and that as a result, the many metaphors we encounter in the medical field are as clear and transparent today, as they were thousands of years ago. Examples are the Chinese words for radius and ulna, 尺骨 (ruler bone) and 橈骨 (bent bone) respectively.

Whereas the meaning of Chinese medical terms may be immediately transparent, the same cannot always be said about their English counterparts which tend to consist of Latin and Greek roots. We will therefore take a closer look at the Latin and Greek medical terms still used in English today and their common structures.

4. Spelling and pronunciation

In the US spelling convention, Greek words which were originally written with 'ae' or 'oe' in English, are written with an 'e', whereas in most former Commonwealth countries, these words are still spelled with 'ae' or 'oe'. Thus, in the US people write *gynecologist*, *anesthetist* and *edma*, whereas in UK spelling these are spelled as *gynaecologist*, *anaesthetist* and *oedema*. US spelling conventions have been followed throughout this book and in the corresponding index.

Word stress and pronunciation varies between health professionals and also between countries. As an example, the word *alveoli* (small air sacs in the lungs) is pronounced by some professionals as 'al-VEE-oh-leye', whereas others may pronounce it as 'al-vee-OH-leye'. See the Reference section for websites and books providing guidance as to the pronunciation of medical terms.

5. Latin and Greek elements in medical terms

Latin and Greek medical terms often contain a combination of elements from either language. Thus, the word *mammo-graphy* contains a form of the word *mamma* (breast) and the Greek *graphein* (to write). Alternatively terms may consist wholly of terms originating from either Latin or Greek. Often, both elements originating from either Latin or Greek may still exist side by side. As an example, the Greek words *ops* and *ophthalmos* (eye), are both used in various medical terms (e.g. *optic* nerve, *ophthalmologist*), alongside terms which contain forms derived from the Latin word *oculus* (eye).

Where medical terms consist of more than one root, a combining form may be inserted in between roots, but only if the second root starts with a consonant. The combining form is usually an 'o', used as a linking vowel. Examples are found in Table 4.1.

Table 4.1 Some examples of combining form in medical terminology

First root	Combining form	Second root	Combination
arthr	-	-itis	arthritis
arthr-	o	-scopy	arthroscopy
psych-	o	-logy	psychology
cyst-	-	-itis	cystitis
cyst-	o	-scopy	cystoscopy

5.1   Common combinations

Medical terms can be a combination of

–   Word root + word root
–   Word root + suffix
–   Prefix + word root + suffix
–   Prefix + word root + suffix
–   Word root + linking vowel* + word root (* usually 'o')

5.2   Common word roots

The most common roots used in medical terms are:

–   Body parts – these come first within the medical term (see Table 4.2)
–   Nouns denoting what is done to these body parts, or what is wrong with these body parts – these nouns usually come last within the medical term, e.g. -*algia* in the term *myalgia* (muscle-pain).
–   Nouns denoting body parts + preposition + verb, e.g. gastr-ec-tomy (stomach-out-cut, See Table 4.3).
–   Prefixes providing information about position, size, color or number of the roots that follow them (see Tables 4.4 and 4.5).

Examples of the various possible combinations will be given in separate tables below.

5.3   Common procedure nouns and verbs

As indicated above, often 'body part nouns' are followed by verbs or nouns denoting what is happening with the body part. Some common procedure nouns and verbs are given in the table below. Please note that these procedure nouns and verbs will come in last position in the medical terms. Examples of the resulting medical terms

Table 4.2 Common nouns denoting body parts

Noun	Meaning	Adjective	Example
abdomen	belly	abdominal	abdominal fat
adip(o)	fat	adipose	adipose tissue
aden(o)	gland	adeno-	adenocarcinoma
caud(o)	tail	caudal	caudal anesthesia
cephal(o)	head	cephalic	cephalic presentation
cervic(o)	neck	cervical	cervical vertebra
chondr(o)	cartilage	chondr(o)	chondrosarcoma
cranio	skull	cranial	cranial nerves
dors(o)	back	dorsal	dorsal root
inguino	groin	inguinal	inguinal hernia
lumb(o)	lower back	lumbar	lumbar spine
mamm(o)	breast	mammary	mammary glands
Mast	breast	-	mastectomy
my(o)	muscle	-	myalgia
neur(o)	nerve	neural	neural system
o(o) or ov(o)	egg	-	oophorectomy
oste(o)	bone	-	osteoarthritis
Sarco	flesh	-	sarcal
spin(o)	spine	spinal	spinal nerves
thorac(o)	chest	thoracic	thoracic surgery
ventr(o)	belly	ventral	ventral surfaces
vertebr(o)	vertebrae; spinal column	vertebral	vertebral column
viscer(o)	internal organ	visceral	visceral fat

may be found in the third column in the table below. Table 3 provides information about terms containing nouns and verbs which describe what is happening to the body parts concerned.

5.4 Common prefixes

Prefixes were often originally prepositions denoting **a position in the body**, e.g. epi (on top), para (alongside), sub or hypo (both meaning 'under'). Prefixes may also provide information about a state (e.g. overactive, underactive, abnormal). See Table 4.4

Table 4.3 Nouns and verbs describing conditions or procedures

Procedure nouns/verbs	Approximate meaning of verb	Examples	Meaning
-ec-tomy	– cutting out	mastectomy; hysterectomy	surgical removal of the breast; surgical removal of the womb
-emia	– in the blood	uremia	urea in the blood
-gram	– result of imaging	angiogram	blood vessel imaging/recording (visible result of the procedure)
-graphy	– process of imaging	angiography	blood vessel imaging/recording (the procedure)
-itis	– inflammation of	arthritis	inflammation of the joint
-logy	study; have knowledge of	neurology	study of nerves
-plasty	– repair	angioplasty	blood vessel repair
-scopy	– looking	gastroscopy; arthroscopy	looking inside the stomach; looking inside the joint
-tomy; (o) tomy	– cutting	gastrotomy	operation on the stomach

Table 4.4 Prefixes relating to position in the body

Prefix	Meaning of prefix	Examples	Meaning
ab	away from	abductor	leading away from
ad	towards	adductor	leading towards
ante	before (Gr)	antenatal	before birth
bi	two	biceps	twoheaded (muscle)
anter(o)	front	anterior	at the front; front
epi	on top of	epidural	
endo	inside		
intra	in between	intracostal	between the ribs
para	alongside	parathyroid	alongside the thyroid
peri	around	perinatal	around birth
post	after	postnatal	after birth
pre	before (Ll)	prenatal	before birth
poster(o)	behind; back	posterior	at the back; behind
inter	between	interpersonal	
meta	beyond; after	metastasis	secondary growth; secondary spread (of cancer)

for some examples. Words marked with Gr originate from classical Greek, while words marked with L originate from Latin.

Other prefixes say something about the size, state, number or color. A small sample of these have been represented in Table 4.5. Where (o) has been added, this indicates that the word originally ended in -o, however the -o may be omitted when the prefix is followed by a word that starts with a vowel sound (an example would be leuk-emia).

Table 4.5 Prefixes relating to size, state, number or color

Prefix	Meaning of prefix	Examples	Meaning
A			
neo	new	neoplasia	new growth (cancer)
dys	abnormal	dysfunctional; dysmenorrhea	
macr(o) (Gr)	large	macroscopic	visible to the naked eye
micr(o) (L)	small	microscopic	visible only using a microscope
poly (Gr)	many	polyuria	[passing] a lot of urine
olig(o) (Gr)	few	oliguria	not [passing] much urine
megal(o) (Gr)	large		
erythr(o)	red	erythrocyte	red [blood] cell
leuk(o)	white	leukemia	'white blood'
cyan(o)	blue	cyanosis	having a bluish color
melan(o)	black	melanoma	black swelling
hyper	higher; over-	hyperglycemia; hyperactive	high blood sugar level; overactive
hypo	underneath; below	hypoglycemia	low blood sugar level
sub	underneath; below	subnormal	
super	higher; over-		
uni	one	unilateral	on one side
ambi	both	ambilateral	on both sides

5.5　Suffixes

These are often adjectival forms such as -al, -ic, -ist, and -iac (e.g. celiac; hypochondriac) but may also originate from nouns such as oma (tumor), scopy (looking). Table 4.6 shows some common roots related to illness. In medical terminology, these roots are usually preceded by a noun denoting which body part is affected. Some authors describe these roots as suffixes, because they usually appear in word final position.

Table 4.6　Some common roots denoting illness – usually appearing in word final position

Procedure nouns/verbs	Meaning of verb	Examples	Meaning
-algia	- pain	myalgia	muscle ache
-patho	- disease	neuropathy	nerve-disease
-rrhaphy	suturing a gap or defect	angiorrhaphy	suturing a blood vessel
-megaly	enlargedness	cardiomegaly	enlarged heart
-rrhea	flow	dysmenorrhea	difficult or painful menstruation
-rrhage		hemorrhage	
-troph(o)	growth; development	hypertrophy	overly developed; grown larger than normal
-blast	developing cell	leukoblast	immature leukocyte, still developing
-cyte	cell	leukocyte	white (blood) cell
-gen(esis)	producing	antigen	producing antibodies
-iasis	state of	candidiasis	state of candida (yeast infection)
-lysis	breakdown; destruction	hemolysis	breakdown of blood cells
-oma	tumor; swelling	adenoma; hematoma	fat (tissue) tumor; swelling consisting of blood
-plasia	formation	(hip) dysplasia	abnormal formation (of hip)
-plasm	result of formation	neoplasm	new growth (cancer)
-osis	abnormal condition	thrombosis	abnormal condition involving blood clots

Summary of main points

Latin and Greek roots often relate to

- body parts
- position in the body
- illness or condition
- number, size or color

Within Latin and Greek medical terms, the body part often comes first, followed by a root or suffix which describes what is happening with the body part in question.

Chinese terms translated from western medicine are more transparent than their English counterparts; while Chinese medical terms with their origins from Traditional Chinese Medicine (TCM) may consist of descriptive metaphors referring to the concept of *yin-yang* and the five elements in medicine: wood, fire, earth, metal and water.

PART II

Interpreting in healthcare settings

Chapter 5

Primary care physicians and General Practitioners

This chapter aims to provide a brief introduction to primary care in their setting. We will start by providing a very brief overview of systems in English-speaking countries, followed by a quick look at the healthcare systems in Chinese-speaking countries. This has been done to help interpreters understand expectations from the side of both health professionals and patients in the interpreter-mediated encounter.

At the time of writing, US primary and secondary (see below) healthcare services are predominantly offered by private providers, and patients mostly pay for this care with the aid of health insurance plans (Sultz & Young 2006). The federal government provides healthcare for some protected populations such as active military personnel and their families; veterans; the merchant marine, and Native Americans living on reservations.

English-speaking countries such as the United Kingdom (UK), Ireland, Australia, New Zealand provide public healthcare to all their residents, which is paid for from general taxation. Canada offers publicly funded healthcare based on the Canada Health Act, and delivered through provincial health insurance (Canadian Healthcare, 2007). All these countries also have a private healthcare sector, catering to those paying from their own funds or holding private health insurance cover.

1. Primary care providers

Primary care is generally provided at a local community level while secondary care is mostly provided by specialist doctors, either in public or private hospitals or in group practices. Primary care doctors specialize in general medicine and family medicine.

Depending on the country, primary care doctors may be referred to as General Practitioners (GPS) or family doctors (UK, Australia, New Zealand) or primary (care) providers (US, Canada), primary care physicians, family physicians (US, Canada). For convenience sake, primary care providers will hereafter be referred to as PCPs.

In most US states, patients receive primary care from either a PCP or from an Advanced Registered Nurse Practitioner (ARNP), depending on the State, while receiving secondary care by public or privately run hospitals, or by group outpatient practices. Outpatient services may be provided by hospitals, or group outpatient practices.

Typically patients see their primary care doctor every time they want medical advice about a new health issue or for preventive care. They also see their primary care doctor for treatment and follow-up of ongoing health conditions such as high blood pressure, diabetes, asthma and chronic obstructive lung disorders.

The distinction between primary care and secondary care services in Hong Kong, Taiwan and Mainland China is not as clear cut as in the States and other western countries. In Hong Kong, the healthcare system operates on a dual-track basis comprising medical services provided by the public and the private sectors. The Hospital Authority of Hong Kong manages public hospitals, specialist and general outpatient clinics. Anyone with a Hong Kong identify card is eligible for public medical services, which are heavily funded by the government, with a subsidized rate of about 95% of the cost (Ko, 2013). There are also privately run hospitals and clinics providing more accessible but relatively costly medical services, usually patronized by those with private health insurance or better financial means to avoid long waits at public medical institutions. Those who cannot afford or do not want to pay for private medical services seek help from outpatient departments or emergency wards of public hospitals even for minor health issues, which would be attended to by PCPs in many Western countries.

Similarly, healthcare services in Mainland China are largely hospital-based and are managed through the Ministry of Health and local governments, supplemented by village doctors and a newly developed system of grassroots providers in urban areas which may be said to be comparable to PCPs (Eggleston 2012). However, unlike in Hong Kong, where many patients choose emergency and outpatient services provided by public hospitals because of their low charges, many people in Mainland China visit secondary and tertiary hospital outpatient departments for relatively minor conditions, primarily due to what Eggleston (2012) describes as their well-funded distrust in the quality of care provided by village doctors and grassroots providers.

In comparison, Taiwan has a more comprehensive and highly accessible healthcare system following its adoption of a National Health Insurance (NHI) system in 1995 (Wu, 2010). The NHI system operates on revenues contributed by employees, employers and the government and is administered by the government. NHI is praised throughout Asia for its accessibility, comprehensive coverage, short waiting times, friendly health professionals and relatively low cost. Under the NHI system, Taiwanese citizens can see any doctor (a GP or a specialist) and may attend any level of hospital care without a referral. However, since popular hospitals can be overcrowded and may charge a higher co-payment, Taiwanese often choose to see a family doctor or a GP for minor health issues or for preventive care and health check-ups (Wu 2010).

2. History taking

When a patient comes in for a visit, the PCP will ask what current problem the patient has come in with. Questions may include the following:

- What is the problem you have come to see me with today? What brings you in today?
- Are you in any pain? If so, what is the pain like? (Note it is important to accurately interpret the nature of the pain, see *Pain* below).
- Are you experiencing any abnormal sensations?
  - Is there any tingling or pins and needles? Any numbness?
  - Any pain or discomfort anywhere in your body?
- Do you have a fever or have you had a fever?
- Did you take your temperature? When and what was it?
- Are other people in the house or in the family sick as well?
- Are other people in the house or in the family (or at school) sick with the same symptoms?
- Have you had any change in appetite?
- Have you developed a dislike or aversion to any particular foods?
- Have you lost weight? Gained weight?
- Do you have a sore throat?
- Do you have to cough?
- Do you bring up any phlegm? What does it look like?
- Do you have a runny nose? What does the discharge look like?
- Do you have an earache/sore ear? Is there any discharge from your ear?
- Do you feel nauseated? Do you have to vomit?
- How are your bowel movements?
- Do you move your bowels regularly?
- Do you get diarrhea?
- Are your stools formed/soft/loose/watery?
- Do you have irritable bowels?

3. Pain

The doctor may ask the following questions about pain:

- Where is the pain?
- When did it start?
- What brings on the pain? What triggers the pain?

- Does the pain shoot down your leg or up your shoulder?
- Does the pain spread or radiate anywhere?
- Does anything make it better?
- Does anything make it worse? ?
- Does your ... feel irritated/tender or sore?

It is important to establish and accurately interpret the precise nature of the pain. Pain can be described as:

- a dull ache
- a discomfort
- a stitch
- superficial or deep-seated
- stinging
- slight/mild/moderate
- heavy – crushing, like a belt is tightened round the chest
- like a knife – sharp/stabbing/piercing/cutting
- recurrent and ongoing/nagging
- pulsating – coming and going like a pulse
- pounding/throbbing – beating or drumming
- hot – like a burning or searing sensation

4.   New patients

When seeing a new patient, the primary care doctor will take the person's history first, including family, social, medical, surgical and obstetric.

The family history will focus on illnesses which may 'run in families' or be hereditary or imply that the individual concerned may have a predisposition (i.e. a tendency or higher than average chance) for developing a certain condition.

Some of the most commonly asked questions would be, "Is there a family history of":

- allergies (e.g. eczema, hives, hay fever, rhinitis/runny nose, conjunctivitis/watery eyes, certain types of medication) or asthma
- epilepsy
- diabetes
- high blood pressure (hypertension)
- certain cancers (such as breast, lung or colon cancer)
- kidney disease

The social history will focus on factors which can contribute to good health or directly, or indirectly, to health problems. Some major factors would be smoking and drinking (alcohol), but stresses related to relationship problems or problems at work are also seen as factors which may lead to health problems. The doctor will ask questions which aim to elicit this sort of information. Some questions are quite sensitive. Questions as to how many cigarettes the individual smokes or how many units of alcohol he or she drinks per day or per week do not always get an honest response, but the health professional usually makes allowances for this.

Commonly asked questions in relation to the patient's social history would include:

- Do you smoke? If so, how much do you smoke? How many packs a day/per week?
- If you have stopped smoking now, how much did you use to smoke and when did you stop smoking? (This question enables the PCP to work out the number of pack years, which is used to calculate cardiovascular and pulmonological risk)
- Do you drink alcohol?
- How much alcohol do you drink and how often?
- If you have stopped drinking now, how much did you use to drink and for how long?
- Do you use (recreational) drugs?
- What type of drugs do you use? (cocaine, heroin, cannabis/marijuana, ecstasy/MDMA, pseudoephedrine, amphetamines, prescription painkillers)
- How often do you take them and in what dosage?
- Are you currently employed?
- Are you experiencing any stress at work? What is causing the stress?
- Are you experiencing any stress at home? What is causing the stress? Any bullying?
- Are you experiencing any stress in your relationships? What is causing the stress?
- What is your home situation like?
- Do you live
    - in your own home
    - in rental accommodation
    - in a trailer park
    - with other people as a boarder or roommate
    - are you homeless?
- how many people live in your house?
- do any of them smoke?
- do you have support at home? (i.e. people who are willing and able to help you and/or look after you)

The medical history may encompass questions about any previous medical problems, which may include:

- heart disease (angina pectoris/chest pain; heart attack; heart failure)
- diabetes (insulin-dependent or non-insulin-dependent)
- circulation problems (thrombosis; bleeding; narrowing of the arteries)
- digestive (ulcers; constipation; diarrhea; gas)
- lungs (tuberculosis; asthma; pneumonia; bronchitis; chronic obstructive lung disease).

The surgical history will focus on past surgery, what this was (or where) and when. This may include procedures such as:

- total hip replacement
- appendectomy ("Have you had your appendix out?")
- cholecystectomy ("Have you had your gallbladder taken out?")
- terminations of pregnancy (this is the medical term for the lay word "abortion")
- C-sections (Cesarean sections)
- laparoscopy (minor operation where the surgeon looks inside the abdomen through a fiber optic tube called a scope)

Obstetric history questions focus on previous pregnancies, deliveries or miscarriages/ terminations of pregnancy. These are discussed in detail in Chapters 12 and 28.

The primary care doctor may also ask questions concerning the patient's mental health. Such questions may include:

- How have you been feeling about life lately?
- Has your appetite changed? Have you lost appetite? Are you eating more than before?
- Have you been feeling down?
- Are you experiencing any stress at the moment? Are you able to sleep?
- Do you hear voices in your head?
- Have you ever been admitted to a psychiatric ward/acute assessment unit/ psychiatric hospital?
- When and what for?
- Are you currently on any medication?

Once again, it is important that interpreters not only interpret exactly what the patient says but also interpret and relay questions to the patient accurately. In order to do so the interpreter needs to be familiar with current medical and healthcare terminology in both languages. In addition, the interpreter needs to be aware of the healthcare systems in both countries. The interpreter also needs to be aware of the cultural differences and different cultural attitudes towards health problems so as to be able to inform the professional of these if necessary.

5. Physical examination

In order to reach a provisional diagnosis, the primary care doctor will examine the patient (or have vital signs, height and weight recorded by their medical assistant) performing certain checks including:

- *Pulse*: The medical assistant may say "*I will take your pulse.*" This may enable the doctor to tell if the pulse is weak or strong (heart is beating weakly or strongly, blood pressure is low or high), if the pulse is slow or fast, regular or irregular.
- *Blood pressure*: The medical assistant may say: "*I will take your blood pressure; your blood pressure is up (higher than normal)/high/low.*" If the blood pressure is 120/80, 120 is the systolic blood pressure, while 80 refers to the diastolic blood pressure. The doctor may ask certain questions in relation to the person's blood pressure. Some of these might be:
    - Do you smoke? How much/how often do you smoke?
    - Do you drink a lot of coffee/strong tea? How much coffee/tea do you drink in a day?
    - How much salt do you take in your food?
    - What medications are you on at the moment? (This includes asthma inhalers)
    - Have you lost a lot of blood/do you have very heavy periods?
    - Is there a family history of kidney problems?
    - Do you feel faint when you get up suddenly?
    - Do you feel any pressure/tightness in your head?
- *Auscultation:* The doctor may use his stethoscope to listen to the person's chest or abdomen. He or she may listen for abnormal breathing sounds or abnormal heart sounds, or for signs that the bowels are working.
  Auscultation of the lungs: The doctor will tell the patient to "*take a deep breath*" and listen to the breath sounds.
- *Auscultation of the heart:* the doctor may count the heart rate by placing a stethoscope at the base of the heart. This may enable the doctor to tell if there are any problems such as heart murmurs (abnormal heart sounds) or irregular heart beat.
- *Percussion:* This involves the doctor tapping the patient's chest and abdomen – listening for "dull" and "hollow" sounds. This does not usually require any interpreting.

- *Palpation:* This involves the doctor feeling for normal/abnormal *"lumps and bumps."* The doctor may feel the lymph nodes or lymph glands (in the neck or groin) to see if they are enlarged. They may also feel the liver. Often the doctor will ask questions such as *"Does it hurt if I press here?"*

6.   Tests or diagnostic studies

Some tests may be performed at the primary care doctor's office, while others are carried out elsewhere. Patients may be given a lab form and told to report to the nearest laboratory for blood tests, or to go to the nearest radiologist service for X-rays or ultrasounds.

Tests still done by primary care doctors include:

- pap smears (to check for cervical cancer)
- blood glucose tests – to test the amount of sugar in the patient's bloodstream
- HbA1c test – to test the patient's blood sugar levels over the past few months
- urine tests – checked for sugar, protein, ketones
- peak flow test – to test the amount of air a patient with asthma is able to breathe out
- electrocardiogram (ECG or EKG) – to record the electrical activity of the heart

Other common tests which the primary care doctor may order and give the patient a referral form for include:

- *chest X-ray* – an X-ray of the chest to examine the structures of the organs in the chest (heart, lungs, windpipe, diaphragm)
- *ultrasound of the abdomen* – a scan using high-frequency sound waves. Some gel is placed on the abdomen and the sensor is moved around to examine organs in the abdomen. Patients may need to have a full bladder, depending on the instructions they are given prior to the ultrasound.
- *blood tests.* Commonly ordered blood tests would include:
  - complete Blood Count (CBC); especially Hemoglobin (see glossary),
  - white blood cells (see glossary) and platelets (see glossary)
  - urea and electrolytes
  - thyroxin and TSH levels – to test the amount of thyroid and thyroid stimulating hormone in the blood
  - Liver function tests – to see if the liver is working normally
  - cholesterol test – see page 256
  - erythrocyte sedimentation rate (ESR) – a blood test mainly used to check if there is any inflammation process going on in the body
  - urine tests – some urine tests may be performed by the primary care doctor, e.g. pregnancy tests; tests which show sugar or protein, the presence of which can be tested by using a simple dipstick

7.   Immunization schedule

Parents who wish to have their children immunized may go to their primary care physician who will examine the child first to ensure that he or she is in a fit state to be immunized. The vaccinations themselves are usually given by the doctor's nurse. Parents are instructed to contact the doctor if the child becomes unwell following the vaccination.

8.   Health education

The primary care doctor has an important role to play in the area of health education. They can explain medical conditions to the patient and also give instructions and advice on how to control the medical condition; how to deal with warning signs; what diet to follow; what exercise to undertake (if any), and where to go for specialist advice. The primary care doctor will also explain what referrals are possible and which associations offer further help and advice.

It is important that the interpreter convey instructions and advice very carefully and accurately. Interpreters may wish to provide the primary care doctor with information on the patient's cultural background where appropriate.

9.   Referrals

On the basis of his/her findings, the primary care doctor may reach a provisional diagnosis and decide to either:

–   treat and observe the patient himself/herself, in which case the patient will be sent home with a prescription and/or instructions and the patient may be asked to come back for a follow-up visit
–   refer the patient to other health professionals more specialized in a particular area. In this case the patient may be referred to
    –   a surgical outpatient clinic if the doctor suspects that the patient's problem may (eventually) require surgery
    –   an internal medicine specialist clinic
    –   the hospital's emergency room
    –   other health professionals out in the community.

In the US some insurance plans will allow patients to self-refer to a specialist, however, most require the patient to have a referral from a PCP. In most other English-speaking countries, General Practitioners will refer patients to a specialist, and self-referral may not be possible.

It will be clear from this chapter that PCPs have a good all-around knowledge of medicine and may often reach a provisional diagnosis but will refer patients to specialist doctors for further investigation and treatment when necessary.

10. Some notes for interpreters and translators

The interpreter should always wait for the patient's answer and not answer "Yes" or "No" as in the case of the interpreter who was interpreting for a pregnant woman. The midwife said: "*Do you have a pain in your abdomen?*" to which the interpreter hurriedly replied "*Yes, yes, yes*," without relaying the question to the patient. The woman was rushed to the delivery room where another interpreter was called in. With the aid of this second interpreter, who did relay all questions faithfully to the patient, it was established that the woman was not in premature labor, as it was first assumed, but merely experienced a burning sensation whenever she was passing urine, because she did, in fact, have a urinary tract infection.

When asked "*Do you drink alcohol?*" the word *alcohol* itself may give rise to confusion. Nurses at a public hospital tuberculosis clinic in New Zealand were told by interpreters that patients from some cultural and linguistic backgrounds did not consider *beer* to be alcohol. Consequently, many of the patients who were told not to drink any alcohol with their anti-tuberculosis medication still drank beer, in the mistaken belief that that was not really alcohol. For this reason, some of the interpreters decided to render the word "*alcohol*" as "*alcohol and beer.*"

As to the number of cigarettes the person actually smokes, even if the interpreter knows that the person smokes two packs a day, he or she will have to interpret whatever the client says. Questions relating to employment are mainly intended to find out if the patient is stressed or depressed or going through financial difficulties. The patient may be unemployed or may have been laid off. Loss of work can lead to the patient going through the various stages of the grieving process (see Chapter 2). Long periods of unemployment may leave some patients depressed.

Accommodation can also be a major factor in health outcomes. Overcrowded housing situations may lead to children picking up bacterial and viral infections from others in the house. Families may have to sleep on moldy mattresses in drafty trailer homes or garages. Many may be subjected to passive smoking by inhaling second-hand smoke exhaled by others in the house. Smoking (active or passive) has been linked to childhood asthma, crib death (SIDS) and lung cancer, so these are important questions.

Patients (and interpreters) may have to wait quite a while in the waiting room before they can go in to see the PCP or GP. Interpreters should take this into account when booking interpreting assignments.

Summary of main points

This chapter has looked at primary care physicians including:

– history taking (medical, surgical, family, social, mental health)
– physical examination
– common diagnostic tests

This chapter has also provided a glimpse of the healthcare systems in Hong Kong, Taiwan and Mainland China.

Chapter 6

Specialty clinics and Outpatient Clinics

Clinics can provide primary care (primary care clinics) or specialty care (specialty or Outpatient clinics). This chapter will look at specialty clinics in the US and Outpatient Clinics in countries which have a publicly funded healthcare system (such as the UK, Ireland, Australia and New Zealand). Most people will see their primary care provider first when suffering from ill health. In many cases, their provider will examine, diagnose and treat the patient. However, if the doctor feels that the patient's condition is outside their area of specialty, or the patient's condition is unstable or not improving, or the doctor feels that another (differential) diagnosis may be possible, the doctor may refer patient to a specialist (in a specialist group practice). PCPs will tell their patients: "I'm referring you to Dr. XXX in neurology." PCPs will email a referral to the specialist. The referral will briefly outline the patient's previous history and the history of the current condition. PCPs refer patients to specialists, who operate clinics that provide the relevant tests (e.g. a neurologist would administer EMGs at her own office). There are imaging clinics that perform mammograms, sonograms, and the like upon referral by a PCP. The tests are administered by technicians, who send the sonogram or whatever to a radiologist or other specialist, who in turn reports back to the PCP on the results.

Seeing a specialist has advantages in that patients get to be seen by a highly experienced doctor. Some US patients find they cannot afford the specialist's fees or that their health insurer will not cover them. In countries with a public health system there is usually no fee payable for attending an Outpatient Clinic (if the patient is a citizen or permanent resident), however, patients may have to wait a while before they get their appointment. In these countries, non-residents may be presented with a bill (invoice) after receiving medical attention. Some Chinese-speaking patients who are not residents say they prefer to be presented with an invoice beforehand (as the Chinese healthcare system may require pre-payment) so they know what amount to expect to pay.

1. Specialty clinics

Some specialty clinics include:

Prenatal   Also called antenatal. Women are referred here for check-up visits during pregnancy. Since Gestational Diabetes (GDM) is increasingly common in many countries, larger hospitals may have dedicated clinics for women with GDM.

Gynecology	Women are referred here if their doctor thinks they may need specialist consultations for gynecological problems.
Neurology	Patients are referred here if their doctor suspects they may problems affecting the central nervous system or peripheral nervous system.
Cardiology	Patients are referred here if their doctor suspects they may have a problem with their heart (e.g. coronary artery disease, heart valve problems or rhythm problems), for pre-operative and post-operative assessment of the heart and Holter monitoring (monitoring heart rate and sometimes also blood pressure over a longer period).
Orthopedics	GPs/PCPs will refer their patients here if they suspect they might have a problem to do with their bones or joints (e.g. osteoarthritis of the hip joint, possibly needing a total hip replacement). Many patients who have fractured (broken) a bone, go here for follow-up visits.
Urology	Patients are referred to the urologist for prostate problems, recurring urinary tract infections, and so on.
Endocrinology	Patients are referred here with problems of the hormone producing system, including hyperthyroidism (an overactive thyroid gland), diabetes and the like.
Family planning	Couples who wish to conceive or those who do not wish to conceive can go to the family planning clinic for advice on contraception, fertility and so on.
Dental	Patients are referred here with major and acute problems concerning their teeth.
Plastic Surgery	Burn patients can be referred to the plastic surgery clinic for surgical repair of badly scarred areas on their bodies (e.g. due to burns); patients can also be referred here for treatment of skin cancers, repair of nerves, tendons and skin, or correction of cleft palates or protruding ears.
Renal	This is a clinic for people who have kidney problems. Some patients may have end-stage renal failure and will need to go on dialysis.

Some specialty clinics provide medical check-ups and assistance for people with chronic conditions such as diabetes or asthma. This may include the following:

Diabetes Clinic	Here patients can consult special diabetes nurses who can teach them how to inject insulin and how to do their own blood sugar readings; in addition, there are dietitians who can offer special dietary advice.
Eye clinic	This clinic treats eye complaints.

2. Staff at specialty clinics

Staff at outpatient or specialist clinics will vary from one state to another, but in general includes registered nurses, specialized ARNPs and medical specialists. Clinics may also employ medical technicians, healthcare assistants and residents training to become specialists.

3. Procedure at specialty clinics

The patient may have been to see his primary care doctor or may have been to the clinic before, and may have been asked to return for a follow-up appointment.

After reporting to the clinic, the patient's weight may be checked. Usually medical staff will want to know the patient's weight for three main reasons:

–   Weight gain may be a sign that the patient has regained his/her appetite, which can be a sign of recovery. Conversely, weight loss may be a sign that the patient has lost appetite and may be deteriorating.
–   Weight gain may be a sign that the patient has too much fluid on board (retaining fluid in his/her body). For this reason weight gain is checked in patients who are pregnant, or patients with heart or kidney problems, amongst other things.
–   Doctors use the person's body weight to calculate the doses of medication that they need to receive. A short, slender woman might be easily overdosed if she received the drug dose prescribed for a much taller and heavier woman. She might possibly experience more side effects.

In addition to weight, the patient's history will be documented and physical examinations and commonly performed tests may be performed (much the same as that for the procedure followed by the primary care provider).

The following procedures may also be carried out at outpatient service facilities:

Imaging:	This may include X-rays; magnetic resonance imaging (MRIs); computed tomography (CTs); (positron emission tomography (PET) scans; ultrasounds; Doppler tests.
Other diagnostic tests:	These may include bronchoscopy, colonoscopy, colposcopy, gastroscopy; eye examinations; lung function testing, hearing testing and many others.

For more information on specific areas of medicine and common disorders and treatment methods, please refer to the relevant chapters.

4.   Some notes for interpreters and translators

There are countries in which the concept of specialty clinics does not exist. In some countries, people 'self-diagnose' their problems to a large extent and go straight to a private specialist without any referral from a primary care provider, as is the case in Taiwan, where patients can see a specialist directly or attend any level of hospital without a referral, as described in the previous chapter. In Hong Kong, a patient can also see a specialist in a private specialty clinic without a referral if the consultation is self-funded.

Alternatively, patients may self-diagnose and then visit a drugstore or pharmacy to buy what *they* think they need (such as antibiotics). This practice is common among people who do not like the idea of seeing a doctor and in some poor areas in Mainland China where people cannot afford the high medical consultation fees, which usually have to be prepaid.

Some countries do not have a system where primary health care is provided by PCPs or GPs and so the whole concept of primary care physicians referring patients on to specialty care clinics may be difficult to convey. Migrants from such countries may present straight to the Emergency Room or Emergency Department at the hospital, with symptoms of what are considered Primary Care types of complaints in countries with a good primary care system.

Patients (and interpreters) may have to wait quite a while in the waiting room before they can go in to see the specialist. Interpreters should take this into account when booking interpreting assignments.

Summary of main points

This chapter has looked at outpatient and specialist clinics including:

- different specialties (medical, surgical, family, social, mental health)
- health professionals involved
- procedures and common diagnostic tests

Chapter 7

Hospitals

Very often interpreters are first called in when the patient has been admitted, or is in the process of being admitted, to the hospital. Due to ongoing changes within the American healthcare system, information in this chapter will be very general. Every hospital has its own culture and its own way of doing things. However, in most English speaking countries, the hospital system can trace its historical roots to Britain and to the hospitals set up by religious orders in Medieval Europe. Some commentators (cf. Risse 1999; Wall, n.d.) describe the broad underpinnings of hospital cultures in countries within northwestern Europe and North America as follows:

- the isolation of the sick, dating back to the isolation of ill people in medieval Europe, in hospitals (literally: guest houses), looked after by religious "brothers and sisters" (monks and nuns);
- the medico-scientific or biomedical approach, in which diagnosis and treatment are based on scientific evidence and cultural beliefs are not taken into account;
- the patient-oriented approach, in which medical staff is focused on the individual patient, rather than on the patient's family.

It needs to be stressed that hospitals can be expected to be uniform and consistent in core matters such as standards of care and professional ethics of medical and nursing staff. However, differences across countries in the three aspects listed above can result in cross-cultural issues which may affect the interpreter and will therefore be discussed in some more detail below.

1. The isolation of the sick

Peculiar, perhaps, to Western culture is the tendency to isolate sick people in hospitals, where they are looked after by health professionals. As Helman states (1990, p. 70), "Patients are removed from the continuous emotional support of family and community and cared for by healers whom they may never have seen before." In most Western countries, people accompany their loved ones to hospitals, stay only during visiting hours, two visitors at a time, and then depart, trusting that their loved ones will be well looked after by those whose job it is to do so. Nurses expect family members to come in to visit only during visiting hours, so as not to disturb the nurses in doing their job in caring for the patients. An exception to this is pediatric specialty hospitals, where parents are considered part of the care team and often stay with their sick child 24/7.

The tendency to isolate sick people in hospitals, and to leave them to the care of professionals, may not be found in all countries. New immigrants from many areas around the world may feel that leaving a sick relative in the hospital, without being there for them, is socially unacceptable. Anybody who left their old parents all by themselves in the hospital overnight might be branded a 'bad' child. For this reason, relatives may request to be allowed to stay with patients in order to look after them. Such requests may be misunderstood in healthcare systems where the isolation of the sick is the accepted norm.

2.   The biomedical approach

In most Western countries, the diagnosis of 'disease' is based on scientific evidence. The word medico-scientific also means that it is medical staff who prescribe treatment on the basis of scientific evidence. As explained in Chapter 3, sometimes patients' attitudes may be based on different cultural and religious belief systems, and this may lead to conflict, mutual misunderstanding and mistrust. Immigrant patients may self-diagnose illness and self-treat their conditions. The diagnosis they reach will be based on their own beliefs as to how the body functions. Similarly, the remedies they choose may be based on scientifically unproven popular beliefs and folk remedies (Helman 1990; Jackson 2006; Camplin-Welch 2007). If the initial remedies do not have the desired effect, sick people may seek help from a wide range of alternative healers such as herbalists, faith healers, clairvoyants and shamans. Often, medical help is only sought as a last resort.

Cases of patients receiving a diagnosis and then leaving the hospital to try alternative healers are not uncommon. In some unfortunate cases, patients have then returned to the hospital when alternative treatments have failed. Interpreters may find that they have to act as cultural liaisons in cases in which hospital staff find it difficult to understand the various cultural and popular beliefs that motivate patients to seek alternative treatments based on deep-seated cultural beliefs.

3.   The patient-oriented approach

In most Western societies (cf. Hofstede 1980), it is the patient who is told that they have a certain condition. The doctor will explain treatment options so as to enable the patient to make a decision based on these treatment options and will obtain the patient's agreement (informed consent) before embarking on any operations or potentially harmful procedures.

This is in contrast with accepted procedure in some other societies where the patient may be the last to know what is wrong and what is going to happen as family members may have decided what is best for the patient. One Pacific Island support worker reported the case of the young woman who needed radical surgery to give her a real chance of surviving her cancer. Her family were outraged and insisted that she seek help and advice from a faith healer. The woman had to literally "go into hiding" from her family in order to have the treatment she wanted.

Situations such as these may give rise to conflict and misunderstanding and may lead to relatives putting pressure on the interpreter, asking that he not interpret the real diagnosis. Relatives should approach medical staff through the interpreter, rather than asking interpreters to breach the interpreters' code of ethics.

4. Hospital staff

In certain areas of the hospital, it may be difficult to differentiate between nursing staff, medical staff and technical support staff as all may be wearing '*blues*' or '*greens*' or even everyday clothing. In this case the interpreter should pay specific attention to name badges in order to know with whom he or she is dealing. In inpatient settings, the contact person for the interpreter will most likely be the charge nurse, while in hospital-based outpatient clinics, the contact will be the check-in or registration staff.

5. Nursing staff

In most English and Chinese-speaking countries nursing staff will mainly consist of Registered Nurses (RNs) and midwives. However, interpreters in the US will work with a range of nursing staff, including:

- Certified Nursing Assistants (CNAs), who have a few months of training and usually perform basic direct care tasks such as changing bedpans;
- Licensed Practical Nurses (LPNs), or Licensed Vocational Nurses who usually have about one year of training and who can do all the tasks of a CNA plus more advanced care such as starting IVs, giving injections, and assessing patient progress.
- In the US Registered Nurses (RNs) can have a two year degree (ASN) or a four-year degree (BSN). They can do all the tasks of lower-level nursing staff, as well as more advanced tasks such as supervising the work of other nurses, operating medical equipment, giving medications, assisting in surgery, and administering care plans. In all other countries, RNs usually have a Bachelor Degree and are able to work under supervision by a doctor.

Advanced Practice Registered Nurses (APRNs) hold advanced degrees and specialize in specific areas of care. Some examples of APRNs include Certified Registered Nurse Anesthetists (CRNAs), Certified Nurse Midwives (CNMs), Certified Nurse Specialists (CNSs), Certified Nurse Specialists for Psychiatric/Mental Health (CNS/PSYCH) or Advanced Registered Nurse Practitioners (ARNPs). Generally speaking, APRNs function semi-independently, providing care under the indirect supervision of an MD.

Because this range of nursing qualifications may not exist in other countries, it may be difficult to find a satisfactory equivalent in Chinese for example, and interpreters may have to paraphrase by adding some information about the nursing professionals' scope of practice.

Midwives	Midwives are health practitioners trained to guide women during pregnancy, as well as during and after childbirth. Different countries and states have different training programs and different legislation determining midwives' scope of practice.
Private nurses	Also known as *private duty nurses,* they attend an individual patient, usually on a fee-for-service basis, and they may specialize in a specific type of disease.
Geriatric nurse	Registered Nurse specialized in nursing elderly patients.
Visiting nurse	A Registered Nurse who works for a public health agency or hospital to promote community health and especially to visit patients in their homes and give them treatment recommended by the treating physician. Also known as a ***public health nurse.***

6.   Medical staff

Interpreters will work with medical doctors, ranging from newly qualified to specializing or qualified specialists/attending physicians.

In Mainland China, medical training is similar to that in the UK, but involves a condensed five-year program, followed by residency training which may range from anywhere between 3 to 8 years, depending on the specialty. Graduates must work as a resident physician for a few years before being able to sit the National Medical Licensing Examination (NMLE) leading to certification as a physician. Graduates can only practice medicine in China once their registration as a physician has been approved by the Chinese Ministry of Health.

In the United Kingdom (UK), Ireland and New Zealand (NZ), medical training tends to involve six years at Medical School, and includes internships for medical students. After graduating from Medical school, 'Junior Doctors' undergo further training in the public hospital system. Doctors training to become medical specialists may be referred to as Registrars. In the UK and NZ, medical specialists may still be referred to as 'consultants' when working in the public hospital system.

The Australian medical training system is undergoing some changes and moving ore towards the US model: doctors training to specialize in a particular area of medicine may be referred to as residents.

In the US newly qualified medical doctors undertake 3–8 years training as a resident, the duration of training depending on their chosen specialty. First-year residents are called 'interns.' In teaching hospitals, residents provide a great deal of the outpatient and most of the inpatient care, although always under the supervision of a more senior physician called the 'attending physician', or just 'the attending.' Residents work in teams, which often rotate from service to service to provide broader exposure to the residents. Attending physicians in inpatient settings work with a team of residents, supervising their work and teaching as they go. In outpatient settings, one resident may be paired with one attending.

Patients in hospitals in the US will also see 'hospitalists'. These are physicians who specialize in the care of acutely ill hospitalized patients. It is a specialty focused on the location of care (the hospital), rather than on a disease (such as oncology), an organ system (such as gastroenterology), or an age group (such as geriatrics).

7. Specialists

Specialists are physicians who have developed a specialized knowledge in a specific area over many years of supervised training in a particular specialty and who have been recognized as a specialist by members of a specific college of specialist physicians (e.g. the American Board of Obstetrics and Gynecology).

8. Other hospital staff

Admitting Staff   Admitting staff is based in the Admitting Department or at the front desk. This clerk ensures that the necessary information required for admission is collected and entered. Admitting staff will ask about health insurance, race/ethnicity, language preference and other demographic data. Also known as Health Unit Secretary.

Chaplain	Most hospitals have chaplains, who may or may not be ordained clergy, but who provide spiritual care to patients of any faith or persuasion. Chaplains may be on staff at the hospital or on call.

9. Other healthcare staff

Dietitian	Hospital meals are prepared by the Dietary Department for all patients. However, dietitians ensure that specific patients receive special individually 'designed' meals in relation to their medical condition.
Lactation Consultant	Usually a nurse or midwife with special responsibility for breast-feeding mothers.
Occupational Therapist or (OT)	A health professional trained to help people to carry out the activities of daily living (ADL), including work activities and self-care activities such as washing, bathing, showering, dressing/undressing, preparing drinks or food and toileting. OTs are also involved with providing adaptations such as orthotics, ramps for wheelchairs, handrails and the like. OTs working in the community may advise on the installation of toilet heighteners, bath planks, wheelchair ramps and support bars on walls.
Pharmacist	The hospital pharmacist checks which medications are in stock, monitors patients' medication charts and assures that nurses have inpatient drug supplies to dispense. Many hospitals also have outpatient pharmacies to serve patients who are being discharged or patients seen at outpatient clinics in the hospital.
Physical therapist	These health professionals are trained to assist patients in regaining mobility following surgery or a serious medical event (such as stroke). They may also be called in to assist with deep-breathing exercises following surgery.
Speech pathologist	Professional involved in treating people who have problems with normal oral communication, usually following some physiological event such as a stroke or head injury. Also called speech language therapist or speech pathologist. See also Chapter 14.

| *Social Worker* | Specially trained professional who assists people who have social, domestic and financial problems as a result of their condition or disability. |

10. Hospital procedures

Hospital procedures can be baffling and confusing to anyone who comes to a hospital for the first time, but particularly so for people who are new to the country as a whole. Hospital procedures vary from country to country and from hospital to hospital. In addition, every department or inpatient unit may also have its own procedures. This book will only present a very general outline of commonly-used procedures.

11. Admissions

11.1 Types – emergency and scheduled

If a patient has a medical emergency that requires immediate care, the patient may be brought by ambulance to a hospital Emergency Department, often called the Emergency Room or 'ER'.

Upon entering the Emergency Department, to the patient will need to be stabilized. Stabilizing involves ensuring that the patient's condition does not get any worse. From there, the patient may be treated and sent home, or he may be admitted to 'a floor' in the hospital for continued care.

An emergency admission can be very stressful for the interpreter, the patient and his or her family. In emergency admission cases, the interpreter may be called in to interpret at odd hours. They may be woken from sleep and may not be feeling quite alert and awake upon arrival in the hospital yet be required to interpret all information with great accuracy. In addition, patients and their families may be very stressed and emotional, which may make it difficult for the interpreter to concentrate and/or remain calm. Furthermore, the interpreter may not have time or opportunity to prepare for the assignment, or for any terminology that may crop up, and there may be very little background information available on the patient and the patient's condition.

It is essential, however, that the interpreter interpret all questions to the patient or the patient's family very accurately. In some cases, the interpreter may note that the medical staff is not getting the complete message because they do not understand specific non-verbal cues, which may mean that they are not able to reach an accurate diagnosis. It is important, in such cases, that the interpreter also serve as a culture broker by clarifying certain non-verbal expressions to the health professional.

In the case of a scheduled admission, the patient has been told beforehand to report to the hospital for a certain procedure or investigation on a certain date.

On the whole, scheduled admissions are less stressful to both interpreter and patient. The interpreter may be told beforehand where the admission will take place and for what reason and therefore typically has time to prepare for the interview. Likewise the patient may be more prepared for the admission and may be less stressed.

12. Admission process

Upon arrival in the inpatient unit for a scheduled admission, one of the nursing staff will show patients where their beds are and where to put clothes and other personal belongings. Some inpatient procedures may be explained and the patient may be shown the layout of the unit. After this, the nursing staff will do some baseline recordings for comparison purposes (e.g. weight, height, blood pressure, temperature, respiratory/breathing rate and heart rate/pulse). Additional baseline recordings may be done, such as a peak flow reading, an electrocardiogram (EKG) or a blood glucose reading, depending on the type of unit and the condition of the patient. The nurse will record these findings in a chart.

The nurse may then proceed to take a nursing history. These questions typically focus on the patient's mental and physical state. It is important for nursing staff to know whether patient are fully aware of the reason for their admission, how they feel about it, whether they have other concerns or stresses in their life (such as worries about employment, benefits, young children at home, relationship problems), the presence or absence of support people, religious or cultural beliefs, and any special needs and/ or habits. The nurse will also ask patients whether they can still cope with the activities of daily living, such as cooking, doing the household chores, gardening, and so on.

Patients are instructed not to bring with them any valuables such as jewelry, laptops or cell phones, because the hospital will not assume responsibility for any stolen or damaged items. If the patient is in possession of money and other valuables, the hospital provides safekeeping facilities.

When the nurse has finished taking the nursing history, a medical staff member may come to see the patient.

13. Most important rooms (from the patient's perspective)

Nurses' station   This is the central area where nurses keep patient records. Medical staff may also be found here, writing up patient notes.

Patient's room   Can be a single, double room or may be a ward containing four or more beds. The patient's room will generally contain a bed-side locker or bed-side table on wheels, a few chairs and a ward-robe. The toilets and showers usually have to be shared with other patients. Some rooms will contain a toilet chair, also referred to as a commode.

Nursery   Found in maternity units, a special room where babies spend their days/nights. The nursery will be kept at an agreeable temperature and may contain equipment for bathing and changing babies.

14.   Discharge

Once patients have completed their stay in hospital, the medical staff will decide on a discharge date and mode. Most commonly, patients are discharged home with follow-up by their primary care provider. Sometime there may be follow-up by staff at the relevant outpatient clinic or patients may be given a referral for a *visiting nurse*.

Interpreters may be needed to interpret specific discharge instructions regarding medications, diet, follow-up and activities of daily living. Some patients may be advised to avoid certain activities of daily living (such as heavy lifting, vacuum cleaning or sexual intercourse) for a certain period of time. Obviously such instructions will need to be interpreted accurately to avoid putting the patient's health in jeopardy. Clarification of different cultural attitudes may be of great importance at this stage. In some cultures, for example, the idea of being told that you are ill and that you have to exercise may well be considered incompatible. The interpreter may need to act as a culture broker and clarify this to the health professionals concerned, interpreting any clarification s/he provides in the patient's language also. Once alerted to any possible issues, the health professional may then be able to address this with the patient.

The next section of the book deals with rehabilitation and physical therapy.

15.   Rehabilitation

Rehabilitation is an important part of medical care – both in the hospital setting and in the community. Rehabilitation has been defined as the process of restoring "personal autonomy in those aspects of daily living considered most relevant by patients or service users and their family caregivers" (Sinclair & Dickinson 1998, p. 27). In general, rehabilitation focuses mainly on restoring a person's physical (and psychological) independence, well-being and quality of life. This section will also touch on geriatrics, because it is common for older patients to need (long-term) rehabilitation relating to chronic conditions (e.g. emphysema), neurological consequences of stroke or after surgery.

Interpreters may work with health professionals who are assisting patients with recovery after heart attacks (cardiac rehabilitation) and strokes or spinal cord injuries (neurological rehabilitation), or those working with patients suffering from long-term disabilities or recovering from cancer surgery. Braddom (2011) provides an excellent overview of rehabilitative care in a wide range of settings.

Interpreting for rehabilitation therapists and geriatricians centers mostly on an accurate exchange of information. The health professional will usually start by assessing what the client's needs and goals are and what the client is still able and willing to do. Once the therapist has made this assessment, he will proceed with a treatment plan, which he will want to discuss with the client and/or the client's family.

16.   Health professionals

Hospitalist – A physician based in a hospital who is in charge of the care of hospitalized patients in the place of their primary care physicians.

Intensivist – A physician who specializes in caring for critically ill patients, usually in an intensive care unit.

Geriatrician – medical specialist specializing in the health of older adults. *Occupational therapist* – health professional who helps people to improve their ability to perform tasks in their daily living and working environments; the abbreviation OT is often used to refer to this profession. See also Hammell (2009).

Physical therapist – Health professional who has completed studies in the treatment of muscular disorders – see also Chapters 7 and 22.

Speech Pathologist – see Chapter 14.

Podiatrist – medical professional specializing in the medical assessment and treatment of disorders relating to foot, ankle and lower leg, including foot and ankle surgery. Their medical title may be abbreviated as DPM – Doctor of Podiatric Medicine.

Nutritionist – provides guidance on nutrition and diet.

Dietitian – Registered or licensed dietitians provide guidance on diets and nutrition.

17.   Physical therapy

Physical therapists have completed a program of studies in the treatment of muscular disorders and may assist clients with a range of treatment options, following an assessment. Rehabilitation physical therapy usually involves exercises to improve the client's strength, endurance and range of motion (ROM), teaching the client to walk with a walking aid (crutches, walker) or teaching the client how to use a wheelchair and transfer from wheelchair to bed, toilet or even to a motor vehicle. Other treatment options may include exercises; electrical stimulation; massage; taping and bandaging or applying heat or cold (ice).

The physical therapist may give the client instructions on certain exercises and may ask the client if they experience any pain while carrying out particular movements. The physical therapist may ask the client to flex (bend) or extend (stretch). Instead of using these words, the therapist may say things like *"Curl up your toes,"* *"Make a fist," "Grab my hand and squeeze as hard as you can."*.

18.   Occupational therapy

Occupational therapists may work with clients in hospitals, nursing homes or in the wider community. Their aim is to help people to improve their ability to perform tasks in their daily living and working environments (activities of daily living, abbreviated as ADL). Where occupational therapists work with people in their own homes, they may recommend that equipment and aids be installed, to help their clients cope with the ADL. Equipment may include ramps so the client can get in/out of his house by wheelchair, raised toilet seats, bath boards, shower seats, anti-slip mats, and handrails.

19.   Some notes for interpreters and translators

MDs will often liaise with other health professionals, such as residents, attendings, house surgeons, dietitians, public health nurses, counselors, diabetes nurse educators and physical therapists. It is important that all questions and answers be interpreted accurately, to ensure that appropriate care can be continued.

You may hear the term inpatient mentioned: An inpatient is a patient who is admitted to hospital under a certain medical team and who stays at least overnight. The medical team in question assumes responsibility for the patient's treatment and discharges him or her back to the care of the primary care provider when treatment has been completed. If the patient is not going to stay the night, they present to the day surgery area in the hospital for their procedure.

We will finish with a brief note about surgical units as opposed to medical units. Some healthcare interpreters may not be familiar with the double meaning of the word *medical*. In hospitals, the word *medical* is often used to denote the opposite of *surgical*. Surgical treatment involves surgery, whereas medical treatment involves non-surgical treatment methods, such as medication, observation, exercise, bedrest, and the like.

20.   English-Chinese glossary

英漢詞彙表

English	Hong Kong & Taiwan	Mainland China
activities of daily life; activities of daily living (ADL)	日常生活活動	日常生活活动
acute admission	急症入院	急症入院
admission to hospital	入院; 住院	入院; 住院
admissions	入院; 住院	入院; 住院
Admitting Clerk	收症員; 入院登記員	入院登记员
Admitting Department	收症部; 入院登記處	住院部
Advanced Practice Registered Nurse (APRN)	註冊專科護理師; 資深護師	高等(执业)注册护士
baseline recordings	基準線記錄	基本生理指标纪录
booked admission	預約入院; 預約住院	预定入院; 预定住院
Chaplain; Priest	(駐院)牧師; 院牧; (駐院)神父	牧师; 神父
checkup	檢查; 健康檢查	体格检查; 体检
family room	家屬室	家属室
Dietitian	營養學家; 營養師; 膳食師	营养指导员; 营养专家; 营养(医)师
discharge	出院	出院
District Nursing Service	地區社康護理服務	地区护理服务
emergency admission	緊急入院	紧急入院
Emergency Department	急症室	急诊科; 急诊科
Emergency Services	急症室服務; 急救服務	急救服务
Geriatric Nurse	老人科護士	老年病护士
Geriatrician	老人科醫生; 老人科專家	老年病科医生; 老年病科专家
Hospitalist	駐院醫生	駐诊医师
Intensivist	深切治療科醫生; 危重病醫學專家	重症监护; 重症专科医师
tests; lab tests	測試; 化驗	检测; 检验

(Continued)

English	Hong Kong & Taiwan	Mainland China
Lactation Consultant; Breastfeeding Consultant	哺乳顧問; 母乳顧問	哺乳咨询师; 母乳喂养顾问
Licensed Practical Nurse (LPN)	登記全科護士	持证执业护士
medical records	醫療記錄; 病歷	医疗记录; 病案; 病历; 病历档案
Medical ward	內科病房	内科病房
Nurse Practitioner(NP)	執業護士; 護理師	执业护士
Nursery	嬰兒室; 育嬰室; 嬰兒護理室	婴儿室
nurses' station	護士當值處; 護士室	护士台
Nursing Assistant	護理助理	护理员; 护理助理
Nutritionist	營養學家; 營養師	营养学家; 营养专家
Occupational Therapist (OT)	職業治療師	作业疗法师
Orderly	病房助理	病房助理
Outpatients' Clinic	門診; 門診部	门诊; 门诊诊所
patient's room	病房	病房
Pharmacist	藥劑師	药剂师; 调剂员
physical examination	身體檢查	体格检查; 体检
Physical therapist; Physiotherapist	活動治療師; 物理治療師	理疗师; 物理治疗师
Podiatrist	足病診療師; 足療師	足病医师
Primary Care Physician (PCP)	全科醫生; 家庭醫生	初级保健医师; 全科医师; 家庭医生
Public Health Nurse	公共衛生護士	公共卫生护士
range of motion (ROM)	動作幅度	可动度; 动度
Registered Nurse (RN)	註冊護士	注册护士
scheduled admissions	預約入院	预定入院
sluice room; utility room; soiled utility	污洗室; 雜物間; 染污物品	杂用间; 染污物品
Social Worker	社工; 社會工作者	社会服务人员
Speech Therapist; Language Therapist; Speech Pathologist	言語治療師	言语治疗师
sterile room; treatment room	無菌室; 治療室	无菌室; 治疗室
Surgical ward	外科病房	外科病房
Visiting Nurse; Home Health Nurse	家訪護士; 家庭保健護士	家庭保健护士
ward	病房	病房
Ward Clerk; Health Unit Secretary (HUC)	病房文員; 病房文書	病房文书

Summary of main points

This chapter has looked at hospital settings, including:

–   admission and discharge procedures
–   health professionals involved in medical care, nursing and allied care and rehabilitation.

Chapter 8

Emergency Departments or ERs

The Emergency Department (ED) is often referred to as the Emergency Room (ER). Some hospitals have been accredited as Trauma Centers, which means they have highly specialized trauma staff, diagnostic equipment and special trauma surgeons. Such hospitals usually have a helipad where helicopters carrying seriously injured patients can land.

Interpreting in the ED may present a real challenge to the interpreter. One of the factors which may make interpreting in the ER a challenge is that accuracy is essential, yet the interpreter may have been called in urgently with little or no preparation time. The best advice that may be given to the interpreter is to interpret both the doctor's questions and the patient's responses exactly and to ask for clarification whenever something is not quite clear. Furthermore, the interpreter may be faced with situations where there have been terrible accidents, instances of domestic violence or acute medical situations. There may be gross injuries, visible blood loss, a very stressed and very ill patient, surrounded by equally stressed relatives (and staff). In addition, the interpreter's services may be required when the doctor tells friends and relatives that the patient has died. The doctor may use phrases such as *"He has passed on"* and *"There was nothing more we could do"* or *"We tried everything we could"* or *"It was very quick"*.

The ER can be full of tension and stress. In spite of all this, the interpreter should try and remain cool, calm and collected, so as to be able to interpret information accurately. The level of accuracy will go a long way to helping the medical staff obtain a clear picture of what has happened, and this in turn will help them reach a correct diagnosis. ***Once the correct diagnosis has been reached, appropriate treatment can be started.*** If correct information is not obtained, or is incorrectly relayed through the interpreter, the consequences may be very unfortunate.

This chapter will list some common reasons for admission to the Emergency Department, as well as some of the most commonly asked questions. Common procedures and diagnostic tests have also been included. What follows, first of all, is a list of some commonly encountered staff in the ED, listed here in alphabetical order.

1.   Emergency Department staff

The first point of contact in ED will be the person at the front desk:

Admitting Clerk/
Health Unit Secretary   Not a clinician. The clerk registers the patient by asking them why they have come in. In the US, all EDs are required by law to accept patients with acute emergencies regardless of their ability to pay or their legal status. The same applies to other English-speaking countries: patients are not expected to pre-pay, but are given an invoice afterwards. The clerk will also check whether the patient has been admitted before and may check the person's medical records. Most hospitals now keep electronic patient records. Names may need to be spelled out.

The clerk will call the Registered Nurse if he/she thinks that the patient needs immediate medical attention (e.g. chest pain, shortness of breath, bleeding, or unconsciousness). The clerk will also give the patient an identification bracelet, usually in the form of a wristband with the patient's name and medical record number on it.

Emergency Room
Imaging specialists   Staff trained in carrying out imaging such as MRI or CT scanning.

Intern/Resident   Doctor undertaking their first professional experience in the hospital system. Interns answer to an Attending Physician and often check with the latter when in doubt.

Radiographers   People who are specially trained in working X-ray equipment. They often come to the ED with portable X-ray equipment to take X-rays of patients who are too ill to be taken to the X-ray department.

Registered Nurse   In the Emergency Department this will be a nurse with experience in **triage** (sorting out who needs attention first) and observation. It may also be a special trauma nurse.

Security Guard   The security guard may often be seen in the ED, as tempers may flare and some of the patients or their friends and relatives may be drunk and cause a disturbance. They often cover the front desk after hours, regulating entry by visitors and others to the hospital's facilities.

Technicians   Are now employed by many EDs to carry out technical duties to provide basic life support. Technicians are also called *Techs*.

Trauma Team	Many hospitals have a special team of doctors and nurses who specialize in dealing with trauma patients. This will include a *trauma specialist or Traumatologist* (a doctor specialized in trauma medicine).

2.   Emergency Department areas

Ambulance Bay	Where ambulance officers (paramedics) load or unload their patients, usually with the aid of stretchers.
Cubicles	Within the triage area, patients are kept in separate cubicles – small spaces with a bed and some equipment such as oxygen. Cubicles are separated from other cubicles by either a wall or a curtain.
Front Desk	Counter manned by the Unit Secretary and possibly also by security guards. All those who present to ED need to report here first. *This is also where interpreters would present themselves.*
Helipad *(or helicopter pad)*	A large open space where the Emergency Services Helicopter (sometimes called a MedEvac Helicopter) can land.
Observation bay *(or holding bay)*	Some patients are given medication and then observed for some time, until the medical staff have decided whether they should be discharged home or transferred to one of the units (to the floor).
Resus room	Resus is an abbreviation for resuscitation, which literally means "bringing back to life." In the ER, seriously ill patients are taken straight into Resus, where they are either stabilized (doctors make sure that the patient does not get any worse) or resuscitated (doctors make sure that the patient stays alive or comes back to life). The process of "resuscitation" may include *cardiac massage* plus administering breaths/oxygen (CPR), administering fluids, blood and medication to the patient, and perhaps defibrillating the patient's heart to restore normal heart rhythm and placing the patient on a ventilator or respirator (breathing machine).
Triage area	Triage refers to the process of sorting out who needs treatment first and/or who is most likely to survive without immediate treatment. Assessment takes place based on the kind of illness or injury, how serious it is, and whether the hospital has the facilities to treat the problem.

	If hospital staff have established that they do not have the facilities to treat the patient, the patient may be transferred to another hospital which does have those facilities. Patients may be transferred by ambulance or by helicopter.
Waiting room	Area outside of the ER proper where patients with less acute medical or surgical problems sit and wait. Once the patient is called in, they go to the triage area for assessment first.

3.   Emergency Department admission

Patients may be taken to the ER by ambulance, often following a distress call or telephone call to the *Emergency Services* (911).

Patients may also *self-refer* (present themselves on their own initiative without referral) or they may be brought in by friends and family. Some critically ill patients may be referred to the ER by their primary care doctor, in which case their own doctor may order an ambulance to take the patient to hospital.

When patients turn up at the ER themselves, ER staff will have no prior knowledge of what condition or problem they are presenting with. In contrast, when patients are referred by their PCP, or brought in by ambulance staff, ER staff will be aware of their condition and history before they arrive. As an example, a primary care doctor who examines a patient with acute chest pain and who suspects the patient is having a heart attack may call the doctors at the ER, write a quick letter of referral and arrange for an ambulance to take the patient to the ER.

4.   Some common reasons for admission to ED

Reasons for admission to ED may include:

- medical problems – See Section 4.1
- trauma (including orthopedic problems) – See Section 4.2
- issues requiring surgical intervention – See Section 4.3

The most common problems for each of these categories are listed below, starting with medical problems.

4.1   Common medical problems

1.   *Anaphylaxis or severe allergic reaction* – This can be a life-threatening response to "allergens" (substances which cause an allergic reaction).

Causes: Allergens include foods (seafood, peanuts, strawberries, chocolate, milk), medications and bee stings.

Symptoms: The body's response is exaggerated, causing all blood vessels to widen, leading to a severe drop in blood pressure. A rash may appear, the person may lose consciousness, and may even die unless action is undertaken quickly. The Emergency Services need to be called.

Questions: Questions may be asked of witnesses, as the patient may be unable to answer any questions. These include

- What happened; where was the patient (garden, kitchen, dining room); what was the patient doing, what was the patient eating, drinking or inhaling?
- Does the patient have any known allergies?
- Do allergies run in the family?

Treatment: The patient will most commonly be given adrenaline/epinephrine, to make the blood vessels constrict (narrow), which will help the blood pressure go up.

2. *Asthma* – Very common, especially among children. In asthma, the bronchi (breathing tubes) become narrow and the patient has problems breathing out. Attacks can be life-threatening.

Causes: Attacks may be triggered by breathing in pollen, dust or other allergens, or by exercise, infections, or breathing in cold air.

Symptoms: The patient's bronchi respond to these triggers with a hypersensitive reaction, becoming narrowed and starting to producing mucus. This makes it difficult for the patient to breathe out, and they may either wheeze (make a whistling sound) or cough when breathing out. Children will often cough a lot, especially at night.

Questions:
- Is there a family history of asthma or hay fever?
- Have you got any allergies or is there a family history of allergies?
- What triggered (brought on) this attack?
- Have you had a similar attack before?
- Are you on any medication? What?
- What was your last peak flow (maximum amount of air the patient is able to breathe out, measured by a small hand-held device called a peak flow meter)?

Treatment: Medication to open up the airways called *bronchodilators*. These may be given as *inhalers* or as *nebulizers* (see Chapter 19). Patients may be given steroids (hydrocortisone) into the vein (intravenously) to help the body overcome this crisis situation.

3. *Bronchitis* – Inflammation of the bronchi (breathing tubes) (see Chapter 19, Page 237).

4. *Chest pain*

Please note: Chest pain means "pain in the chest" and should always be interpreted as such. It should never be interpreted as "heart pain," as chest pain may have a range of causes.

Causes: Chest pain may originate from:
– the stomach – Stomach acid may cause a burning sensation behind the breast bone. This is usually referred to as heartburn, which is often due to reflux (see below).
– the esophagus – Stomach acid can go back up the esophagus and cause a burning sensation there. This is usually referred to as reflux. If reflux causes inflammation, the doctors will use the word *esophagitis* (inflammation of the esophagus).
– the muscles between the ribs – Caused by too much coughing or by a torn muscle (e.g. due to playing racket sports).
– the lungs – Inflammation of the pleura (the outer lining of the lungs) or by an embolism (very large blood clot) in the lungs. The pain will then be *associated with* breathing.
– the heart muscle – If the heart muscle does not get enough oxygen, because the arteries to the heart muscle are narrowed or even completely blocked, the patient will experience pain in the chest, possibly radiating (spreading) into the jaw, neck or arms. This is called *angina pectoris*.

Questions asked may include the following:
– When did the pain start?
– Have you ever suffered stomach complaints or a stomach ulcer?
– Have you been playing any sports recently?
– Have you had a (chest) cold recently?
– Have you been coughing a lot?
– Have you brought up any phlegm?
– Have you ever had any problems with your heart?
– Do you have to sleep propped up with pillows or sitting up in bed?
– Do you get any swelling of the ankles?
– Can you walk half a mile without getting breathless or without getting pain in the chest?
– Can you walk up the stairs without getting breathless/without getting pain in the chest?
– Is there a family history of heart problems?

- Have you ever had angina? Have you ever had a heart attack?
- What is the pain like? (dull, sharp, heavy, crushing, like a belt around the chest?
- just a "niggling" pain or very slight pain?)
- Does the pain spread into the neck or arms?
- Have you ever had surgery on the heart?
- Is there a family history of coronary artery disease (problems with the blood-vessels going to the heart muscle itself)
- Do you take any medication for your heart? What is it called? What dosage do you take? How often?
- Do you carry any medication with you to relieve pain in your chest? What type of medication is it?

Medication: The patient may be given medication such as an antacid drink to neutral-ize stomach acid. Alternatively, the patient may be given oxygen to see if this relieves the pain. If pain persists the patient may be given a special spray under the tongue. This spray may help to open up the *coronary arteries* which supply the heart muscle with oxygen.

Tests: The doctor may order certain tests such as:
- *Chest X-ray* – to look at the structures in the chest, especially heart and lungs
- *Blood tests* – these can show signs of infection or evidence of damage to the heart muscle
- *EKG or ECG (Electrocardiogram)* – to check the electrical activity in the heart – an EKG might show that the patient has had or is having a heart attack

5. *Congestive heart failure (CHF)* – Heart is not able to pump blood properly. The doc-tor may never mention the term heart failure, but may say things such as: "You have some fluid in the lungs" or "We need to give you something to get rid of some extra fluid"

Questions asked:
- Do you have to sleep sitting up or propped up with pillows at night?
- Do you get swelling of the ankles?
- Do you frequently have to urinate or pass water at night?
- Do you get short-of-breath on exertion?

Medication: Diuretics are frequently given to help the body get rid of excess fluid by increasing urine output. As a result, there is less fluid for the heart to pump around the body.

Digoxin is a drug that may be given to strengthen the pump action of the heart.

6.   *Chronic obstructive pulmonary disease (COPD),* also known as *chronic obstructive respiratory disease (CORD).* COPD patients are people with a long history of breathing disorders which cause obstruction of the airways, making breathing difficult and forced. This includes long-standing asthma, chronic bronchitis, and emphysema (see Chapter 19 for more information).

7.   *Coughing up blood or hemoptysis (hemo: blood; ptyo: to spit)*
–   There can be many different reasons why the patient is coughing up blood: bronchitis; an abscess in the lung; tuberculosis (Tb) or lung cancer.
–   Tuberculosis is now making a comeback in some countries.

Please refer to Chapter 19 for some commonly asked questions and common tests related to breathing problems.

8.   *Cerebro-vascular accident (CVA) or stroke* – An "accident" involving the blood vessels in the brain (cerebro: brain; vascular: to do with the blood vessels). A stroke can be due to a blood clot obstructing the blood supply leading to part of the brain. A stroke can also be due to a bleed in the brain (brain *hemorrhage*). Without oxygen, the affected part of the brain will stop functioning or function less well.

Symptoms may include: Paralysis (inability to move); paresis (weakness); aphasia (inability to speak or to understand speech); blurred vision; hemianopia (half-sided loss of vision).

Questions:
It is often necessary to obtain a "history" from the patient's relatives as the patient may be unable to speak, or patients may have no recollection of what happened while they were having the stroke.

Important questions to the patient's relatives would include:
–   Does the patient smoke or has he ever smoked? How much? For how long?
–   Has the patient ever had a TIA (transient ischemic attack), also called a ministroke or a warning stroke? The symptoms are similar to those of a real stroke, but do not last very long.
–   Was the patient able to move all his/her limbs before the attack?
–   How long was the patient unconscious?

Questions to the patient would include:
–   Did you black out?
–   Can you move your arms/legs?
–   Do you have blurry vision? Can you see me if I stand on this side?
–   Are you experiencing any abnormal sensations, such as numbness, tingling, pins and needles?

Tests might include:
- CT scan or MRI scan of the brain.
- Shining a light in the patient's eyes to check the reaction of the pupils.
- Checking the patient's pulse, blood pressure and breathing rate.

9.   *Diabetic Coma* – A life-threatening condition, a deep level of unconsciousness. A diabetic coma can be caused by either a very low blood sugar level (*hypo*glycemia where hypo means "below," glyc- means glucose or sugar, and (h)emia means in the blood) or by a very high blood sugar level (*hyper*glycemia where hyper -just like *super*- means "too much"). As the patient will be unconscious, it will not be possible to take a history from the patient. See also Chapter 25.

If relatives or friends are present, they might be asked the following questions:

- Does the patient inject insulin or did he take tablets for his diabetes?
- Did the patient take his normal dose this time?
- Did the patient eat his normal breakfast/lunch/dinner/snack?
- Does the patient have a fever/infection/cold?
- Has the patient just undergone surgery/been in a stressful situation/had an accident/exercised to excess? (Stress may raise the body's blood sugar levels.)

Treatment:
- The patient may be given *glucose* or glucagon,if the coma is caused by a low blood sugar. Glucagon injections will help to raise the blood sugar quickly. Patients may also be given *sodium bicarbonate* and *insulin*, if the coma is caused by a high blood glucose level. This will be given to treat *metabolic acidosis*.

Once the patient is out of the coma, he or she will almost certainly be kept in the hospital for observation and to try and get the patient's diabetes under control again.

10.   *Heart attack or myocardial infarction (MI)* – blood supply to part of the heart muscle is cut off completely, usually due to a blockage of the coronary artery.

Questions: please refer to the section on *Chest pain* above.

Treatment:
The patient will usually be transferred to the coronary care unit or CCU for observation. The patient will be placed on a heart monitor and will have frequent blood tests. Blood pressure and pulse will be recorded frequently.

Medication may include:
- Medication to relieve pain and anxiety
- Medication to prevent ventricular fibrillation (ventricles quiver but do not contract). A diuretic to get rid of excess fluid in the bloodstream

- Anticoagulants (medications to prevent clotting)
- Thrombolytic medications to dissolve clots
- Beta-blockers to reduce the effect of stress hormones on the heart
- Antiarrhythmic medications to encourage normal heart rhythm
- Medications to reduce blood pressure and blood volume, including *ACE inhibitors and angiotensin* receptor blockers

11.   *Heart failure* – please see *congestive heart failure* above.

12.   *Hyperemesis gravidarum* – Excessive vomiting during pregnancy which may lead to dehydration or loss of electrolytes

Questions will include:
- Are you able to keep down foods and fluids?
- How much have you vomited over the last 24 hours?
- Are you still passing urine? What color is your urine (dark, concentrated, light)?
- Have you got a headache?

If the doctors find that the woman is dehydrated, they may admit her for treatment and observation. They may put her on an intravenous drip with electrolytes to restore her fluid and electrolyte balance.

13.   *Meningitis* – inflammation of the meninges, the outer lining of the brain and spinal cord.
Patients will complain of fever, neck stiffness and severe headache. The cause may be a viral infection or a bacterial infection (serious).

Questions may include:
- Have you taken your/his/her temperature? What was it?
- Have you had the chills? (high fever/feeling hot then cold and shivering)
- Have you vomited at all?
- Any convulsions/seizures?
- Have you (he/she) been more irritable than usual?
- When the baby cries does it sound normal? Any high-pitched cry?
- Does the baby cry when you change his/her diaper?
- Have you noticed any blotches/red spots on the skin? (meningitis rash)

Tests:
- Lumbar puncture or spinal tap (to check for presence of bacteria in the spinal fluid)
- CT scan of the brain

Treatment:
- Antibiotics to treat the bacterial infection
- Medications to stop convulsions (anticonvulsants)

14.   *Miscarriage* – Bleeding during pregnancy associated with fetus and placenta coming away

Questions:
–   Any woman who comes in with vaginal bleeding will be asked if she is pregnant; What was the first day of your last period?
–   Have you been feeling nauseated?
–   Have your breasts felt tender? Do they still feel tender now?

Diagnostic tests:
–   A blood test to check HCG (human chorionic gonadotropin, a pregnancy hormone) levels in the blood. Ultrasound scan of the lower abdomen
–   Vaginal examination

Treatment:
Incomplete abortion: If the fetus has died and has come away from the womb or if some products of conception (fetal or placental tissue) are still inside the womb, a dilatation and curettage (D & C) may be needed. The woman will usually be given general anesthesia and the doctor will open up the neck of the womb and scrape the lining of the womb clean. Any remaining products of conception may result in a risk of infection or molar pregnancy, a form of cancer.

Complete abortion – If the fetus has died and the scan shows that the womb and the cervix are empty, a D & C may not be necessary. A blood test will be taken to check on HCG levels and repeated later on to ensure that there is nothing left inside the womb.

15.   *Peritonitis* – Inflammation of the peritoneum – the inner lining of the abdomen. *Causes*: Infection by bacteria. Peritonitis may develop in people with appendicitis or in patients who are on continuous ambulant peritoneal dialysis (CAPD).

Symptoms: Fever, chills, pain in the abdomen; guarding (muscle defense by abdominal muscles).

Questions:
–   Does it hurt when I press here?
–   Are you feeling nauseated/have you vomited?
–   Do you have diarrhea?
–   When did the pain start? Where did the pain start?
–   Have you had a fever? Have you had chills?

Treatment:
Sometimes laparoscopy or laparotomy to find the cause.

16.   *Shock (anaphylactic shock; hypovolemic shock, neurogenic shock; septic shock)- not enough blood to vital organs and tissues; very low blood pressure; can be life-threatening)*

Anaphylaxis – see under anaphylaxis, under medical problems, above.

Hypovolemic shock: The amount of circulating volume (blood and fluid) is very low. The heart cannot pump enough blood around the body and this may cause vital organs to stop working.

Neurogenic shock – caused by damage to the nervous system

Septic shock – caused by infections in the blood stream, bacteria may multiply very fast and overwhelm vital organs; very serious and life-threatening. Septic shock may be associated with peritonitis or meningitis or other serious infections.

Causes: Severe and prolonged blood loss; severe vomiting. and diarrhea; dehydration; burns; serious life-threatening infections.

Symptoms: Low blood pressure; weak, thready pulse; sweating, cold and clammy skin; rapid breathing; paleness; loss of consciousness.

Tests: Blood tests (complete blood count – CBC); CT scan (to see where bleeding is); echocardiogram.

Treatment: keeping person warm; replacing lost blood and fluids; medication to increase blood pressure; urinary catheter; Swan Ganz catheter (into the heart) to check cardiac output.

Outlook: Possible complications include damage to kidneys, heart and brain and possible death.

17.   *Vomiting up blood*

Causes: This can be due to a variety of causes, including an ulcer in the stomach (peptic ulcer) or in the first part of the small intestine (duodenal ulcer); varicose veins in the esophagus (esophageal varices), which often occur in patients with cirrhosis of the liver; irritation of the lining of the esophagus by reflux of stomach acids into the esophagus (reflux esophagitis); taking aspirin or NSAIDS (non-steroidal anti-inflammatory medications) which can irritate the lining of the stomach.

Questions:
– Do you have a history of ulcers?
– Do you have a history of taking of aspirin or NSAIDS on an empty stomach?
– Have you been feeling nauseated before eating, during meals, after meals?
– Have you been experiencing pain in the stomach before, during, or after meals?
– How much alcohol do you drink? For how many years have you been drinking?
– How frequently do you drink?
– Have you ever been diagnosed with hepatitis (B or C) or cirrhosis of the liver?

Tests and Treatment:
- urgent *endoscopy* (*gastroscopy* or *esophagogastroscopy*) to find the cause of the bleeding or to treat the cause (in some cases)
- *laparotomy* (surgery on the abdomen)

4.2   Trauma

1.   *Assault*

Questions:
- Who assaulted you (man, woman, young, old)
- What with? Blunt weapon: wood, or sharp weapon: switchblade, kitchen knife, machete; what material was it made of: iron bar, wooden club.
- Where did they hit you?
- With what force did they strike/hit/stab you? Did you black out?
- Where is the pain?
- Is there any pain associated with breathing?

2.   *Burns*
It is very important to determine how "deep" the burn has gone.
1st degree burn: superficial only, skin is reddened
2nd degree burn: deeper, skin is blistered
3rd degree burn: underlying tissues burned (including muscle), tissue may be blackened

Questions:
- How did you burn yourself: water, oil, fire (wood fire/electrical fire)?
- What type of first aid did you get? (10 minutes under cold running water? Creams?)

Treatment:
- IV fluids (intravenous fluids) and a high-protein diet
- Dressings and saline baths
- Skin grafts (mesh)

3.   *Drowning or near-drowning*
Questions:
- How long was the patient under water?
- Did he/she drown in fresh water or salt water?
- Did he/she breathe or have a heart beat when he/she came out of the water?
- How cold was the water?

Diagnostic tests:
- Neurological observations: response; pupillary reaction; pulse/blood pressure
- Temperature: undercooling (hypothermia); to what extent

Treatment:
- CPR (cardiopulmonary resuscitation) followed by artificial respiration (patient placed on a ventilator)
- Drug treatment (given intravenously)
- Warming up with a special thermal blanket and/or pre-warmed intravenous fluids
- Monitoring of blood gases (oxygen etc.)

4. *Drug overdose – see poisoning*
Can be accidental or intentional (suicide attempt)

5. *Falls*

Questions:
- How did you fall? Did you stretch out your arms to try and break your fall?
- Did you fall on your head/neck/back?
- Did you black out or lose consciousness at all?
- Can you feel your toes/legs? Can you move your toes/legs?
- Where does it hurt? Does it hurt when you breathe in/out? Did you fall from a moving vehicle? How fast was it moving?

6. *Head injuries*

Questions:
Some questions will be the same as those for falls and accidents.
- Can you squeeze my hand? Can you push my hand away with your foot? Can you grimace?
- Can you lift your hand up?
- What is your name? Do you know where you are? What is today's date?

Diagnostic tests:
- Neurological observations: response; pupillary response; pulse/blood pressure; level of consciousness (LOC).
- Giving the patient instructions and checking whether he is able to respond to these
- CT scan or MRI scan of the brain.

Treatment:
May include urgent surgery on the skull if there is bleeding inside the skull or into the brain; the aim is to reduce pressure and swelling on the brain.

7. *Poisoning – can be accidental or intentional*
Some common medications (e.g. Paracetamol®(acetaminophen), aspirin, tranquilizers and antidepressants) may cause serious problems if taken in excess. It is absolutely

essential to find out exactly what was taken, as each drug acts in a different way and may cause damage in different ways and to different parts of the body.

Questions:
- What was taken (ingested)/when/how much/by what route (mouth, inhaling, huffing, sniffing inhalants, or injecting intravenously)?
- Was anything done to induce vomiting?
- Did the patient take or drink anything (e.g. milk) to counteract the poisoning?
- What/when/how much?

Diagnostic tests:
Blood test (drug levels)

Treatment: This can include:
Gastric lavage (emptying stomach out by means of tube and then flushing it clean with water).

Antidotes – Drugs to reverse the action of the first drug (e.g. Narcan (naloxone) to counteract narcotic overdose

Charcoal – Charcoal can absorb what was ingested and stop it from being absorbed into the body.

8. *Road traffic accident (RTA)*
Also known as motor vehicle accident (MVA), motor vehicle traffic collision (MVTC); car wreck, motor vehicle collision (MVC), road traffic collision (RTC), road traffic incident (RTI).

Questions may include:
- Where were you sitting (driver seat, front passenger, rear seat passenger)?
- Were you wearing a seat belt?
- Were you thrown clear of the car?
- Did you have an airbag?
- Did the car have side-intrusion bars?
- Did the car roll?
- How fast was the car going at the time of impact?
- Did you black out/lose consciousness at all?
- Can you remember what happened just before the accident?

Diagnostic tests:
Blood tests; imaging such as X-rays/CT scans/ultrasound scans/MRI scans; exploratory surgery to check for internal injury or problems medical staff are not aware off.

Treatment:
Urgent surgery may be required, especially to stem any internal bleeding.

9.   *Shock (all types)* – see pages 91–92.

10.   *Orthopedic problems*

These usually relate to broken bones (fractures) or to dislocations (e.g. dislocated shoulder); sometimes they relate to *avulsion fractures*, in which a small piece of bone has been torn off, usually due to pull of the surrounding muscles or tendons.

Questions:
–   How did the accident happen?
–   Do you have osteoporosis?
–   Where does it hurt?
–   Have you had surgery before? (Followed by all the common pre-operative questions as per Chapter 10).

Diagnostic tests:
X-rays; CT scans; MRI scans.

Treatment – see Chapter 20.

4.3   Surgical problems

Some of the most common surgical problems (problems requiring surgical treatment) are:

1.   *Appendicitis:* Inflammation of the appendix (see also Chapter 26)

Questions:
–   When did the pain start? Where did the pain start? Where is the pain now?
–   Do you feel nauseated? Have you vomited? Have you had diarrhea?
–   Have you had the flu or a viral infection?

Diagnostic tests and treatment:
–   Palpitation (rebound tenderness); blood tests; ultrasound scan
–   Laparoscopy and laparotomy and possibly an appendectomy (surgical removal of the inflamed appendix)

2.   *Collapsed lung:* Air (pneumothorax) or fluid or blood (hematothorax) has entered the space between the pleurae, and the lung has collapsed as a result. This may be the result of a broken rib, a stab wound, or an asthma attack where air cannot be breathed out.

Diagnostic tests:
-   Chest X-ray shows a white-out (area where there is little or no air movement or gas exchange); patient very short of breath

Questions:
-   Do you have asthma?
-   What were you doing when your lung collapsed?
-   Were you assaulted/stabbed? What with? How long was the knife? How far did it go in?

Diagnostic tests:
X-ray.

Treatment:
Drains to drain fluid/blood:
-   Chest tube (also called chest drain or thoracic catheter) to keep the lung expanded
-   Pleural tap: To drain fluid from the space between the pleura layers with a long hollow needle

3.   *Perforated stomach ulcer*

Questions:
-   Where is the pain? When did the pain start? Does the pain radiate anywhere?
-   Do you have stomach ulcers or duodenal ulcers?

Diagnostic tests: Laparotomy (to check for damage and repair at the same time)

Treatment: Surgery to repair the perforation and stop the bleeding.

4.   *Sub-acute bowel obstruction* – Bowels are almost completely blocked and food cannot pass through. Normally the patient vomits up fecal fluid and bowels do not function at all. This may be due to the presence of tumors in the abdomen (bowel cancer, ovarian cancer) or to the patient having swallowed something large (e.g. a whole orange) without chewing.

Questions:
-   What did you eat before this happened?
-   Have you had previous abdominal surgery?

Treatment: Drip and suck: IV drip (to keep the patient hydrated) and nasogastric tube to drain fluid out of the gastrointestinal tract.

5.   English-Chinese glossary

英漢詞彙表

English	Hong Kong & Taiwan	Mainland China
1st degree burn	一級燒傷; 表面燒傷	一度烧伤
2nd degree burn	二級燒傷; 中度燒傷	二度烧伤
3rd degree burn	三級燒傷; 深度燒傷	三度烧伤
Accident and Emergency Department (A&E); Emergency Department (ED); Emergency Room (ER)	急症室	急诊室; 急诊科
ACE inhibitors	血管緊張素轉換酶抑制劑	血管紧张素转化酶抑制剂
allergens	過敏原; 致敏原	过敏原; 致敏原
ambulance bay	救護車專用車位	救护车专用车位
anaphylactic shock	過敏性休克	过敏性休克
anaphylaxis; severe allergic reaction	嚴重過敏反應	严重过敏反应
angina pectoris	心絞痛	狭心症; 心绞痛
angiotensin receptor blockers (ARBs)	血管緊張素受體對抗劑	血管紧张素受体拮抗剂
anti-arrhythmic drug	抗心律不齊藥物	抗心律失常药
anticonvulsant	抗痙攣劑; 抗抽搐劑	抗惊厥剂; 抗抽搐剂
anticoagulant	抗凝血劑	抗凝剂; 抗凝血剂
antidepressant	抗憂鬱劑; 鎮抑劑	抗抑郁药
antidote	解藥; 解毒劑	解毒药; 解毒剂
aphasia	失語	失语 (症)
appendectomy	盲腸切除術; 闌尾切除術	阑尾切除术
appendicitis	盲腸炎; 闌尾炎	阑尾炎
appendix	盲腸; 闌尾	阑尾
asthma	哮喘	气喘; 哮喘
avulsion fracture	撕裂骨折	撕脱骨折; 扭伤骨折
beta-blocker	β-阻斷劑	β-受体阻滞剂
black out	昏迷	昏迷
blood pressure	血壓	血压
bowel cancer	腸道癌; 大腸癌	肠癌
breathing rate	呼吸率	呼吸率; 呼吸频率
bronchitis	支氣管炎	支气管炎
bronchodilator	支氣管擴張劑	支气管扩张药
cardiopulmonary resuscitation (CPR)	心肺復蘇法	心肺复苏术

(Continued)

English	Hong Kong & Taiwan	Mainland China
cerebrovascular accident (CVA); stroke	腦血管破裂; 腦栓塞; 腦中風; 中風	中風; 脑卒中
charcoal	(藥用) 炭	(药用) 炭; 炭末 (吸附剂)
chest X-ray	X-光胸肺檢查; 胸肺 X-光顯影	胸部X射线检查; 胸透检查
chills	寒顫; 畏寒; 發冷	寒战; 畏寒; 发冷
chronic obstructive respiratory disease (CORD); chronic obstructive pulmonary disease COPD	慢性呼吸道阻塞症; 慢性阻塞性肺病	慢性呼吸道阻塞症; 慢性阻塞性肺病
cirrhosis of the liver	肝硬化	肝硬化
collapsed lung	肺萎陷	肺萎陷
complete blood count (CBC)	血常規; 全血指數; 血細胞數量檢查	全血 (细胞) 计数; 血常规
congestive heart failure (CHF); heart failure	充血性心臟衰竭; 心臟衰竭	充血性心衰竭; 心衰竭
continuous ambulant peritoneal dialysis (CAPD)	持續流動式腹膜透析 (俗稱「洗肚」)	持续流动式腹膜透析
convulsion	抽搐; 痙攣	痉挛; 惊厥; 抽搐
coronary artery disease	冠心動脈心臟病; 冠狀動脈病; 冠心病	冠状动脉疾病; 冠心病
Coronary Care Unit (CCU)	冠心病護理病房; 冠心病加護病房	冠心病监护病房; 冠心病医护单位
CT scan	電腦斷層掃描; 電腦斷層攝影; 電腦掃描	CT扫描
diabetic coma	糖尿病昏迷	糖尿病昏迷
dilatation and curettage (D&C)	宮頸擴張與刮除術; 子宮擴刮術; 刮宮術	扩张宫颈和刮宫术; 宫颈扩张子宫刮术
dislocation	脫臼	脱臼
dressing	包紮; 敷料	包扎; 敷料
duodenal ulcer	十二指腸潰瘍	十二指肠溃疡
Electrocardiogram; ECG; EKG	心電圖	心电图; 心动电流图
electrolyte	電解質; 電離質	电解质; 电解物
embolism	栓塞	栓塞
Emergency Department (ED)	急症室	急诊室; 急诊科
Emergency Room (ER)	急症室	急诊室; 急诊科
endoscopy	內窺鏡檢查	内窥镜检查; 内腔镜检查
esophageal varices	食道靜脈曲張	食道静脉曲张; 食管静脉曲张
esophagitis	食道炎; 食管炎	食管炎

(Continued)

English	Hong Kong & Taiwan	Mainland China
esophagogastroscopy	食道胃 (上消化道) 內窺鏡檢查 (俗稱「照胃鏡」)	食管胃镜检查
fracture	骨折	骨折
front desk	前臺; 接待處	前台; 服务台
gastric lavage	胃灌洗; 洗胃	洗胃
gastrointestinal tract	腸胃道; 腸胃管; 消化道	胃肠道; 消化道
gastroscopy	胃內窺鏡檢查; 胃鏡檢查	胃镜检查; 胃窥镜
guarding	(腹壁) 緊張	(腹壁) 紧张
hay fever	花粉過敏; 花粉症	花粉过敏症
hematothorax/haemothorax	血胸; 胸腔積血	血胸
hemianopia	偏盲; 一側視力缺失	偏盲; 一侧视力缺失
hemoptysis	咳血; 咯血	咳血; 咯血
hepatitis	肝炎	肝炎
huffing; sniffing inhalants	口吸吸入劑; 鼻吸吸入劑	口吸吸入剂; 鼻吸吸入剂
human chorionic gonadotropin (HCG)	人體絨毛膜促性腺激素	人类绒毛膜促性腺激素
hyperglycemia	高血糖; 血糖過高; 多糖症	高血糖; 高血糖症
hyperemesis gravidarum	妊娠劇吐; 妊娠嘔吐	妊娠剧吐; 恶性孕吐
hypoglycemia	低血糖 (症); 血糖過低	低血糖 (症)
hypothermia	低溫症; 體溫過低	体温过低; 低体温
hypovolemic shock	血容量過低休克	血容量过低休克
Imaging specialist	影像專家	成像专家
inhaler	吸入器	吸入器
insulin	胰島素	胰岛素
intra chest wall drain (ICWD); chest tube	胸膜腔引流; 胸管; 胸腔引流管; 胸腔導管	胸管; 胸腔管; 胸腔导管
Junior Doctor; Foundation Medical Officer; Intern	初級醫生; 實習醫生	初级医生; 实习医师
laparoscopy	腹腔 (內窺) 鏡檢查	腹腔镜检查
laparotomy	剖腹 (手) 術	剖腹术
lumbar puncture	腰椎穿刺 (抽腦脊液)	腰椎穿刺 (术)
meningitis	腦膜炎; 腦脊膜炎	脑膜炎; 脑脊膜炎
metabolic acidosis	代謝性酸中毒	代谢性酸中毒
miscarriage	流產; 小產	流产; 小产
MRI scan	磁力共振掃描	磁 (性) 共振成像; 磁振造影扫描

(Continued)

English	Hong Kong & Taiwan	Mainland China
myocardial infarction (MI); heart attack	心肌梗塞; 心臟病猝發; 心臟病發作	心肌梗死; 心肌梗塞; 心脏病发作
nasogastric tube	鼻胃管	鼻胃管
nebulizer	噴霧器; 霧化器	喷雾器; 喷洒器; 雾化器
nonsteroidal anti-inflammatory drug (NSAID)	非類固醇類消炎 (止痛) 藥物	非类固醇抗炎药; 非甾体抗炎药物
numbness	麻木; 麻痹; 無感覺	麻木; 麻痹
observation ward; observation unit; holding ward	觀察病房	观察病房; 观察病室
Orderly; Certified Nurse Assistant (CNA)	病房助理; 註冊護理助理	病房助理; 持证护理员
osteoporosis	骨質疏鬆 (症)	骨质疏松 (症)
ovarian cancer	卵巢癌	卵巢癌
palpitation	心悸; 心律急促	心悸
paresis	輕度癱瘓	轻瘫
peak flow	(肺) 活量	(肺) 活量
peak flow meter	肺活量計	肺活量计
peptic ulcer	消化性潰瘍; 胃潰瘍	消化性溃疡; 胃溃疡
perforated stomach ulcer	穿孔性胃潰瘍	穿透性胃溃疡
'pins and needles'	發麻	发麻
pleura	胸 (肋) 膜; 肺膜	胸 (肋) 肺膜
pleural tap; thoracentesis/Chest Tapping	胸膜腔穿刺放液術	肺膜腔
pneumothorax	氣胸	气胸
pupillary reaction	瞳孔反應	瞳孔反应
Radiographer; Radiation Technologist	放射技師	放射科技术员
rebound tenderness; point tenderness	按壓後放鬆疼痛; 點壓痛	按压痛; 点压痛
reflux	反流; 倒流	反流; 倒流
Reflux oesophagitis; gastroesophageal reflux	反流性食道炎; 胃食道反流	反流性食管炎; 胃食管反流
Registered Nurse	註冊護士	注册护士
Registrar; Resident; Resident Medical Officer	專科培訓醫生	专科培训医生
Resus room; Resuscitation Room	急救室	抢救室; 复苏室
saline bath	鹽水 (浸) 浴	生理盐水 (泡) 浴; 盐水浴
security guard	保安員; 護衛員	保安; 警卫

(Continued)

English	Hong Kong & Taiwan	Mainland China
seizures	抽筋; 癲癇發作	抽搐; 癫痫发作
shock	休克	休克
skin graft	植皮; 皮膚移植; 表皮移植	皮肤移植; 皮片移植
spinal tap	脊椎穿刺; 抽脊髓液	脊椎穿刺; 脊椎抽液
stress	壓力; 緊張	紧张状态
subacute bowel obstruction	亞急性腸阻塞; 亞急性腸梗阻	亚急性肠梗阻
thready pulse	絲脈 (脈搏微弱)	丝脉; 细脉
thrombolytic drug	血栓溶解藥物	溶栓药
tingling	發麻; 麻刺感	发麻; 麻刺感
transient ischemic attack (TIA); mini stroke; warning stroke;	短暫性腦缺血症; 「小中風」	短暂性脑缺血症; 微卒中
trauma team	創傷小組; 外傷小組	创伤小组; 外伤小组
triage area	分流區	检伤分类区; 分诊处
tuberculosis (TB)	(肺) 結核	(肺) 结核
ultrasound scan	超聲波掃描	超声波扫描
ventilator	呼吸器; 人工呼吸機	呼吸器; 呼吸机
ventricular fibrillation	心室顫震	心室纤颤; 心室颤动
X-rays	X光; X射線	X (射) 线

Summary of main points

This chapter has looked at Emergency Departments including:

- health professionals involved
- three main reasons for admission into the ER, including
    - medical conditions
    - trauma
    - surgical problems

Chapter 9

Informed consent

Informed consent forms or Agreement to Treatment forms are used in all hospitals. The informed consent procedure is a legal requirement for all invasive and/or potentially harmful procedures. It involves an agreement between the patient and the health professional and means that the patient is consenting to a certain procedure, having been informed what is to be done, what is involved, and what the potential risks and complications are.

The procedure involves the medical professional explaining the intended operation or procedure to the patient. The outcome of the doctor's explanation should be for the patient to understand what is going to be done, why, how, who is going to do it, what the risks will be, and what the expected result will be.

The informed consent form is a legal document. It protects both the patient and the health professional. The patient cannot undergo a potentially risky procedure without being fully aware of the possible risks. Also, the patient cannot have limbs, body parts or even tumors removed without having given his or her express consent. The health professional is protected in that, if the outcome of the procedure is not good, he or she can state that the patient was aware of the risks and had agreed to the procedure.

There are circumstances in which "informed consent" cannot be obtained in writing and from patients themselves, for example:

- The patient is unconscious, but in need of urgent surgery.
- The patient is a minor "under the age of consent". Consent procedures will vary from country to country and state to state. Typically in such cases, the "consent" form is signed by the parents or legal guardians of the child.
- Patients are under the influence of mind-altering substances (e.g. alcohol, drugs) or sleep-deprived to such an extent that they are incapable of reaching an informed decision.
- The patient is *non compos mentis* (mentally incapable of reaching an informed decision). This may be the case if a patient suffers from Alzheimer's dementia or is otherwise intellectually challenged or under the influence of mind-altering substances. This can be quite a hazy area, and psychiatric assessment may be required to gauge whether the patient is capable of giving informed consent.

If the patient is not capable of giving informed consent himself/herself, the medical staff will try to get hold of the patient's next-of-kin to act in the patient's best interests and sign the informed consent form on the patient's behalf.

In an emergency, where immediate action needs to be taken, consent may be obtained over the phone. If time does not permit this, doctors may proceed with treatment, providing they are acting in the best interests of the patient and death or permanent harm will result if they do not intervene. Note that if a doctor knows that the patient would not have consented but proceeds with intervention nonetheless, he or she could be held liable in some countries. As an example, if an adult patient tells the doctor that he refuses a blood transfusion for religious reasons (e.g. if the patient is a Jehovah's Witness), and the doctor gives the patient blood all the same, the doctor has acted against the patient's consent and can be held liable. In the US, doctors must obtain a court order in order to treat a minor against parental wishes. In emergency cases, doctors may proceed with urgent treatment without waiting for a court order, however parents may later proceed with a claim against medical staff (University of Virginia 2013).

1.   Issues which might arise for interpreters during the informed consent process

Ideally, the doctor/professional should explain the following:

- *What* they aim to do (the procedure)
- *Why* they think this procedure is necessary or desired
- *How* the procedure will take place
- *Who* will undertake the procedure (i.e. an experienced person or a trainee)
- *What* the *expected outcomes* are
- *What side-effects* or *risks* could be involved. This is often expressed as a percentage of patients who have experienced harmful side-effects (morbidity rate), or who have died (mortality rate)
- Whether there are *any alternatives*/other options to the proposed treatment

However, in practice the whole informed consent process may be fraught with issues which may catch the interpreter unawares. These may include, but are by no means limited to the following:

- Some medical staff expect the interpreter to do a sight translation of the form and even complete it on behalf of the patient, rather than interpreting for the medical staff who are taking the patient through the informed consent process.
- Some medical staff may want to absent themselves during this process, leaving the interpreter "in charge".

- Some medical staff orally convey certain risks and side-effects to the patient which are interpreted by the interpreter. They may then add other issues in writing to the informed consent form, without either mentioning or clarifying these. An example would be where the medical practitioner mentions "post-operative infection" as a possible side-effect, but then writes down "death" on the form, without mentioning this. The interpreter is then caught in a difficult situation (see also mention of Duty of Care in Chapter 2).
- In most cases, surgical consent will be obtained before the anesthesiologist takes the patient through the informed consent for the anesthesia, but it may happen that the surgeon rushes through the informed consent process while the anesthetic agents are already starting to take effect. This means the patient is no longer able to give "informed" consent.
- Medical practitioners may also rush through the informed consent process for other reasons, leaving interpreter (and patient) to feel that the process has not been properly administered.
- The interpreter may find himself interpreting for the patient and his family, with the family answering or asking questions on behalf of the patient. This may particularly be the case in situations where the question of whether the patient is capable of giving informed consent is borderline. The interpreter may need to convey different "voices" simultaneously without being fully aware who is saying what, and may feel he is losing control of the interpreting process.
- In the US "next-of-kin" is legally defined as a person's closest living blood relative. Patients may not nominate a "next-of-kin;" they may, however, create other legal documents to nominate a surrogate decision-maker.

Other issues pertain to the particular type of legal English often used in informed consent forms. In the US, best practice discourages interpreter from sight translating legal documents such as a consent form. Interpreters are encouraged to interpret for a provider as he/she orally consents a patient. Doctors may use legal English when orally consenting a patient and this may pose problems for the interpreter. The interpreter needs to be aware of cross-linguistic and socio-pragmatic issues in conveying the linguistic features of the legal English often used in these forms. Prominent features of legal English may include:

- the passive voice ("we transferred the patient" -> "the patient was transferred")
- nominalizations (turning a verb into a noun, e.g. "to heal" -> "recovery/healing")
- words originating from the Latin or the Greek, rather than from Old English (deceased rather than dead)

Both the passive voice and nominalizations are grammatical structures which can leave the listener confused as to "who did what". An example of the use of the passive voice in a medical context would be: "Mrs Z *was noted* to have diffuse swelling of the right arm". This sentence would be easier to understand if it read: "I/the nurse/Doctor X saw that Mrs Z had widely-spread swelling of the right arm". An example of the use of nominalization would be: "Intubation proved to be very difficult," when we could say: "*I* found it very difficult to intubate *him*," which tells us *who* intubated *whom*.

Both the passive voice and nominalizations can prove problematic for English-Chinese interpreters and translators as neither of them are common linguistic devices in the Chinese language. In Chinese, the use of passives is arguably associated with unpleasant happenings (e.g Baker 1992). The use of nominalization as a grammatical structure to avoid specifying the agent carrying out a certain action is equally problematic for English-Chinese interpreters/translators. Chinese is a non-inflectional language and the turning of a verb into a noun by nominalization is not available as a linguistic device in the Chinese language, although there are some words which can function as both a verb and a noun, just like in English.

In other words, the interpreter may have to decide what the text really means, but must at the same time leave ambiguities ambiguous. If the text is intended to have a double meaning, the interpreter must convey the double meaning. When dealing with either the passive voice or nominalizations, the Chinese interpreter can either supply a more generic subject equating to "we" or simply omit the subject, which is allowed in Chinese especially in spoken Chinese. Please see Tebble (2003), Meyer (2003) and others for a detailed analysis of medical discourse. Suggested further readings include Faden & Beauchamp (1986), Hunt & Voogd (2007), Simon, Zyzanski & Durant (2006).

Summary of main points

The informed consent process requires accurate and impartial interpretation of all relevant information, but may in practice be fraught with issues, leaving the interpreter in a difficult dilemma.

Chapter 10

Pre-operative and post-operative procedures

1. Pre- and post-operative procedures

The words pre-operative and post-operative refer to what happens before (pre) and after (post) procedures such as operations (surgery). The interpreter may also hear these abbreviated as pre-op and post-op.

Pre-operative procedures and questions

There are a number of procedures which are commonly carried out prior to surgery. Similarly, there are a number of questions which are commonly asked prior to the patient having surgery. Many of these procedures and questions are necessary to prevent things from going wrong during or after surgery (e.g. fasting prior to surgery reduces the risk of stomach contents being inhaled into the lungs by the unconscious patient). Most of the questions below may be asked by nursing personnel or anesthetic assistants, while others will be asked by the anesthesiologist (see next page).

Some commonly asked pre-operative questions (directed at the patient):

- Have you had any previous surgery? (meant to check whether everything went okay and how you responded to the anesthetic)
- Where and when and what for? (meant to trace the information needed, and to learn something about your general health status)
- Do you have any allergies? (Medication, seafood, latex, bandaid. Allergies may cause life-threatening reactions which lead to the patient going into a severe allergic reaction known as *anaphylactic shock*). Sometimes common substances which may cause severe allergic reactions are included in the question:
- Are you allergic to:
    - aspirin
    - antibiotics
    - bee stings
    - blood and blood products
    - plasma expanders (used to treat low blood pressure)

- iodine (commonly used in contrast dye, for instance during angiography procedures)
- penicillin
- bandaids (any color)
- sulfa drugs (antibacterial *sulfonamides*)

NB: A common answer to this question is: "Not that I am aware of," or "Not as far as I know," which is "translated" into the medical notes as *nil known* or NKDA for no known drug allergies.

- When did you last have anything to eat or drink (if the patient has something in his/her stomach, the contents may be accidentally "aspirated"/inhaled into the lungs while the patient is unconscious.
- When did you last urinate, void or pass urine (pee/go weewee/pass water) – a full bladder may empty itself while the patient is relaxed/unconscious; or it may be accidentally "perforated" during surgery.
- Are you Hepatitis B positive/HIV positive?
- Do you drink (alcohol)? How much/how often? (People who consume a lot of alcohol may require more anesthetic to "go under"; they may also require more pain relief after surgery.)
- Do you have any crowns/caps/loose teeth/bridges or plates in your mouth? (This is an important question as the anesthesiologist wants to be sure he does not run the risk of knocking out any loose teeth when he or she inserts the breathing tube or, worse still, push the loose teeth down into the airways with the breathing tube!)
- Do you wear dentures? (This question is asked for the same reason as the previous question – the patient will have to leave both pride and dentures behind with the rest of his belongings.)
- Do you wear make-up (lipstick/blusher) and/or nail-polish (the anesthesiologist can gauge the patient's well-being partly from looking at the color of lips and finger nails – in some private hospitals patients are allowed to go to the operating theatre wearing make-up!)
- Have you removed all your hairpins/rings, earrings, etc.? (These metal objects can lead to electric shock and burning when the doctor is using the cauterization equipment during the operation, or they may quite simply slip off people's fingers and get lost; staff can place any valuables in an opaque plastic bag with the rest of the patient's belongings. The bag will have the patient's name on it.

The anesthesiologist will visit the patient before the patient goes into the operating room. The main reason for this visit is to check whether there are likely to be any problems with the anesthetic. The anesthesiologist does this by looking the patient over (eye-balling) and by asking the patient if he had any problems with previous anesthesia.

The anesthesiologist will look at any aspects of the patient's build that may need to be taken into account when administering anesthesia. If the patient has a very short thick neck, for example, the anesthesiologist may have to use a shorter breathing tube.

In addition to looking at the patient, the anesthesiologist may ask questions such as:

- Have you had previous surgery?
- Did they perform the surgery under general anesthesia or under regional anesthesia?
- What type of regional anesthesia was used: an epidural, a spinal block, local anesthetic injected under the skin, an arm block, etc.?
- Did you experience any side-effects or after-effects from the anesthetic?
- What type of side-effects did you experience? (e.g. headache, pain in the back, vomiting, drowsiness)
- Do you have any preferences (type of anesthetic)?
- Do you have a latex allergy?

In addition, the anesthesiologist will probably like to decide what type of anesthetic would be best for this patient in view of the patient's medical history and current condition and to discuss options, benefits and possible side-effects or risks with the patient.

Intra-operative: During surgery and anesthetic

Main types of anesthesia

- General Anesthesia
- Regional Anesthesia: epidural, spinal block, caudal block, arm block, superficial local anesthesia

NB: No matter what type of anesthetic is used, the patient will almost always have a small needle inserted into a vein. This enables the anesthesiologist to administer medication, blood or fluids quickly, should this be necessary. The interpreter may be involved in interpreting while the patient is being given anesthetic and after the patient has returned from the operating room.

General Anesthesia or GA
Basically, in general anesthesia, the patient is given a combination of drugs intravenously. These drugs have different effects on the body. Most commonly they include:

- something to put the patient to sleep (a hypnotic)
- a muscle relaxant – this will relax all muscles in the body, including the breathing muscles, so the anesthesiologist will have to look after the patient's breathing.

He can do this by putting in a breathing tube and connecting the patient to a ventilator or breathing machine. Anesthesiologists may also use a laryngeal mask (inflatable silicone mask and rubber connecting tube which cover the opening of the windpipe).

– something to suppress the patient's reflexes
– a pain killer (long-acting/short-acting; strong or less strong)

For very short procedures, the anesthesiologist may induce sleep by putting a mask over the patient's face. The patient will breathe in the anesthetic gas and fall asleep.

Epidural Anesthesia and Spinal Anesthesia

The anesthesiologist will ask the patient to sit on the edge of the bed and bend forwards, making a curved back. For some patients, this is really difficult, and in those cases, the anesthesiologist may ask the patient to lie on his side, with a curved back.

In the case of epidural anesthesia, the anesthesiologist will then insert a hollow needle and check whether he has found the correct space. Once he has found the right space, the anesthesiologist will inject the anesthetic into the epidural space. The epidural space is the outermost part of the spinal canal. All nerve roots exiting or entering the spinal canal pass through the epidural space on their way out of or into the spinal canal.

After this, he will insert (through the needle) a very narrow tube and attach this catheter to the patient's back with tape. The catheter can be used to give the patient additional anesthetic if required. All spinal nerves which exit the spinal canal will pass through the epidural space first. By putting the anesthetic into the epidural space, the spinal nerves are anesthetized at the point of exit.

For spinal anesthesia, the anesthetic is injected into the spinal canal itself and mixes with the spinal fluid. By putting the anesthetic into the spinal space, the spinal nerves are anesthetized below a certain level (see Figure 17.1 in Chapter 17).

The purpose of this type of anesthesia is to block messages from the brain to the body and vice versa at a certain point. If the patient is to have knee surgery, the anesthesiologist can ensure that the patient does not feel any pain from the waist down (the pain signals do not reach the brain, and the patient does not feel any pain). If the brain sends a message such as *"Move that leg,"* that message is blocked as well.

The nurses will test the effectiveness of the anesthetic using different methods.

Some nurses apply an ice cube to the skin and ask the patient if he can feel the cold. Some nurses use cotton soaked in ether (which will also feel cold) and ask the patient if he can feel that.

Nerve Blocks

For surgery on the fingers or hand, anesthesiologists may prefer injecting anesthetic into the bundle of nerves going into the patient's arm. This type of anesthesia is called an arm block.

The anesthetic is injected into the underarm, into the "plexus" or bundle of nerves going into the patient's arm. Once the block takes effect, the patient may feel as if his arm has been replaced by a heavy block of wood. The arm will feel heavy, and the patient will lose all sensation or feeling in that arm.

Local Anesthesia
The anesthesiologist or doctor will inject the local anesthetic agent into the superficial tissues under the skin, through a very fine needle. If adrenaline has been added to the local anesthetic, the blood vessels will contract and skin may start to look very pale. The adrenaline is added to ensure that the anesthetic agent stays in place, therefore lasting a bit longer. It also helps to reduce bleeding.

Post-Anesthetic Care Unit or Recovery Room

After surgery, most patients spend some time in the Post-Anesthetic Care Unit (PACU) or Recovery Room, before going back to the floor.

Those who may have developed complications or who are showing signs of instability go to the Intensive Care Unit. These are usually patients who need special attention for a longer period of time, before being able to return to a normal nursing environment. It is standard procedure for patients to spend some time in the Intensive Care Unit after certain types of procedures (e.g. after coronary artery by-pass surgery).

When the patient is in the PACU, he will still be sleepy and it is not very likely that interpreters will be called in to interpret here.

For the sake of completeness, though, we will mention some of the most common pieces of equipment that will be used in the PACU and some of the most commonly performed observations.

IV drip – most patients will still have an intravenous needle (or luer) in their veins. Fluid can be given through plastic tubing, straight into the patient's vein. There are several reasons why patients are left with intravenous lines (or IVs) connected after surgery:

- They can be used to give extra fluid quickly, if needed.
- They can be used to give the patient medication accurately and quickly, for immediate effect, if need be.
- They can be used to give the patient a blood transfusion, if the patient needs this.

Some related terms:
Long lines – this term refers to the fact that the intravenous catheter (inside the patient's vein) is pushed almost as far as the patient's heart. Long lines can be

used to monitor blood pressure at a point just before the blood flows back into the patient's heart.

Arterial lines – these lines are inserted into the patient's artery and can be used to take arterial blood from the patient or to monitor the patient's blood pressure; arterial lines can also be used to take blood samples from the patient.

Bleeding lines – these are usually inserted into a large vein and closed off with a little cap.

Central venous lines – are usually put into the patient's large hollow vein, just below the collar bone (subclavian vein). However, sometimes central venous lines are lines inserted into the jugular vein (in the neck), or long lines inserted into the vein in the crook of the arm. Central venous lines can be used to monitor central venous pressure (CVP). Central venous lines are also used to give patients intravenous nutrition (IVN) or total parenteral nutrition (TPN – which means by-passing the bowels), containing fats, carbohydrates, sugars, vitamins, minerals and trace elements.

Position of IV (IntraVenous) lines
IV lines are usually put into the veins on the back of the patient's forearms or hands. Occasionally, they are put into the crook of the patient's arm. They can also be inserted into the patient's neck vein (jugular vein) or in a larger, more central vein (e.g. a subclavian catheter inserted in a large vein close to the heart, below the collar bone).

Pain pump – also known as PCA *pump* for *patient controlled analgesia.* The PCA involves an infusion pump which delivers pain relief from a syringe filled with a pain-killing solution. The syringe is placed in a chamber. The syringe is connected to tubing which connects on to the patient's IV line (or spinal catheter, see below). A push button is connected to the chamber and the patient can give himself a dose of pain killer before painful procedures, such as turning.

The amount of pain killer the patient is allowed to have (either continuously or intermittently) is prescribed by the anesthesiologist and programmed into the PCA pump by nursing staff. The prescribed dose cannot be exceeded, as the pump will refuse to give the patient more than the patient is allowed to have.

Pain pumps may also be connected to the nerve block catheter, e.g. an intrathecal pain pump will be connected to a spinal catheter and anesthetic drugs will be delivered straight into the spinal fluid.

Various types of monitoring equipment used in PACU
Monitoring equipment used in the PACU may include:

- *EKG dots* – three or four dots are usually attached to the patient's chest, sometimes to the shoulder or shoulder blades if there is no room on the chest. These dots are connected to leads which connect to an EKG monitor which shows the patient's heart beat and pattern of electrical activity in the patient's heart.

– *Blood pressure cuff and stethoscope* or
– *Automatic blood pressure monitoring* or
– *Invasive blood pressure monitoring equipment* – arterial line connected to a "transducer"

The blood pressure cuff and stethoscope may still be used for monitoring the patient's blood pressure by hand, using an inflatable cuff and a mercury manometer.

If the patient needs to have his blood pressure measured very frequently, automatic blood pressure monitors such as the Dynamap® may be used. A cuff is placed around the patient's arm. The cuff is connected to monitoring equipment. At set intervals, the cuff fills with air and the patient's blood pressure reading will show up on the screen of the monitor.

Thermometer – used to check whether the patient's temperature is within normal range. The thermometer is usually a *tympano-thermometer*, which is held briefly inside the patient's ear, until it bleeps, or a *forehead thermometer* which scans across the forehead ending on the temple.

Oximetry – pulse oximeters are used to monitor to what extent red blood cells are saturated with oxygen. Usually they consist of a little machine, with a cord and a finger clip with a red LED light in it. The finger clip is placed over the patient's nail and used to measure the oxygen saturation in the small arteries in the tip of the finger.

Drains – drains are often left in to drain the surgical site of excess fluid which might hamper recovery and healing.

Types of drains:

Vacuum drains – most drains are of the vacuum type: they actively drain wound fluid from within the body.

Harmonica drains – tiny drains shaped like a harmonica.

T-drains or T-tubes – used to drain bile (usually dark green-brown in color) from the body. They look like a T-junction, hence the name. These passive drains are usually connected to a simple catheter bag.

Chest drains – chest drains are used in patients who have had a collapsed lung or blood in the lung. They are taped securely and connected to one or two big glass jars which are half-filled with water. Chest drains are often connected to suction and thus are seen to be bubbling.

Urinary catheter – also called indwelling catheter or Foley catheter. Urinary catheters drain urine from the patient's bladder.

Irrigation systems – (continuous) bladder irrigation systems may be used in patients who have had surgery on the prostate. These patients will have a three-way "balloon" catheter inserted, which serves a dual purpose. The balloon is blown up and puts pressure on the space inside the prostate to stop the bleeding. The catheter will also drain urine from the patient's bladder. The catheter is irrigated with a saline (salt water) solution from time to time, to stop the catheter from getting blocked.

Once the patient is breathing consistently by himself, and temperature, blood pressure and heart rate are normal, and there is no uncontrolled bleeding or oozing from the wound, the patient is escorted back to the floor.

Possible complications after surgery

- Vomiting and nausea
- Patient breathing very slowly or very superficially
- Patient losing a lot of blood, either via the drains or straight into the gauze dressing which has been placed over the wound; bleeding can be a slow ooze or trickle. If the patient loses a lot of blood, he may need a blood transfusion, or he may need to go back to the operating room
- Blood clot forming in the lower leg (deep vein thrombosis)
- Rise in body temperature
- Patient is unable to pass urine
- Patient is unable to have a bowel movement within a few days of surgery – bowels usually "go on strike" for a few days after surgery, especially after surgery in the abdominal area.

Commonly asked questions after surgery

- Most of the questions asked after surgery are aimed at ensuring that there are no complications from surgery and that all systems (e.g. the renal system and gastro-intestinal system) are working normally again. Questions may include:
- Have you urinated/passed water? How much/How often?
- Have you passed gas yet?
- Have you had a bowel movement yet?
- Are you in any pain? Where does it hurt?
- Would you like some pain relief? What type of pain relief would you prefer? (injection into the muscle/tablet/suppository/intravenous (IV) pain relief)?
- Are you feeling nauseated? Have you vomited?
- Are you feeling drowsy?
- Can you move your toes? Any tingling/pins-and-needles?
- (After epidural): Have you got full movement and sensation in the legs?

2.   English-Chinese glossary

英漢詞彙表

English	Hong Kong & Taiwan	Mainland China
anaphylactic shock	過敏性休克	过敏性休克
arm block	臂神經阻斷麻醉	臂神经丛麻醉
arterial line	動脈導管	动脉导管; 动脉插管
balloon catheter	球囊導管	气囊导管
bladder irrigation system	膀胱灌洗系統	膀胱冲洗系统; 膀胱灌注系统
bleeding lines	血液導管	血液导管
blood clot	血塊; 血凝塊	血块; 血凝块
caudal block	脊尾神經麻醉	骶管麻醉
cauterization	烙法; 燒灼 (術)	烙术; 烧灼术
central venous line	中央靜脈導管	中心静脉导管
chest drain	胸腔引流	胸腔引流
deep vein thrombosis	深層靜脈栓塞 (血栓)	深层静脉血栓塞
denture	假牙	假牙; 义齿
ECG dots	心電圖電極	心电图电极
epidural anesthesia	硬膜外麻醉	硬膜外麻醉
general anesthesia (GA)	全身麻醉	全身麻醉
analgesia drain	止痛引流	止痛引流
hypnotic	安眠藥; 催眠藥	安眠药; 催眠药
intravenous nutrition (IVN)	靜脈營養	静脉营养
invasive blood pressure monitoring equipment	侵入性血壓監察儀器	侵入性血压监护仪
IV drip	靜脈滴注	静脉滴注; 静脉点滴
local anesthetic	局部麻醉	局部麻醉
long line	長導管	长导管
nerve block	神經阻斷麻醉; 封閉麻醉	神经阻滞麻醉; 封闭麻醉
oximetry	血氧定量法	血氧定量法
patient controlled anesthesia/analgesia (PCA); pain pump	病患自控式麻醉; 病患自控止痛法	病人自控麻醉; 病人自控镇痛
'pins and needles'	發麻	发麻
plasma expander	(血) 漿膨脹劑	血浆膨胀药; 血浆增容药
post-operative	手術後	术后

(Continued)

English	Hong Kong & Taiwan	Mainland China
post-operative care unit (PACU)	手術後護理病房	术后监护病房
pre-operative	手術前	术前
pulse oximeter	(脈搏) 血氧計	脉搏血氧计
regional anesthesia	局部麻醉	区域麻醉
sphygmomanometer	血壓計	血压计
spinal anesthesia	脊髓麻醉	脊髓麻醉
spinal canal	髓管	椎管
spinal fluid	脊髓液	脊髓液
sulfa drugs	磺胺類藥	磺胺类药物; 磺胺药类
T-drain; T-tube	T形 (引流) 管; T型管	T形 (引流) 管; T型管
total parenteral nutrition (TPN)	腸胃道外營養療法; 全靜脈注射營養	全肠外营养; 全静脉营养
transducer	變換器; 轉導器	转换器
urinary catheter	導尿管; 尿管	导尿管
vacuum drain	真空引流	抽吸引流

Summary of main points

This chapter has touched on pre- and post-operative care settings; it has also touched on some of the knowledge competent health interpreters need to possess to interpret in these settings. It has also offered a brief overview of:

–   types of questions asked before and after surgical procedures
–   types of anesthesia
–   equipment used in pre- and post-operative care

Chapter 11

Intensive care

Intensive care units or ICUs are units which specialize in the care of seriously ill or potentially seriously ill people, who require round-the-clock nursing and medical attention. Patients are monitored closely and treatment is generally aggressive. Life support systems are often used. Sometimes patients are deliberately paralyzed and sedated by drugs and thus unaware of their surroundings. Patients may be placed in a medically induced coma (or artificial coma) to help them recover.

Intensive care units may vary in their specialty and in the age group they serve. There are special ICUs for newborn babies (usually called Neonatal Intensive Care Units, abbreviated as NICU) and special ICUs for children (usually called Pediatric Intensive Care Units, abbreviated as PICU). Some ICUs focus on a specific group of patients. There are Neurological Intensive Care Units for patients with neurological problems or head-injuries. CardiacCare Units focus on patients who need round the clock monitoring for their heart condition.

The three main reasons for admission to an ICU are:

- monitoring
- rest
- treatment

A wide range of patients may be admitted to an ICU, including the following:

Major trauma: Patients who have multiple life-threatening injuries following assaults, accidents or falls.

Respiratory System: Severe asthma attacks; pneumonia; pulmonary embolism; near-drowning; severe lung contusion; respiratory arrest; also: patients who are making a slow recovery from anesthesia.

Heart and cardiovascular complications (such as those following cardiac arrest or heart attacks): heart shock; arrhythmias (irregular heart rhythm); congestive heart failure (CHF); different types of shock (septic shock, anaphylactic shock, cardiogenic shock or heart shock), aneurysms; diffuse intravascular coagulation; hemorrhages

Neurological: Brain hemorrhages (bleeding into the brain): head injury (as a result of assault, traffic accident, or fall)

Renal: Renal failure (kidney shutdown)

Obstetric Problems: Pre-eclampsia (please refer to Chapter 28); hemorrhages (bleeds) before or after childbirth

Burns: Patients with deep and/or extensive burns who suffer from swelling of the airways, shock, loss of protein and electrolyte imbalance and who need special dressings and pain relief

Major surgery: Patients recovering after major surgery, such as extensive abdominal surgery or radical head and neck surgery, or any other surgery where the patient's condition is compromised (serious)

Equipment

The amount of equipment and the extensive use of technology sets ICUs apart from other patient care areas. Equipment is used for diagnosis, monitoring and treatment of patients.

Some of the most commonly used equipment found in the ICU includes:

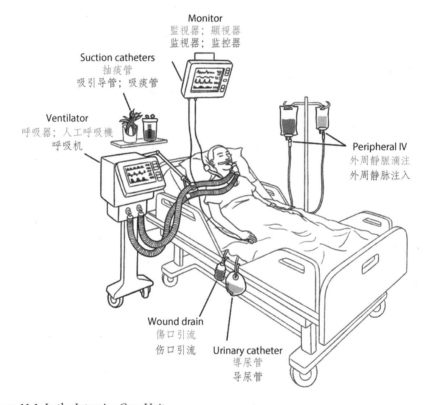

Figure 11.1 In the Intensive Care Unit
深切治療部內
重症监护室內

1. Ventilator

The ventilator or respirator is sometimes referred to as a breathing machine and is used to maintain breathing for the patient.

Intubation is the name of the process whereby a tube is inserted into the patient, either

- through one nostril, down the throat, through the vocal cords into the windpipe (nasotracheal tube), or
- through the mouth, down the throat, through the vocal cords into the windpipe (oro-tracheal tube) or
- through a special incision called a tracheostomy straight into the windpipe (endo-tracheal tube).

Nasotracheal tubes may be used in children. Endotracheal tubes are used in patients who need to be intubated for longer periods of time. The endotracheal tube is often referred to as the *"trach"* (pronounced "trake'). The trach is a relatively short and curved tube, which can usually be removed for cleaning purposes or replaced with a clean trach.

Intubated patients are often unable to cough up their own phlegm, so suctioning tubes are used to suction off these secretions.

As mentioned previously, patients in the ICU are sometimes paralyzed and sedated – they are unconscious, due to an induced coma (a level of deep uncon-sciousness, brought about by drugs), and need help with their breathing for that reason. Patients who have fractured their spine at neck level may be unable to breathe because the nerve supply to the breathing muscles has been interrupted. In other instances, the patient may simply be unable or too weak to breathe in by himself.

Usually, staff will try to wean the patient off the ventilator gradually, whenever possible.

The ventilator can be set in such a way that the patient is helped with any sponta-neous attempts at breathing. If the patient makes a small attempt at breathing in, this triggers the ventilator, which will then deliver a "full breath" to the patient. The patient can then be extubated (i.e. the breathing tube can be removed).

2. *Monitoring equipment*
Most ICU patients will be attached to a variety of monitors, each of which delivers important information.

Monitors may include:

- monitors showing information about cardiac and pulmonary (lung) pressures (using a Swan Ganz Catheter in the heart)
- an electrocardiograph (ECG) or EKG monitor which shows heart rate and rhythm
- a pulse oximeter which shows the amount of oxygen in the patient's blood (oxygen saturation)
- a temperature probe, which monitors the patient's body temperature

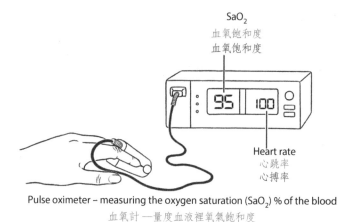

Pulse oximeter – measuring the oxygen saturation (SaO$_2$) % of the blood

血氧計 —量度血液裡氧氣飽和度

脉搏血氧測定仪 —量度血液氧气饱和度

Figure 11.2 Pulse oximeter

血氧計

脉搏血氧測定仪

3. *IV pumps*

Intravenous lines or IV lines are very often used to administer medication to the patient – in many cases the rate at which medication is administered is very important and "pumps" are used to ensure that the patient gets exactly the right amount of medication in exactly the right amount of time.

IV pumps are pumps which accurately regulate the amount of fluid administered to the patient. The IV fluid often contains medication, either in an IV fluid bag or in a syringe.

Where patients are conscious, *PCA (patient controlled analgesia) pumps or pain pumps* may be used to provide the patient with a consistent amount of basic pain relief. These pumps enable the patient to administer some pain relief when he wants it or just prior to painful procedures such as being washed or turned.

4. *Lines and tubes*

The term "*lines*" generally refers to long narrow plastic tubes inserted into blood vessels for various purposes. Tubes may be inserted into the body for drainage of fluid or sometimes for the administration of fluid.

The various lines and tubes used in ICUs (and other services) may include:

- *Intravenous lines or IV lines:* used for administering fluid, medication and nutrition, and also for monitoring pressures inside the patient's heart, lungs and major blood vessels. Common IV lines include:
- *peripheral lines* – inserted into peripheral veins, usually on the hands or forearms, occasionally in veins on the foot; peripheral lines in the stomach and bowels. The

IV lines may be used to give the patient fluid, glucose and electrolytes (such as sodium and potassium). Medication may be added to the IV fluid. Blood may also be given through a peripheral line.

–   *Central Lines* – inserted into the jugular (neck) vein or into the subclavian vein (under the collar bone). Central lines may be used to give the patient complete nutrition, known as total parenteral nutrition (TPN) or intravenous nutrition (IVN).

–   *Arterial Lines* – inserted into arteries; arterial lines are often connected to a monitor for monitoring various types of blood pressures; they are also used for taking arterial blood samples.

–   *Drains* – may be used to drain fluid away from the body for specific reasons. See Chapter 10 for a list of drains.

–   *Nasogastric tubes* may be inserted through the nose, down the esophagus into the stomach to drain away stomach juices (and other fluid produced in the gastrointestinal tract).

–   *Chest Drains* or chest tubes – may be used to drain air, fluid or blood from the lungs, to enable the patient to breathe better.

–   *Urinary Catheters* – also called indwelling catheters (IDCs). IDCs are used to drain urine out of the bladder into a container. In the Intensive Care Unit, the urine usually drains into a urine meter, which enables staff to measure exactly how much urine the patient produces.

1.   Staff

The staff in the ICU is especially trained to look after patients who need intensive care. Staff is ever-present and there is usually one nurse assigned per patient. This nurse will be the contact person for interpreter and family.

The medical staff will usually consist of intensive care specialists (sometimes known as intensivists – specialists in providing intensive care) and intensive care residents.

In some smaller centers, anesthesiologists and medical/surgical specialists provide medical back-up for nursing staff.

2.   Some notes for interpreters and translators

Interpreting in the ICU will usually take place during interviews between the patient's relatives and medical staff. Sometimes informed consent may need to be obtained from relatives for procedures or for permission to switch off the support systems. On some occasions the interpreter may have to interpret for a semi-conscious patient (who may just be waking up from sedation), to convey messages to and from medical and allied staff.

3. English–Chinese glossary

英漢詞彙表

English	Hong Kong & Taiwan	Mainland China
anaphylactic shock	過敏性休克	过敏性休克
aneurysm	動脈瘤	动脉瘤
arrhythmia	心律不整; 心律不齊	心律不齐; 心律失常
breathing machine	人工呼吸機	呼吸机
cardiac arrest	心動停止; 心跳驟停	心动停止; 心搏停止
cardiogenic shock (heart shock)	心原性休克	心原性休克
chest drain	胸腔引流	胸腔引流
congestive heart failure (CHF)	充血性心臟衰竭	充血性心衰竭
Department of Critical Care	重症監護部; 危重病加護病房	危重病人护理病房
diffuse intravascular coagulation	彌漫 (散播) 性血管內凝血	播散性血管内凝血
electrocardiograph/ Electrocardiogram (ECG) monitor	心電圖監察器	心电图监察器
endotracheal tube	氣管內導管	气管内导管; 气管内插管
heart attack	心臟病發作; 心臟病猝發	心脏病发作
High Dependency Unit	加護病房; 重症護理病房	加护病室; 重症护理病房
Induced coma	引發性昏迷	引起性昏迷
Intensive Care Room	深切治療室; 深切治療病房	重症监护室
Intensive Care Unit (ICU)	深切治療部	重症监护室
intravenous nutrition (IVN)	靜脈營養	静脉营养
intubation	導管插入	插管法
IV fluid	靜脈輸入溶液	静脉输液; 静脉注射液
IV line	靜脈導管	静脉导管
IV pump	靜脈泵	静脉泵
major trauma	重大創傷	重创伤
nasotracheal tube	鼻氣管導管	经鼻气管插管
nasogastric tube	鼻胃導管	经鼻胃管; 鼻饲管

(Continued)

English	Hong Kong & Taiwan	Mainland China
Neonatal Intensive Care Unit (NICU)	初生嬰兒深切治療部	新生儿 (重症) 监护病房
orotracheal tube	口氣管導管	口腔气管插管
patient controlled anesthesia/ analgesia (PCA); pain pump	病患自控式麻醉; 病患自控式止痛法	病人控制式麻醉
peripheral lines	外周導管 (靜脈點滴)	外周管
Preeclampsia/Pre-eclampsia	先兆子癇	先兆子癇; 子癇前期
pulmonary pressures	肺壓	肺压
pulse oximeter	(脈搏) 血氧計	脉搏血氧计
respirator	人工呼吸機	呼吸器; 呼吸机
septic shock	敗血性休克	败血症性休克; 感染性休克; 脓毒性休克
Swan Ganz catheter	氣囊漂浮心臟導管	气囊漂浮导管
temperature probe	體溫探針; 溫度探針	温度探针
total parenteral nutrition (TPN)	腸胃道外營養療法; 全靜脈注射營養	全 (胃) 肠外营养; 全静脉营养
ventilator	呼吸器; 人工呼吸機	呼吸器; 呼吸机

Summary of main points

This chapter has touched on intensive care settings; it has also provided an overview of the knowledge competent health interpreters need to possess to interpret in these settings. It has also offered a brief overview of:

- types of cases requiring treatment in the ICU
- equipment encountered in ICU settings

Chapter 12

Obstetrics

Adapted from a contribution by Maureen Kearney, RN, RM

This chapter aims to present a brief overview of obstetric care, to give healthcare interpreters an idea of what tests are done and what questions are asked. This chapter will mention some of the complications of pregnancy, which are discussed in more detail in Chapter 28. Problems of sick newborns will be discussed in Chapter 13.

Women may be able to choose from a variety of healthcare providers to care for them during pregnancy. These include midwives; primary care doctors; and obstetricians (specialists dealing with pregnancy and childbirth) and Ob/Gyns (specialists in obstetrics and gynecology).

Similarly, women may be able to choose from a variety of locations in which to deliver their baby, including a hospital, a birthing center, or their own home.

The woman discusses these options with her practitioner, who will also take into account her past obstetric history, her diet, any current health or pregnancy-related problems.

Prenatal care is very important. The first visit is done to obtain all the relevant information early on in the pregnancy, and further check-ups are done to ensure that mother and baby continue to be healthy and that baby continues to grow well in respect to its gestation or age. If there are any problems, it is vital that these be detected and treated as early as possible, to ensure the best possible outcome for mother and baby.

The practitioner may encourage the woman to attend birthing classes, so that the woman knows what to expect and feels confident about the coming birth. Classes are usually offered through the hospital or birthing center where the woman expects to deliver.

1. Prenatal care

Once her pregnancy has been confirmed, the woman will generally visit one of the above-mentioned practitioners for her first visit. This first visit will be a very thorough visit (as described below). After this, visits generally increase from once a month (first two trimesters, from week 1–28), to once every two weeks (week 28 to 36), to once a week (after week 36) as the expected date of delivery approaches. Obviously, this schedule may vary, depending on how the pregnancy progresses.

During the first prenatal visit the woman may be:

- Booked in for delivery in the hospital (even though she may express the wish to deliver elsewhere). It is important that the woman is booked into a hospital, just in case it becomes necessary to transfer the woman there in the course of delivery.
- History will be recorded. This is a very important part of the first visit and will include:

Obstetric History
- The first day of the last menstrual period (LMP)
- Past child-bearing experiences
- Previous terminations of pregnancy (abortions)
- History of repeated miscarriages (spontaneous abortions)
- Complications in previous childbirth

Social History
- Planned/unplanned pregnancy?
- Wanted/unwanted pregnancy?
- Support from partner/family
- Response of mother and whole family to the pregnancy
- Financial support
- Environmental factors (housing, heating, diet, and so on)
- Age – is it a teenage pregnancy?
- Is the woman over 35?
- General health (practitioner will give advice on this if necessary)
- Exercise
- Cigarette smoking, use of alcohol and drugs (practitioner will discuss these with the woman if necessary)

Menstrual History
- The practitioner will try to determine the date on which the woman started her last menstrual period (LMP). The practitioner will then add 9 months plus 7 days to the first day of the LMP to arrive at the approximate due date, or Expected Date of Delivery (EDD).
- The practitioner will discuss the woman's normal cycle and amount of bleeding and will find out if any pain is associated with this menstrual cycle.
- The practitioner will discuss the woman's contraception history with her.

Medical History
- The woman's past health is very important, as medical conditions may affect the pregnancy. These may range from severe heart conditions to common urinary tract infections. Some of the more common medical conditions are asthma; epilepsy; diabetes; high blood pressure or hypertension; mental

health problems; heart disorders (including rheumatic fever) and any other condition for which the woman may be taking medication.

Family History
-   Certain conditions are genetic in origin while others are familial (occurring in certain families) or racial (confined to certain races) or social (influenced by social conditions). It is important to know the woman's family history and that of her partner, if they know of them, so the caregivers can be more aware of any risks to the baby. Obviously, if either the father or the mother has been adopted, this information may not be available. There is increasing evidence to suggest that Asian women (including Chinese) have a greater likelihood of developing Gestational Diabetes Mellitus than Caucasian women. Women are also more likely to develop GDM if their own mothers had gestational diabetes while carrying them.

-   *Physical Examination*. The practitioner will carry out a thorough physical examination of the woman, which may include height and weight; blood pressure; and height of the fundus (the top of the womb)
Diagnostic tests may include:

-   Urine test for glucose/sugar (this may be a sign of gestational diabetes) and protein (this may be a sign of pre-eclampsia)
-   Blood tests for hemoglobin (to check for anemia and thalassemia); complete blood count (CBC) or full blood count (FBC); blood group and Rhesus factor (Rh factor); antibodies in the blood (rubella, hepatitis B); VDRL (to check for venereal diseases such as syphilis) and glucose tolerance tests
-   Vaginal speculum (vaginal smear) (cells are checked for cervical cancer) and vaginal swabs (check for infection, e.g. chlamydia)
-   Baby's heart beat (depending on how long the woman has been pregnant)

2. Follow-up visits

Once all the above information has been recorded during the booking visit, further prenatal check-ups are usually less involved. The following would be checked during a typical check-up:

-   mother's general well-being
-   blood pressure
-   weight
-   urine test for sugar and protein
-   abdominal palpation (feeling the mother's abdomen). Feeling and measuring the baby's growth is an important factor in determining whether baby's growth equals its *gestation* or age.

–   checking fetal movements. It is very important that the mother be aware of the baby's movements and that she feel at least 10 movements a day (this becomes more significant after approximately 25 weeks).
–   checking if mother has any swelling in face, hands and feet (signs of pre-eclampsia)
–   checking baby's heart beat

Other tests may be done during the prenatal period if the practitioner, or the woman, think these are necessary or desired. These may include (in more or less chronological order):

–   ultrasound – Imaging with the aid of high-frequency sound waves, usually done by a radiographer. The ultrasound can show the baby on the screen and can detect growth and abnormalities (if any). A 3D-scan will show the developing fetus (baby) in 3D. Scans may be done right through pregnancy.
–   Chorionic villus sampling (CVS) – Usually done between 9 and 11 weeks, when a sample of early placental tissue is taken to check for abnormalities.
–   alphafetoprotein (AFP) – Test done at approximately 13 weeks to identify potential congenital abnormalities (birth defects), such as spina bifida or chromosomal problems such as Down Syndrome.
–   amniocentesis – Usually done between 16 and 18 weeks. Some amniotic fluid is taken from around the baby. This is withdrawn with a needle which is inserted through the abdominal wall under ultrasound guidance. The amniotic fluid is then tested for abnormalities. This is a very accurate test which can also tell the sex of the baby.
–   cardiotocograph (CTG) – Can record the baby's heart beat via an abdominal disc which has been strapped to the mother's stomach. The heart beat will show up on a graph. The same graph can also record any contractions (or tightening) the mother may have. It can show the strength of these contractions and how often they come.

3.   Term of pregnancy

As a large proportion of infants admitted to the NICU are premature, it is necessary to understand what is meant by 'term pregnancy' so as to understand the implications of preterm delivery or premature birth.

A normal term of pregnancy is 40 weeks from the first day of the last menstrual period (LMP). The estimated date of confinement (EDC) or expected date of delivery (EDD) is calculated by adding 9 months and 7 days to the date of the LMP. The number of weeks of gestation is calculated accordingly. A pregnancy is regarded as term when it reaches 36 to 38 weeks. Once the pregnancy passes 40 weeks it is regarded as post-term. Any gestation before 36 weeks is treated as preterm, therefore delivery before 36 weeks' gestation would be regarded as pre-mature birth.

However, classification based on the date of the LMP may, sometimes, be inaccurate. Many women have irregular menstrual periods which can make LMP quite unreliable, while other women may not remember, or may conceal, for a variety of reasons, their actual date of LMP. As a result, ascertaining gestation can be very difficult, and gestation could be different from the actual size and development of the fetus. Thanks to ultrasonography the maturity of a pregnancy can now be assessed quite accurately. Ultrasound uses high-frequency sound waves to reflect the image of the fetus in the mother's abdomen, enabling healthcare professionals to measure the actual size of the fetus. Comparing these measurements to a standard measurement gives a fair indication of how mature the fetus is.

The biparietal diameter (BPD) of the fetal head offers a reliable parameter in *ultrasonography* to assess how far along the pregnancy is, because the head of the fetus grows at a fixed rate. The head-abdomen ratio (H:A ratio) is another measurement done to ascertain duration of pregnancy. Since head and abdomen grow at different rates, the H:A ratio is usually larger in early pregnancy and lower in late pregnancy when the abdomen grows faster than the head.

Most babies are delivered near term, that is, after a pregnancy of around 40 weeks. However, some babies are delivered pre-term and some post-term. Most pre-term deliveries, and some term or post-term deliveries, may cause problems for babies. The more pre-term the infant, the more problems can be expected. Please see Chapter 13 for more detail.

4. Labor and childbirth

Childbirth is a major life experience. Labor is described as the process by which the baby, placenta and membranes are expelled through the birth canal. Normal labor occurs spontaneously at "term" (38–42 weeks of pregnancy), with the baby presenting head first and face down. It is considered normal for the woman to deliver between 37 and 42 weeks.

Note: the interpreter may need to stay close to the mother and interpret the health practitioner's comments and instructions during childbirth. If the interpreter feels faint, he or she may have to sit down.

There are three stages of labor:

- *Stage one:* The cervix (or opening of the womb) dilates (opens), beginning with regular rhythmic contractions of the uterus. Dilatation of the cervix is complete when the cervix opens to 10 cm.
- *Stage two:* The baby is born. This stage begins when the cervix is fully dilated and finishes when baby is born.

–   *Stage three:* In this stage, the placenta (afterbirth) and membranes detach from the wall of the uterus and are expelled. This stage also involves the control of bleeding. It begins after the birth of the baby and ends when the placenta and membranes have been expelled.

5. Common terminology

–   *Contractions or tightening:* The pain of the contractions comes and goes and is mostly felt in the lower abdominal and upper stomach areas, due to the muscles in the wall of the womb squeezing and relaxing.
–   *Drip:* An intravenous line inserted into a vein, usually in the back of a hand, so fluids can be given straight into the blood.
–   *Entonox:* A form of pain relief which is inhaled by mouth: it consists of nitrous oxide mixed with oxygen.
–   *Epidural:* Injection of local anesthetic into the epidural space near the base of the spine. See Chapter 10.
–   *Fetal scalp electrode (FSE):* This is a clip which is attached to the baby's head via the vagina. The lead is plugged into a machine which will accurately record the baby's heartbeat.
–   *Meconium:* Baby's first, greenish-black bowel movement. When the baby has passed a bowel movement while still in the uterus, the amniotic fluid around the baby will become a greenish color. When amniotic fluid appears this color it is a sign that baby has been distressed at some stage. Meconium in the amniotic fluid also means an increased risk of infection. If meconium has been observed, a fetal scalp electrode will be used.
–   *Membranes ruptured* (waters leaking or waters have broken or the bag of waters has broken): The amniotic fluid (waters) is contained within two layers of membranes around the baby, which protect the baby from any infection. These membranes should not rupture (break) until labor has begun. Women are often unsure as to whether the membranes have ruptured. They describe feeling wet as though they have passed urine. Once the waters have broken, baby will need to be delivered within a certain time-frame, because there is a risk of infection once the protective amniotic sac has ruptured.
–   *Narcotics:* Are sometimes still given as pain relief.
–   *Perineum:* The area between the lower vagina and the rectum. The perineum is stretched, particularly when the baby's head is born. In order to avoid having it tear, the obstetrician may make a small cut in it in a procedure called an episiotomy, to allow for baby's head to pass through. After a tear or episiotomy the perineum is repaired with dissolving sutures (stitches).

- *Position:* Refers to the way the baby's head is lying and is assessed by feeling (by vaginal examination) the sutures and fontanelles on baby's head.
- *Bloody show:* A sticky discharge of mucus (slime) and blood, that appears usually early in labor. This is a plug of mucus that was situated in the opening of the cervix during pregnancy, protecting the baby from infection. Once the cervix begins to soften and dilate, this mucus comes away.
- *Vaginal examination:* This is done by the practitioner to assess whether the cervix is changing and is the most accurate way of assessing progress in labor.

6. Postnatal checks

At one and five minutes after birth, the practitioner will check the appearance, pulse, grimace, activity, respiration (APGAR) score. Appearance involves the baby's complexion or skin color (pink, pale, blue). Pulse relates to baby's heart rate. Grimace relates to baby's reflex to stimulation (none, grimace, crying). Activity relates to muscle tone (none, some, flexion), and respiration relates to breathing (none, weak, strong). A score of 0, 1 or 2 is given for each aspect. Best outcome would be a total score of 9 or 10 overall, while an overall score of < 3 means the baby needs immediate medical attention.

A thorough baby check is done after birth, including listening to the baby's heart and lungs, testing the baby's reflexes, hips and so on. This thorough check is repeated at six weeks by a pediatrician. Any baby that is feeding well and sleeping well should thrive.

The following are typical baby tests:

- *Feeding* – It is important to know whether baby is going to be fed on formula or breast-milk. The practitioner will check how much baby drinks and how often, and if there are any problems.
- *Skin* – The practitioner will check for spots, rashes, marks, skin infections, and so on.
- *Head* – The practitioner will check fontanelles, ears, eyes, nose, mouth and so on, for any signs of infection, redness and so on.
- *Cord* – The practitioner will check whether this is drying or moist. The practitioner will also check for redness, an offensive smell, or whether the cord has fallen off (usually around the fifth day).
- *Bottom* – The practitioner will check for redness, diaper rash, spots or thrush.
- *Urine and bowel function* – The practitioner will check whether baby is passing urine and having bowel movements normally.
- *Sleeping pattern* – The practitioner will check baby's sleeping pattern and give advice if necessary.
- *Crying or agitation* – The practitioner will check for crying, agitation or any unusual behavior.
- *Growth* – The practitioner will check baby's height and weight.

7. Postnatal care

The postnatal period is also called the *puerperium*. This is the period between birth and 6 weeks after birth. The mother may or may not stay in the hospital for the first few days. This is a time of great physical, emotional and psychological change. It is important to establish a bond between mother and baby and to establish breastfeeding. Although breast-feeding is a natural process, lots of help and support are often needed.

Postnatal checks and care of the mother generally include:

- *Physical check on mother* – Mothers generally need to visit the obstetrician's office for postpartum care.
- *General well-being* – Does mother feel well?
- *Breasts* – Breasts are checked for red, painful areas, lumps or any other problems.
- *Nipples* – Nipples are checked to ensure that there are no blisters, cracks, bleeding areas, etc. Are the nipples coping with the breast-feeding and the constant sucking from baby?
- *Fundus* – The fundus is the top of the uterus. After the baby is born, the fundus should be at umbilicus (belly-button) level. From there on, the fundus drops a bit each day (approximately 1 centimeter), until it finally returns to the pelvis, under the pubic bone. This process is called involution, and feeling the level of the fundus forms part of the postnatal check.
- *Vaginal discharge or lochia* – The vaginal discharge begins as fresh bleeding. Over a period of time (different for each woman), the lochia changes into a whitish discharge. Some women may bleed on and off for up to six weeks.
- *Legs* – Women are encouraged to be up and about early after the birth of their babies to stimulate a good blood flow through the legs and thereby avoid the formation of blood clots (thrombosis).
- *Urine* – After birth, women will pass urine in larger quantities and more frequently than usual, in order to get rid of the excess fluid they have been carrying during pregnancy. Urinary tract infections can be common after birth so the practitioner will check that there is no pain, stinging or unusual smell associated with the urine.
- *Sleep* – The mother will be encouraged to sleep when her baby sleeps, as overtiredness is very common in the postnatal period.
- *Nutrition* – The woman needs to eat regular, nutritious meals and snacks, especially if she is breast-feeding. There is some evidence to suggest that ginger in the mother's diet may contribute to prolonged jaundice in breastfed infants, especially when these were born prematurely (Weng, Chiu & Cheng, 2012).
- *Hydration* – The woman needs to be encouraged to drink lots of fluid, especially if she is breast-feeding, as the baby will take a lot of fluid away from her.

- *Bowel function* – Often mothers do not have a bowel movement for a few days and may find themselves constipated. Their practitioners may advise them to take gentle laxatives or to eat high fiber foods and to drink a lot of fluids.
- *Postnatal exercises* – These should be started in a gentle way, soon after the birth. The so-called pelvic floor exercises," which aim to strengthen the pelvic floor muscles, are especially important. Abdominal exercises and other exercises can be introduced later.
- *Postpartum blues* – Major emotional and hormonal changes can occur postnatally. It often takes 6 to 12 weeks to return to a normal emotional state. "Blues" or "feeling down" can occur at any time between 3 and 10 days after birth. "Blues" are most common on the fifth day after birth. This is a normal reaction to childbirth, and it affects approximately 60% of women. Signs are tearfulness and a feeling of panic. The first days after birth are a time of great hormonal changes, with progesterone levels dropping to almost zero, and tearfulness usually settles down after 24 hours.

8.   English-Chinese glossary

英漢詞彙表

English	Hong Kong & Taiwan	Mainland China
alphafetoprotein (AFP)	甲 (種) 胎 (兒) 蛋白	甲胎蛋白
amniocentesis	羊膜穿刺抽液術 (俗稱「抽羊水」)	羊膜穿刺术
anemia/anaemia	貧血	贫血
APGAR test	阿帕嘉試驗	阿普加评分试验
biparietal diameter (BPD)	胎兒雙頂徑; 胎兒頭骨橫徑	两顶骨间直径; 双顶 (间) 径
cardiotocograph (CTG)	胎心宮縮圖	胎心宫缩图
cervical cancer	(子) 宮頸癌	子宫颈癌
childbirth	分娩	分娩; 生产
chlamydia	衣原體	衣菌体
chorionic villus sampling (CVS)	絨膜絨毛抽樣檢驗法	绒膜绒毛取样; 绒毛取样 (法)
contractions	宮縮	宫缩
delivery	生產; 分娩	生产; 分娩
Down Syndrome	唐氏綜合症	唐氏综合症
drip	靜脈滴注	静脉滴注; 静脉點滴
epidural	硬膜外	硬膜外
Entonox	安桃樂 (俗稱「笑氣」)	安东诺克斯; 一氧化二氮-氧混合气
expected date of delivery (EDD)	預產期	预产期

(Continued)

English	Hong Kong & Taiwan	Mainland China
fetal/foetal scalp electrode (FSE)	胎兒頭皮電極	胎儿头皮电极
fundus	宮底	宫底
gestational diabetes	妊娠性糖尿病	妊娠糖尿病
Hemoglobin/Haemoglobin	血色素; 血紅素	血红蛋白
hepatitis B	乙型肝炎	乙型肝炎; 乙肝
labor/labour	分娩; 生產	分娩; 生產
last menstrual period (LMP)	上一次經期	末次月经
Lead Maternity Carer (LMC); Primary Maternity Caregiver	產婦專責護理人員	产妇专责护理人员
lochia	惡露 (分娩後的子宮陰道分泌物)	恶露
meconium	胎糞	胎便; 胎粪
membranes ruptured	胎膜穿破	胎膜破裂
NICU	新生兒深切治療部	新生儿重症监护病房
perineum	會陰	会阴
postnatal	產後	产后
postnatal blues/Post partum depression	產後抑鬱症	产后抑郁症
preeclampsia	先兆子癇; 子癇前期	先兆子痫; 子痫前期
prenatal/Antenatal care	產前護理	产前保健; 产前护理
puerperium	產後期; 產褥期	产褥期; 产后期
Rhesus Factor	獼猴因子	Rh因子; 猕 (猴)因子
rubella	風疹	风疹
show	見紅	见红; 现血
spina bifida	脊柱裂	脊柱裂; 脊椎裂
spontaneous abortion	自然流產	自然流产; 自发 (性) 流产
syphilis	梅毒	梅毒
termination of pregnancy	終止懷孕; 終止妊娠	终止妊娠
thalassemia/thalassaemia	地中海貧血	地中海贫血
ultrasonography	超音波檢查; 超聲波檢查	超声检查
ultrasound scanning (USS)	超音波掃描; 超聲波掃描	超声扫描
vaginal discharge	陰道分泌物	阴道分泌物; 阴道溢液
vaginal smear	陰道塗片	阴道涂片
vaginal speculum	陰道鏡; 陰道窺器	阴道镜; 阴道窥器
vaginal swab	陰道拭子	阴道拭子
venereal disease	性病; 花柳病	性病; 花柳病

Summary of main points

This chapter has offered a brief overview of:

–   the three stages of pregnancy
–   health professionals involved in the period leading up to, during and after childbirth
–   common procedures and diagnostic tests

Chapter 13

Child health

Adapted from a contribution by Dana Lui, RM,
Nurse Specialist – Neonatal Advanced Practice

Interpreting in the area of child health may be very rewarding but can also be extremely taxing. The parents' strong emotional involvement may place additional strains on the interpreter. Sometimes interpreters will need to interpret for children. They will need to make sure they convey information in appropriate language. It is important to remain calm and collected during the interpreting assignment, but equally important to seek debriefing from a counselor or supervisor after difficult interpreting situations.

1. Neonatal Care

Newborn infants are classified as neonates from the day of birth to one month of age. Newborn services provide health care for this group of babies. Other health professionals may provide follow-up services. This section will focus on delivery of care within the Neonatal Intensive Care Unit (NICU), as these units provide immediate care for sick neonates as soon as they are born.

1.1 Levels of Care

In most countries neonatal care can be divided into three levels:

Level 1 is the basic care provided to all newborn babies and is often called a well baby nursery This generally refers to mother crafting like feeding, bathing, changing diapers, looking after the umbilical cord, etc.

Level 2 or intermediate care is provided in the special care nursery to sick newborn infants who require close observation and special management.

Circumstances for admission to intermediate neonatal care may include:

- Babies of low birth weight. Low birth weight babies weigh less than 5 pounds 8 ounces or 2.5 kilograms at birth, regardless of gestational age. Low birth weight babies may be preterm, born before 37 weeks gestation, or small for gestational age (birth weight below tenth percentile for gestational age). Some babies are both preterm and small for gestational age. This includes babies who are born at less than 31 weeks' gestation who do not need ventilation support.

- Babies with respiratory distress (breathing problems) as a result of prematurity, e.g. birth asphyxia, meconium aspiration or infection. These babies may be admitted to the NICU depending on the severity of the problem.
- Babies with suspected or clinical signs of infections such as pneumonia, meningitis, urinary tract infection or umbilical infection.

Level 3 care is intensive care delivered to newborn infants who are extremely premature (under 31 weeks' gestation), who have a low birth weight (less than 2 pounds 12 ounces or 1250 grams), who require ventilation support or blood transfusions, or who cannot be appropriately cared for at level 2. Level 3 units are mostly located in academic teaching hospitals (tertiary hospitals) which have maternity units and which serve as teaching units or research centers. Level 3 care units are referred to as neonatal intensive care units (NICU) and have easy access to most of the back-up services, such as laboratory and radiology services.

Other conditions that would make it necessary for a baby to be admitted for intermediate or intensive neonatal care could include:

- hypothermia (low temperature)
- hypoglycemia (low blood sugar level)
- jaundice
- congenital abnormalities
- gastro-intestinal problems, such as feeding problems severe enough to cause clinical concern, bile-stained vomit, or other signs suggesting bowel obstruction
- convulsions
- cardiovascular problems

Occasionally, babies are admitted for social issues or for terminal care when deemed appropriate after consultation between health professionals of different disciplines.

1.2   Asphyxia

The most serious problem a term infant can face at delivery is birth asphyxia. Asphyxia means respiratory failure. In a newborn, this may be the result of anoxia (a complete lack of oxygen) or hypoxia (not enough oxygen, i.e. less than normal oxygen concentration). Anoxia and hypoxia could be the result of events before birth (antepartum), during birth (intrapartum) or after birth (postpartum).

Antepartum hypoxia may be caused by maternal hypoxia; poor functioning of the placenta; intrinsic problems of the fetus, such as severe anemia resulting from hemolysis (break down of red blood cells); hemorrhage (bleeding) or clotting defects.

These may all lead to chronic hypoxia of the fetus. If the fetus (baby) is already compromised prior to labor, going through labor may cause even more distress.

Intrapartum hypoxia may be due to cord compression (circulation of blood through the umbilical cord is compressed); fetal dystocia (where the fetus presents in a position which makes delivery difficult); acute bleeding or meconium aspiration, which can predispose the baby to asphyxia. Meconium aspiration occurs when the baby passes stools before being born. The fetus inhales these stools into its airways, thereby making the process of breathing impossible or difficult at birth.

Postpartum hypoxia may be due to hyaline membrane disease (infant respiratory distress syndrome), or surfactant deficiency, which results in the baby's air sacs (or alveoli) being unable to expand, thus making breathing a very difficult process. This disease is more prominent in preterm infants (especially less than 32 weeks' gestation, although some term infants may have this problem as well).

The effect of asphyxia on the body of the newborn infant can be very serious. Before birth, the baby receives oxygen through the umbilical cord, in other words, supplied by the mother however, after birth, baby is supposed to breathe for itself. If the baby is not getting enough oxygen, the baby's body may revert back to fetal circulation (circulation as it was before birth). That is, as the baby cannot get oxygen through its lungs, the baby's blood once again by-passes the lungs via various channels that would normally close after delivery (see also Patent Ductus Arteriosus, page 222). This condition is called persistent fetal circulation or persistent pulmonary hypertension.

Persistent fetal circulation is very dangerous for the baby. Fetal circulation was helpful for the baby while it was getting its blood supply directly from the mother, but if it persists when the baby's blood supply is disconnected from the mother's blood circulation (i.e. when the umbilical cord is clamped), the baby can be in real danger.

Hypoxia after birth means that all of the baby's body will be deprived of oxygen, with the brain cells affected worst of all. The infant may develop seizures as a result of hypoxia and end up in a condition called hypoxic-ischemic encephalopathy, where the brain is suffering the effects of insufficient oxygen supply. In order to deliver oxygen to the tissues of the body, the infant will need intubation (insertion of a breathing tube) and ventilation (receiving air and oxygen through a breathing machine).

1.3 Premature delivery

Sometimes babies need to be delivered prematurely because labor starts too early. If the baby is very premature, the obstetrician will try to suppress the spontaneous onset of preterm labor by giving the mother medication. At the same time the mother will receive corticosteroid drugs which help the fetal lungs mature.

If the baby's lungs are a bit more mature, the baby will have a greater chance of survival even when it is born too early. If the woman's membranes (or 'waters') do rupture prematurely, antibiotics are also given to protect both mother and fetus from infection. If there are signs of infection (e.g. if the mother develops a high temperature) delivery may be allowed to proceed, because infection will be dangerous to both mother and child.

Most of the time, it is not clear why labor starts prematurely. In some instances, if the woman starts to bleed or if she shows signs of an intrauterine infection, it may be necessary to deliver the baby quickly in order to save both mother's and the baby's lives. Another serious condition, known as pre-eclampsia (previously known as gestational proteinuria and hypertension), may also make it necessary to initiate premature delivery (especially if this condition is worsening). It is the mother's condition which determines how urgently the baby is delivered. Sometimes there is no time to give the mother the corticosteroid drugs. As a result, the lungs of the preterm baby may be so immature that the baby cannot survive.

Sometimes the baby is delivered prematurely because there are signs that the baby is at risk. Signs could include poor growth and reduced movement. Often a difficult decision has to be made on the balance of either delivering the baby too early or leaving a compromised (at risk) baby inside the uterus.

1.4 Problems of prematurity

Premature birth will result in a baby who is not yet ready for independent life. Such problems are foreseeable, given that all organs and systems of the infant are immature. These problems can include:

1. *Respiratory problems*
At 24 weeks' gestation the fetal lungs have developed to a stage where they could be functional. Gas exchange is possible as the air sacs start to form. Prior to this period the fetus is not viable (cannot live). However, while all the necessary tissues are there at 24 weeks the ventilation system is still very primitive. By giving the mother corticosteroids before the baby is born, baby's lungs are helped to mature more quickly. Infants born before 32 weeks' gestation are likely to develop hyaline membrane disease (HMD) because of the lack in production of surfactant (a substance lining the air sacs). This leads to respiratory difficulties. After delivery an endotracheal tube can be passed down the trachea (windpipe) of the baby and positive pressure can be administered to deliver oxygen-enriched air to expand the air sacs, thus making gas exchange possible and keeping the premature baby alive. This process is called ventilation. Artificial surfactant can be given directly into the baby's lungs to counteract HMD. Giving antenatal corticosteroids, maintaining the preterm baby on a ventilator (breathing machine) and early administration of surfactant enable a lot of extremely premature babies to survive. The more premature the infant, the longer it needs to stay on ventilation.

Ventilation helps preterm babies to survive, but it is has limitations and can cause complications. One has to remember that in order for gas exchange to take place in the lungs, the respiratory system has to have developed to a stage where the basic organs and tissues are in place.

If an infant is less than 24 weeks' gestation, the infant may not survive despite the best machines available. One can also imagine that when positive pressure is constantly being pumped into these babies' lungs, a hole can be inadvertently created, causing a pneumothorax to develop. Pneumothorax means the presence of free air in the thoracic (chest) cavity between the layers of lung coverings (pleural layers). As free air occupies space, it stops the lungs or the air sacs from expanding, making gas exchange ineffective. Pulmonary hemorrhage (bleeding in the lungs) can also occur due to the fragile nature of preterm infants' lung tissue. This fragility can result in the rupture of blood vessels under pressure, the side-effect of the surfactant, or because of clotting defects resulting from prematurity.

Small preterm babies may need to stay on ventilation for a long time. The pressure exerted by the ventilator on the immature lungs can cause damage to the lung tissues, leading to a condition called chronic lung disease, where lung tissues become fibrotic and lose their elasticity. Worst of all, giving a preterm baby increased oxygen over a prolonged period of time, can be toxic and cause blindness.

2.   *Hypothermia*

In hypothermia, body temperature is low. Normal body temperature is between 96.8 and 98.6 degrees Fahrenheit (36 to 37 degrees Celsius). Normal term babies need to be kept warm by keeping them in a warm environment with appropriate clothing and bedding, as they tend to lose heat much faster than an adult.

A preterm infant has little or no subcutaneous tissue for insulation to preserve body heat. At birth, these infants leave the warm environment of the uterus wet, because they have been surrounded by amniotic fluid. In these babies the organs for heat production, the muscles, are underdeveloped, and therefore heat production is basically ineffective or non-existent. In addition, most of these infants need resuscitation at birth. It is essential, therefore, that they be dried immediately as heat loss through evaporation, conduction and convection can be very dramatic within a short time. To prevent heat loss and maintain a normal temperature, premature babies will be placed and nursed on a heat table or in an incubator. A heat table is an open crib with an overhead radiant heater with control for adjustment of the temperature according to the baby's temperature. The incubator is a transparent box that a baby can be nursed in almost naked so that observation is possible and warmth can be provided.

A cold baby needs more energy and oxygen to maintain its body heat, therefore when a baby is sick, a low temperature will only further compromise the baby' health as its body systems shut down.

3. *Hypoglycemia*

In hypoglycemia, blood sugar levels are low. A preterm baby has very little fat and muscle, so its ability to store energy is poor, and any sugar in the blood is used up very quickly. If a baby is cold it will also need more energy in order to keep itself warm. As all tissues and cells need energy to function properly, a low blood glucose (sugar) level means problems. Again, the brain cells will be the worst affected. A baby will start to have seizures if the blood sugar level drops down too low. A term infant who is healthy and who sucks well will be offered the breast or a bottle of formula as soon as possible after birth. A preterm or sick infant will typically be started on an intravenous infusion of glucose water.

4. *Blood problems*

All newborn organs and systems are immature, including the organs and systems that produce blood. Most sick preterm infants will be anemic (have low levels of red blood cells) as they may have bled before birth and may have a comparatively low blood volume. Therefore, newborns may require more frequent blood tests to assess their clinical condition, and blood transfusions may be necessary to compensate for their anemia. Newborn babies may also have low levels of white blood cells (leukocytes) and platelets (thrombocytes). As white cells are responsible for fighting infection, a decreased white cell count or a decreased white cell response makes the baby more vulnerable to infection and/or may make the effects of infection more profound. A reduced platelet count increases the chance of bleeding, both internally and externally, which can lead to life-threatening events or very poor outcomes. Newborns are particularly vulnerable to pulmonary hemorrhage (bleeding into the lungs) and intraventricular hemorrhage (bleeding into the brain).

5. *Infection*

Sepsis is another term used for wide-spread infection. When a baby is preterm, the immune system is also immature. Response to infection may be delayed or inadequate, therefore making an infection that would be harmless to an adult or term infant very severe. In addition, because premature infants are so small, infection can spread throughout the whole body in a very short time. Most preterm neonates will receive antibiotic cover (protection) straight after birth to prevent any infections from entering the body. Simple measures like hand-washing are very important in preventing infection and cross-infection. Aseptic techniques are necessary for all traumatic procedures, such as blood taking, so as to minimize the chance of introducing infection. Nursing an infant in an incubator (special bed for very sick newborns) also provides a protective environment.

6. *Cardiac problems*

One cardiac problem specific to very preterm neonates is Patent Ductus Arteriosus (PDA). PDA is the persistent opening of the duct between the aorta and pulmonary arteries, an opening which normally closes after birth. This duct is open in fetal life so that oxygenated blood that comes in from the mother (through the umbilical cord) can by-pass the lungs. After delivery, the neonate should be able to breathe and supply its own oxygen, so this duct normally closes. In some cases, however, the duct remains open. This causes problems for both the lungs and the heart and makes a sick neonate even sicker. In order to close the PDA a special drug may be given. If this drug does not work, or if it gives rise to too many side-effects, an operation can be done to ligate (tie) the duct. In most cases, the neonate then improves instantly.

7.   *Intraventricular hemorrhage (IVH)*

IVH is bleeding in the head of the preterm neonate. Because the brain of a preterm baby is immature, the blood vessels in the brain are very fragile and can easily break and bleed. IVH occurs most often in the first week of life, typically during the first three days after birth. There are four stages of IVH. Grade I bleeding is bleeding limited to the germinal matrix (primitive tissue), while Grade II bleeding is bleeding into the ventricles (cerebrospinal fluid chambers of the brain). Both Grade I and Grade II bleeding will cause minimal brain damage once they have resolved. In Grade III bleeding there is bleeding into the ventricles, causing distention of the ventricles. Grade IV bleeding is bleeding into the brain tissue surrounding the ventricles as well. Both Grade III and Grade IV hemorrhages can lead to quite severe brain damage and to long-term disabilities.

8.   *Necrotising enterocolitis (NEC)*

NEC is an inflammation of the gut specific to preterm babies. The wall of the gut breaks down as infection sets in. This can lead to perforation of the intestines within a short time if left unrecognized and untreated. If the infection is recognized early enough, and if the baby is given antibiotic cover and left without feeding for two weeks, the condition can generally be cured. If perforation occurs an operation will be necessary to remove the necrotized (dead) portion of the gut. Occasionally, a premature baby may die from this condition.

9.   *Jaundice*

Many newborn babies will have jaundice (yellowish discoloration of skin and mucous membranes). This is a direct result of the breakdown of red blood cells. Most term infants are able to handle and get rid of this jaundice through their liver, and for this reason the condition is described as physiological (normal). However, in a preterm infant liver function is immature, as is the processing of bilirubin (the bile pigment which causes the jaundice). Placing these infants under phototherapy (UV light treatment) helps to break down the bilirubin so that it can be passed out via urine and stools, thus reducing the jaundice. If the bilirubin level is too high it can cause brain damage. In order to avoid this, a blood exchange transfusion may be necessary.

10. *Feeding intolerance*

When a preterm baby is born its gut may not be ready for feeding, as digestive enzymes may be absent or deficient, absorptive ability may be very limited, or the gut may not be moving as yet. If the infant was hypoxic at birth, the gut may take an even longer time to recover, because the body attends to the major organs (e.g. brain, heart, lungs and kidneys) first.

The mother's breast milk is the best choice of food for preterm babies as it is more easily absorbed and contains antibodies important for fighting infections. In the initial days, when breast feeding is not possible, mothers are encouraged to express their milk regularly so as to establish lactation (breast milk production). Breast milk can be frozen for up to 3 months, so that it can be used later when the infant starts to feed. If the baby is unlucky enough to develop necrotizing enterocolitis, introduction of feeding needs to be more cautious and slow.

1.5 Admission process

When a preterm or sick infant is admitted to the NICU, ventilator support will usually be necessary. Umbilical lines (intravenous lines in the umbilical vein) may be inserted to deliver fluid to the baby. Umbilical lines also provide access for blood sampling and blood pressure monitoring. Antibiotics will be started after blood samples have been taken. Once stabilized the baby will be weaned from the ventilator (breathing machine) and encouraged to breathe, with some support, on its own. Continuous Positive Airways Pressure (CPAP) is an alternative means in which to help the infant breathe spontaneously. A tube is passed down the nose of the baby to just above the throat and a small amount of pressure is delivered to keep the airways open. Oxygen may also be given through this tube. As the baby grows or improves, CPAP may be stopped and the breathing tube removed (extubation) and head box oxygen (oxygen provided in a "box" around baby's head space), or nasal prong oxygen (oxygen through prongs in the nostrils), will be given instead. This also allows easy handling of the baby by its mother.

Feeding is started when the baby's respiratory status improves. Baby will receive small but regular feeds via a nasogastric tube (stomach tube inserted through the nose), or orogastric tube (stomach tube inserted through the mouth), so that the baby does not need to suck. If baby tolerates these feeds, both volume and frequency will increase. When this happens, intravenous infusion of nutritious fluids can be decreased and finally stopped.

When the baby's condition improves, or when it reaches a certain weight, or when it passes a certain gestational age, the infant will be transferred from the NICU to the special care nursery until it can be discharged (allowed to leave the hospital).

In the special care nursery, the baby needs to show that it is able to feed effectively and gain weight (particular if the baby was born very premature) before going back to the well-baby nursery or going home. Generally preterm infants have to reach a weight of 2.5 kilograms (or 5 pounds 8 ounces) or have to be close to term before discharge planning is organized. Prior to discharge, the mother may need to learn to be totally responsible for the care of her baby, with the backup support of the unit. Some babies may go home on oxygen and with an apnea mattress which helps alert parents to baby's apnea (not breathing).

1.6   Some common diagnostic tests

Blood tests

Åstrup	See blood gases
glucose	serum sugar level
electrolytes	important minerals which are part of the biochemistry of the blood, including sodium (Na), potassium (K), calcium (Ca)
blood culture	to check for infection
blood gases	to check the biochemistry of the blood so as to gain information about the respiratory status
chromosome study	to rule out congenital abnormalities
complete blood count (CBC)	checking the number of red blood cells, white blood cells, platelets, packed cell volume, and toxic ratio/left shift
full blood count (FBC)	See Complete Blood Count
genetic study	See chromosome study
groups and Coombs test	to check for hemolytic disease (breakdown of blood)
Phenylketonuria (PKU)	screening for a metabolic disorder which can lead to brain damage if it goes undetected.
SBR	serum bilirubin level
thyroid function tests	to check levels of thyroid hormones
urea, creatinine	Tests to check kidney function

Radiological studies (examinations by X-ray)

abdominal X-ray	to assess abnormalities in the abdomen
chest X-ray	X-ray to assess condition of heart and lungs

Ultrasonography (examinations by sound waves)

cranial ultrasound	ultrasound of the head
echocardiogram	ultrasound of the heart
renal ultrasound	ultrasound of the kidneys

Urine tests

culture and microscopy	to detect infection; find out what organisms are causing infection

Other tests

endotracheal aspirate culture	to detect infection in the airways
gastric aspirate	to detect infection in the stomach
lumbar puncture	obtaining cerebrospinal fluid to check for meningitis
spinal tap	same as lumbar puncture
TORCH study	to detect congenital infection
viral study	to detect viral infection

2. Pediatrics

Pediatrics (child medicine) is a specialized area of healthcare. In children, the body's defense system is still developing, and this means that they are very susceptible to a large range of infectious diseases. In addition, children are often not aware of the dangers of particular situations and may be involved in a wide range of accidents, ranging from accidental poisoning (e.g. taking their parents' medication or drinking household cleaning liquids) to falls or (near-) drowning accidents in swimming pools or small creeks.

Sadly, sometimes children become the victims of abuse (physical or sexual) or neglect (not receiving appropriate care) or they become victims in car accidents, especially when they have not been strapped into child safety seats, booster seats or seat belts.

In this chapter we will look into some of the most common childhood illnesses. Please refer to the Chapter 8 on Emergency Departments for further information on accidents.

2.1 Child health professionals

A doctor specializing in child health is called a *pediatrician* and the children's area of a hospital is referred to as the *pediatric* unit. Family practice doctors also take care of children.

A child's pediatrician will check for normal growth and development, making sure that the child reaches its developmental milestones at the right stages in its development. Pediatricians also provide parents support and education. Parents are often given a book in which they can record milestones in the child's development, such as the first smile, the first steps (unaided), the first words, etc. Dates for (repeat) immunizations are also recorded in this book. If health providers have reasons for concern, they may refer the parents to a child specialist or to a special child development clinic. Health providers may also refer so-called *at-risk* children to other services.

2.2   Immunization

Immunization means "giving immunity to." We have immunity (defense) against certain diseases when we have enough antibodies (comparable to specially-trained defense troops) in our body to fight off an attack of these illnesses.

Sometimes doctors talk about *passive immunity* and *active immunity*

Passive immunization occurs when the child/patient becomes immune to something without having to fight the infection him/herself. Breastfeeding mothers give their children passive immunization against certain disorders by passing on their own antibodies via their breast milk.

Children usually have passive immunity during the first 5 or 6 months of life, because their mother's antibodies still circulate in their bodies. Patients may also be given passive immunity against certain diseases by being injected with the antibodies.

We get active immunity against certain diseases by actively fighting off a (small) attack ourselves. Health professionals can help us get "active immunity" by injecting us with a small amount of "vaccine" leading to a small attack on our immune system. The process of injecting the vaccine to help us develop antibodies against a certain disease is called *vaccination* or *immunization.*

Childhood immunization programs exist throughout the United States.

It is important that children be taken to the doctor whenever their next immunization is due. The doctor will check the child to make sure the child is in good health and able to develop the antibodies. If the child is not well, the doctor will delay the immunization until the child is well again.

2.3   Possible childhood health problems

1.   *Attention Deficit Hyperactivity Disorder* (ADHD) – A combination of hyperactive behavior and the inability to concentrate on anything for more than a few seconds or minutes (flitting from one thing to the next).

Causes: Research into a number of potentially contributing factors continues.

Symptoms: An inability to sit still and listen.

Diagnosis: Observation of child and taking history (parents describe behaviors)

Treatment: Drug treatment may be prescribed.

2.   *Autism* (*Autism Spectrum Disorder or ASD**) – Children with ASD may be anywhere on a continuum from very severe autistic tendencies to high-functioning with much less severe autistic tendencies (formerly referred to as Asperger Syndrome). Some children with ASD may have poor (or no) verbal skills and may have trouble relating to or understanding other people. They may avoid eye contact and go through repetitive movements such as rocking backwards and forwards or hand flapping.

Alternatively, children with this syndrome may have advanced (verbal) skills, but have poor social skills and be unable to understand nonverbal language. This may mean they have trouble making friends or understanding other people. The Diagnostic and Statistical Manual of Mental Disorders, commonly known as the DSM-5 (APA 2013) offers a wealth of information on ASD.

Causes: Research into a number of potentially contributing factors, including genetic, continues.

Symptoms: Repetitive movement; flapping; rocking; behaviors as described above.

Diagnosis: Observation of child and taking history (parents describe behaviors)

Treatment: Behavioral therapies; speech therapy; occupational therapy; some doctors prescribe diets free of gluten, casein or soy.

*ASD may also be an abbreviation for Atrium Septum Defect, a hole in the wall between the atria of the heart.

3.   *Asthma* – Refer Chapter 19 for more information.

Symptoms: During an asthma attack, a child will be unable to get enough air into his lungs, as the airways swell and close down. This can be fatal. Children with chronic asthma will often have a dry cough, rather than a wheeze.

Treatment: During an asthma attack, if the child is unable to speak, he or she should be taken to hospital by life support ambulance immediately. In the hospital, the child may be given intravenous or inhaled steroids and special asthma bronchodilator medication through a nebulizer to open up the airways.

4.   *Bronchiolitis* – Virus infection of the smallest air passages in very young children.

Causes: The infection, usually caused by a virus, often follows a runny nose or sore throat and cough.

Symptoms: Wheezing; coughing; shortness of breath, which may lead to difficulty in feeding.

Diagnosis: Chest X-ray; listening to lungs.

Treatment: Oxygen, feeding through a nasogastric tube; oxygen.

5. *Bronchopneumonia* – Infection of the bronchi and alveoli (little air sacs).

Causes: Infection of the upper airways spreads into the bronchi (breathing tubes) and alveoli; may be caused by either bacteria or a virus.

Symptoms: Cough, fever, shortness of breath; *whiteouts* (areas of no air movement) on the X-ray; loss of appetite.

Diagnosis: Chest X-ray; listening to lungs.

Treatment: Oxygen, bedrest, antibiotics.

6. *Cerebral Palsy* – Damage to parts of the brain which control muscle movement, balance and posture.

Causes: Doctors think this damage usually takes place while the baby is still in the uterus, during birth, or shortly after birth, for instance in some very premature children.

Symptoms: Babies may be floppy and stiff, show a lack of head control; children may adopt particular postures and have spasticity of the muscles. Some, but definitely not all, children with cerebral palsy also have epilepsy (see Chapter 17), problems with hearing, eyesight, or an intellectual disability.

Diagnosis: Testing reflexes and movement by pediatrician.

Treatment: Physical therapy to encourage movement, posture, head control and balance; *speech therapy* to encourage movement of the mouth.

7. *Chest infection* – Infection of the bronchi (breathing tubes) and lungs (refer *bronchiolitis* and *bronchopneumonia sections above*).

8. *Chickenpox* – A very contagious viral infection (varicella zoster virus).

Causes: Viral infection.

Symptoms: Skin rash with crops of blisters (filled with fluid), accompanied by slight fever and a feeling of unwellness. Chickenpox is contagious until all the blisters have crusted over (formed scabs).

Diagnosis: Physical examination.

Treatment: Calamine lotion for itchiness; ensuring that blisters do not get infected. Immunization is available.

9. *Child abuse* – Includes any instances of physical abuse, neglect, emotional abuse/ neglect, mental cruelty, poisoning or sexual abuse.

Treatment: Children need to be protected. Children depend on adults to ensure their health and well-being. In most states, suspicions of child abuse are reported to Child Protective Services, a state agency that will investigate the charge; provide support and education to families where appropriate; bring in police support to deal with the abuser; and remove the child from the abusive situation if necessary.

10. *Convulsions* – Refer section on *Seizures* below

11. *Crib Death* – Also known as *Sudden Infant Death Syndrome (SIDS)* or *cot death*, crib death occurs when the young baby suddenly stops breathing, for no apparent reason.

Cause: In spite of ongoing research, it is still not known what causes crib death. Factors that may possibly contribute to crib death include smoking (around children or during pregnancy); bottle-feeding; cold (air) temperature; low birth-weight; placing baby's head on an adult pillow (obstructing baby's airway); adults rolling on top of baby while bed sharing, and possibly many other as yet unidentified factors.

Symptoms: Baby suddenly stops breathing, for no apparent reason. This is followed by cardiac arrest and the child dies.

Treatment: Prevention is the key, including no smoking and using an apnea mattress under baby (alarm will sound when the baby stops breathing).

12. *Croup* – A viral infection of the voice-box and windpipe.

Causes: Viral infection.

Symptoms: Stridor (a rasping noise) when the child breathes in; shortness of breath and respiratory distress; in-drawing of the chest.

Diagnosis: Physical examination

Treatment: In serious cases admission to hospital; steroids, nebulized adrenaline (epinephrine).

13. *Cystic Fibrosis or mucoviscoidosis* – Production of thick mucus in the airways.

Causes: Inherited gene.

Symptoms: Production of very thick mucus which results in frequent lung infections. The thick mucus also stops digestive enzymes produced by the pancreas from going to the bowels, so there is a problem in absorbing food (malabsorption). The child's sweat will contain a lot of salt, and he/she will have loose stools and may not put on any weight or only gain weight slowly.

Diagnosis: Testing in early pregnancy.

Treatment: Ongoing physical therapy (at home) to treat and prevent chest infections, antibiotics, pancreas enzymes with every meal to help absorb food, genetic counseling for couples who are known to carry the gene and who want to have children.

14.   *Diabetes* – Even very young children may develop Type I diabetes mellitus, a condition in which the child's *pancreas* does not produce (enough) insulin. Without insulin, sugar cannot get into the cells, but remains in the blood. There is another type of diabetes, called Type II diabetes, which used to be seen in adults only, but is now diagnosed in children as young as 9 or 10 (refer Chapter 25 for more information).

Cause: Type 1 diabetes is an autoimmune condition, where the body attacks its own insulin-producing cells in the pancreas. Type II diabetes usually follows the pathway of insulin resistance (see Chapter 25).

Symptoms: The cells do not get (enough) sugar to burn for energy, so the child feels weak and tired. The child will have a high blood glucose level (as the sugar cannot get out of the blood and into the cells). The kidneys start leaking sugar into the urine, which in turn draws more fluid from the body into the urine; the child will be very thirsty and urinate very frequently.

Diagnosis: Fasting blood glucose test; glucose tolerance test.

Treatment: Special diet; insulin, either injected or through insulin pump; regular blood sugar testing; changing lifestyle; diabetes education. Diabetes in children poses a special challenge as children are still growing and are generally active (playing sports, running around) which means diet and insulin dosages have to be adjusted all the time to accommodate growth and activity levels.

15.   *Ear infection or otitis media* – Infection of the middle ear.

Causes: Infections travel from nose/throat area to the middle ear via the Eustachian tubes.

Symptoms: Fever, pain in the ear, difficulty hearing (everything sounds 'muffled'), enlarged lymph nodes in the neck, sometimes also a sore throat or runny nose. Otitis media can lead to complications such as glue ear, where fluid remains in the middle ear, making hearing difficult, or a perforated eardrum/burst eardrum, where fluid in the middle ear leads to pressure on the eardrum that can eventually cause it to burst.

Diagnosis: Checking ear with the otoscope (see Chapter 23).

Treatment: Antibiotics for bacterial infections; viral infections clear by themselves. *Ear tubes* (tiny ventilation tubes) may be inserted in the eardrum if children have repeated ear infections, allowing the fluid to drain without damaging the eardrum. An *adenoidectomy* (surgical removal of the adenoid – lymph tissue in the roof of the throat) may be performed if the doctor feels that repeated ear infections are due to a very large adenoid. Ear infections often lessen in frequency as the child grows and the Eustachian tubes get larger, allowing for better drainage of the middle ear.

16. *Eczema* – Also known as atopic dermatitis, is an inflammation of the skin.

Causes: Often caused by hypersensitive reactions and common in people with a family history of asthma or hayfever.

Symptoms: Inflammation and/or redness of skin.

Diagnosis: Physical examination; history.

Treatment: Topical creams (including corticosteroid ointments).

17. *Encephalitis* – Inflammation of the brain tissue.

Causes: Infection; can occur as a complication of measles or mumps.

Symptoms: Headache, fever, drowsiness, unconsciousness, tremors, seizures and convulsions.

Diagnosis: CT scan, screen for viruses, blood tests, electroencephalogram or EEG, lumbar puncture (spinal tap) to test the cerebrospinal fluid.

Treatment: Good nursing care; fluids.

18. *Epilepsy* – Uncontrolled activity of (part of) the brain. There are many different forms of epilepsy; what they have in common is that the child has no control over what happens.

Causes: See Chapter 17.

Symptoms: May be mistaken for febrile convulsions (see below).

Diagnosis: EEG (electro-encephalogram), skull X-ray, CT scan; temperature.

Treatment: Depends on the type of epilepsy; sometimes anticonvulsant drugs are used, and very occasionally brain surgery.

19. *Febrile convulsions* – Results in a loss of consciousness when a child's temperature goes up.

Causes: Sudden rise in temperature.

Symptoms: Staring without seeing, drooling, stiffness, jerking and shaking of body and arms/legs (fits/convulsions).

Diagnosis: History taking, physical examination.

Treatment: Cooling the child by removing clothing, sponging with a wet cloth, giving paracetamol.

20.   *Fetal Alcohol Syndrome* (FAS) – Occurs as a result of the mother drinking alcohol during pregnancy, leading to a range of effects on the baby's heart, skeleton, and neurological/mental development).

Causes: Alcohol consumption during pregnancy.

Symptoms: Various problems involving heart, skeleton, neurological and mental function, including underdeveloped midface (such as small eyes, short nose, thin lips), possibly neurological defects, problems with attention, learning and behavior.

Diagnosis: History, echocardiogram; physical examination, observation of behavior.

Treatment: Special education, social support, nurturing environment. Early diagnosis is important.

21.   *German Measles* – refer section on Rubella below.

22.   *Heart Murmurs* – Abnormal heart sounds.
Murmurs may be innocent (e.g. flow murmurs) or may indicate that there is something wrong inside the heart.

Causes: A flow murmur is an innocent murmur caused by the blood flowing rapidly through the heart, especially if the child has a fever. Other causes include narrowed valves (blood makes extra sound as it goes through the narrowing), a hole in the heart (a hole in the wall separating the left from the right atrium or the left from the right ventricle), a narrowing of the aorta called coarctation of the aorta, and patent ductus arteriosus (PDA). The ductus arteriosus is a by-pass which exists before the child is born, to make sure that oxygen-enriched blood from the mother by-passes the lungs and goes straight to the aorta. Soon after birth this by-pass closes up. If this by-pass does not close up, doctors say it is still "patent" (open) and they can hear the blood flow from the aorta to the pulmonary artery all the time. This can be heard as a continuous murmur.

Symptoms: Abnormal heart sounds.

Diagnosis: Chest X-ray, echocardiogram or cardiac ultrasound, electrocardiogram (EKG), cardiac catheterization and angiography (contrast X-ray of the blood flow through the heart and the blood vessels in the heart).

Treatment – Heart surgery if there is a defect which causes serious problems or which may lead to damage later on.

23.   *Hernia* – Occurs when the contents of the abdominal cavity protrude through a weakness in the wall of the abdomen. Commonly found near the belly button (*umbilical hernia*) or in the groin (*inguinal hernia*).

Cause: Weakness in the abdominal wall, sudden build-up of pressure inside the abdomen from sneezing, pushing, or heavy lifting.

Symptoms: Slight bulge by the belly button or in the groin.

Diagnosis: Hernia can be felt (like a lump).

Treatment: Sometimes hernias heal by themselves (spontaneously); sometimes surgical repair is necessary, especially if the contents of the abdomen get stuck in the opening of the hernia and cause further problems.

24.   *Impetigo* – Also known as *school sores, are boils* (skin infections).

Causes: Usually caused by a type of skin bacteria called *staphylococci* (*staph* for short).

Symptoms: Areas on the skin become red, painful and swollen. Pus may form in the center.

Diagnosis: Physical examination.

Treatment: Antibiotics, antiseptic soap and nasal cream to kill the staphylococci on the skin and in the nose.

25.   *Leukemia* – Literally means "white blood" due to there being too many immature white blood cells in the blood. In children, the most common form of leukemia is acute (sudden) lymphoblastic leukemia or ALL. In this type of leukemia, the bone marrow produces too many lymphoblasts (immature young lymphocytes). Lymphocytes are a type of white blood cell which are involved in fighting infection. Another form of leukemia called myeloid leukemia usually occurs in slightly older children (see Chapter 20).

Causes: Research continues, but recent studies suggest genetic and environmental factors (including infections) impacting on the immune system.

Symptoms: Frequent infections; paleness and tiredness; enlarged liver, spleen and lymph glands. Children may also have anemia (lack of red blood cells) and a shortage of platelets, leading to a tendency to bleed.

Diagnosis: Blood tests; bone marrow test.

Treatment: Chemotherapy to kill the leukemic cells, blood or platelet transfusions, antibiotics, bone marrow transplant, radiotherapy to head and spine to prevent leukemic cells from "hiding out" in those places. Once the child is "in consolidated remission" (no leukemic cells in the blood for a while), maintenance treatment is given for another couple of years.

26.   *Measles* – Viral infection in childhood.

Cause: Viral infection spread by airborne droplets.

Symptoms: Fever, runny nose; red and watery eyes; *intolerance of light*; cough; small white spots in the mouth (Koplik's spots); red *rash* all over body, starting from the forehead and behind the ears and soon spreading all over the body. Complications include *viral pneumonia, encephalitis, secondary bacterial infections* (e.g. *bronchopneumonia*) and middle ear infections.

Diagnosis: Physical examination, history.

Treatment: Keeping child home for 10 days.

27.   *Meningitis* – Infection of the meninges, the protective layer surrounding the brain.

Cause: Viral or bacterial infection.

Symptoms: Fever, headache and neck stiffness, drowsiness, floppiness, refusing feedings, high-pitched cry when changing diapers, unconsciousness, restricted movement of the head (e.g. impossible to lower the chin onto the chest; raising the legs hurts), meningitis rash.

Diagnosis: See Chapter 17.

Treatment: Good nursing for viral meningitis, hospital admission and immediate course of intravenous antibiotics for bacterial meningitis.

28.   *Mumps* – Viral infection affecting the parotid gland

Cause: Viral infection.

Symptoms: Painful swelling of the parotid gland (which produces saliva) just in front of the ear, slight fever. Complications include viral pancreatitis, orchitis (painful swelling and inflammation of the testicles), viral meningitis

Diagnosis: Physical examination, history.

Treatment: No specific treatment; child is usually okay after about two weeks.

29.   *Pyloric stenosis* – See Chapter 26

30.   *Rheumatic fever* – An immune response in which symptoms mimic a rheumatic condition but may also involve heart valve damage. In some people, a strep throat (throat infection by special strain of Streptococcus bacteria) is followed by inflammation of the joints and heart valves. In these people, the bacteria also cause antibodies to 'attack' the body's own joints and heart valves. Occasionally, rheumatic fever involves myocarditis (inflammation of heart muscle).

Cause: A very aggressive type of Streptococcus ("strep") bacterium.

Symptoms: Sore throat, which may be followed by fever; joint pains (arthritis); carditis (inflammation of the heart); palpitations; heart murmur; chest pain; high temperature; a high ESR (indicating inflammation); tiredness on exertion. Complications include heart valve disease (usually the mitral valve, sometimes also the aortic valve, the tricuspid valve and the pulmonary valve).

Diagnosis: Blood tests to check for streptococcal infection/antibodies, throat swab to test for streptococcal infection, ESR (erythrocyte sedimentation rate), EKG (electrocardiogram), chest X-ray, echocardiogram to check for valve defects

Treatment: Bed-rest until ESR and temperature are normal; regular antibiotics to prevent repeat infection especially before dental treatment and before surgery; some patients may need heart valve replacement surgery and penicillin before surgery and before dental treatment.

31.   *Rubella or German measles* – Airborne infection caused by a virus.

Cause: Viral infection spread by airborne droplets.

Symptoms: Very light rash, birth defects to the unborn child if the mother is infected within the first three months of pregnancy.

Diagnosis: Physical examination.

Treatment: Keeping the child home for a few days. Children are normally immunized against rubella; all girls should be immunized to prevent them from contracting rubella if they get pregnant later on in their lives.

32.   *Scarlet fever* – An acute infection of the throat.

Cause: Special strain of *streptococcus* bacteria (*streptococcus pyogenes*).

Symptoms: Cough; sore throat; fever; enlarged tonsils; all-over body rash, starting behind the ears and spreading all over skin. Complications include middle ear infections, sinusit is, rheumatic fever and acute glomerulonephritis (infection of the *glomeruli*, the tiny blood filters in the kidneys).

Diagnosis: Throat swab.

Treatment: Antibiotics.

33.   *School Sores* – Please see Impetigo, Chapter 13, page 154.

34.   *Seizures* (*convulsions*) – Uncontrolled shaking and jerking of the body, arms and legs.

Causes: High fever, sudden increase in body temperature, epilepsy, cerebral palsy (if brain damage present), brain tumor.

Symptoms: Shaking and jerking of the body. rigid face, no response when child is called by name.

Diagnosis: As causes may vary, it is important to identify the cause and treat accordingly.

Treatments: Depends on the cause, e.g. reducing body temperature in febrile convulsions.

35.   *Tonsillitis* – inflammation or infection of the tonsils (the lymph tissue on either side of the throat).

Cause: Usually a bacterial infection.

Symptoms: Sore throat, cough. Complications include *upper respiratory tract* infections.

Diagnosis: Throat swab to check for bacteria.

Treatment: Antibiotics, tonsillectomy (if the infections are frequent.).

36.   *Vomiting and diarrhea* – Often occur together, though not always.

Causes:

–   Congenital blockage somewhere in the gastrointestinal tract can be the cause in newborn babies in the first few days after birth
–   Regurgitating food is usually of no significance, especially if only very small amounts of milk are brought up. Regurgitation can also be due to a hiatal hernia, a condition in which the top of stomach does not close properly and food goes back into esophagus (reflux)
–   Pyloric stenosis, in which case there may be projectile vomiting
–   Emotional upsets can lead to vomiting, especially if the child feels unable to talk about what is upsetting him/her
–   Motion sickness when travelling by bus, boat, car
–   Too much food (especially at birthday parties, etc)
–   Gastroenteritis (inflammation of the lining of stomach and bowels, which may be caused by a virus or by food poisoning); stomach ache and diarrhea
–   Appendicitis – often starts with vomiting and pain around the belly button; pain later moves to upper right-hand part of the abdomen

Diarrhea usually accompanies vomiting in gastroenteritis or in food intolerances [e.g. lactose intolerance or *gluten* (a wheat protein) intolerance in *celiac disease*. Both can lead to dehydration and a disturbance of the electrolyte balance.

Symptoms: Throwing up meals, runny stools.

Diagnosis: Checking fluid balance, taking a stool sample.

Treatment: The main complication of diarrhea and vomiting is *dehydration* and a change in the body's *electrolyte balance*. A lot of children around the world still die from dehydration as a result of vomiting and diarrhea. This is why vomiting and diarrhea should always be taken seriously in children. Parents should make sure the child still passes good amounts of urine and should give the child *rehydration fluid*. This can be bought from the pharmacy or made at home. In serious cases children will be admitted to the hospital and given *intravenous fluids*.

3. English-Chinese glossary

英漢詞彙表

English	Hong Kong & Taiwan	Mainland China
active immunization	自體免疫法	主动免疫
adenoidectomy .	增殖體切除術	增殖体切除术
Anemia/anaemia	貧血	贫血
angiography	血管造影術	血管造影 (术)
anoxia	缺氧	缺氧 (症)
antibodies	抗體	抗体
apnea	窒息症	呼吸暂停; 窒息
appendicitis	盲腸炎; 闌尾炎	闌尾炎
arthritis	關節炎	关节炎
Asperger Syndrome	亞氏保加症; 阿斯伯格綜合症	阿斯伯格綜合症
asphyxia	窒息	窒息
asthma	哮喘	气喘; 哮喘
Åstrup	阿斯特拉普 (氏) 血液氣體分析	阿斯特拉普 (氏) 血液气体分析
atopic dermatitis	特異反應性皮炎	特应性皮炎; 异位性皮炎
attention deficit hyperactivity disorder (ADHD)	注意力失調過度活躍症; 專注不足多動症	注意力缺陷多动障碍; 注意力不足过动症
autism spectrum disorder (ASD)	自閉症譜系障礙; 自閉症	孤独症
bag of waters	羊水囊; 羊膜囊	羊水囊; 羊膜囊
bilirubin	膽紅素	胆红素
blisters	水泡	水疱
blood culture	血液細菌培養	血培养 (基)
blood gases	血液氣體; 血氣	血气; 血内气体
bone marrow	骨髓	骨髓

(Continued)

English	Hong Kong & Taiwan	Mainland China
bronchiolitis	小支氣管炎	(毛) 細支气管炎
bronchopneumonia	支氣管肺炎	支气管肺炎
calamine	爐甘石洗劑 (皮膚科藥)	炉甘石洗剂 (皮科用药)
carditis	心臟炎	心 (脏) 炎
cerebral palsy	大腦麻痹	大脑性瘫痪; 脑瘫
cerebrospinal/Cerebral spinal fluid	腦脊髓液	脑脊 (髓) 液; 脑脊液
chemotherapy	化學療法; 化療	化学疗法; 化学治疗; 化疗
chest infection	胸部感染	胸感染
chest X-ray	胸部X-光攝影	胸部X射线检查; 胸透检查
chickenpox	水痘	水痘
chromosome study	染色體研究	染色体研究
chronic lung disease	慢性肺疾病	慢性肺病
clotting	凝結	凝固
coeliac disease; celiac disease	乳糜瀉	乳糜泻
complete blood count (CBC)	血常規; 全血指數; 血細胞數量檢查	全血 (细胞) 计数; 血常规
congenital abnormality	先天不健全; 先天異常	先天性异常; 先天性畸形
continuous positive airway pressure (CPAP)	持續正氣壓呼吸機	持续正气压呼吸机
contrast X-ray	造影劑X光檢查	造影剂X光检查
convulsions	抽搐	惊厥; 抽搐
cord compression	臍帶壓迫	脐带压迫
corticosteroid drugs	類固醇藥	皮质类固醇药
cot death	嬰兒猝死症	婴儿暴亡症; 摇篮症
cranial ultrasound	頭顱超聲波掃描	颅超声
creatinine	肌酸酐	肌酸酐; 肌酐
cross-infection	交叉感染	交叉感染; 交叉传染
croup	喉氣管支氣管炎; 義膜性喉炎	喉气管支气管炎; 义膜性喉炎
CT scan	電腦斷層掃描	电脑断层扫描; CT掃描
cystic fibrosis	囊性纖維化	纤维囊泡症; 囊性纤维化
diabetes	糖尿病	糖尿病
distention	膨脹	膨胀; 扩张
echo cardiogram/Echocardiography	心臟超音波檢查; 超聲波心動圖	超声心动图
eczema	濕疹	湿疹

(Continued)

English	Hong Kong & Taiwan	Mainland China
electroencephalogram/ Electroencephalography (EEG)	腦電圖檢查	脑电图
electrolytes	電解質	电解质
encephalitis	腦炎	(大) 脑炎
endotracheal aspirate culture	氣管吸取液培養	气管内吸取液培养
endotracheal tube	氣管導管	气管内插管; 气管内导管
epilepsy	癲癇症	癫痫症; 羊癫疯; 羊角风
erythrocyte sedimentation rate (ESR)	紅血球沉降率	红细胞沉降率; 血沉
Eustachian tube	耳咽管; 歐氏管	欧氏管; 咽鼓管
express milk	擠奶	挤出母乳
febrile convulsions	發熱性痙攣; 發熱性抽搐	高热性惊厥; 发热性惊厥
feeding intolerance	喂哺不耐受	喂哺不耐受
fetal/foetal alcohol syndrome (FAS)	胎兒酒精綜合症	胎儿酒精综合症
Fetal/foetal dystocia	胎兒難產	胎儿难产
fibrotic	纖維化; 結締	纤维变性
full blood count (FBC)	血常規; 全血指數; 血細胞數量檢查	全血 (细胞) 计数; 血常规
gastric aspirate	胃抽吸術	胃抽吸
German measles	德國麻疹	风疹; 德国麻疹
germinal matrix	生殖細胞間質; 生殖細胞基質	生发基质
glomeruli	腎小球	肾小球
grommets	中耳導管	鼓室通气管
Groups and Coombs test	血型及庫氏試驗	血型及库姆 (氏) 试验; 抗球蛋白试验
heart murmur	心臟雜音	心 (脏) 杂音
Hemolysis/Haemolysis	溶血	溶血
hernia	疝 (俗稱「小腸氣」)	疝
hyaline membrane disease (HMD)	肺透明膜病	肺透明膜病
hypoglycemia	低血糖 (症); 血糖過低	低血糖 (症)
hypothermia	低溫症; 體溫過低	体温过低; 低体温
hypoxia	低氧; 缺氧	低氧; 缺氧
hypoxic-ischemic encephalopathy	缺氧缺血性腦病	缺氧缺血性脑病
immune system	免疫系統	免疫系统
impetigo	膿疱瘡	脓疱性皮炎; 脓疱病
incubator	(嬰兒) 保溫箱	(婴儿) 保温箱
intraventricular hemorrhage (IVH)	腦室間出血	脑室内出血

(Continued)

English	Hong Kong & Taiwan	Mainland China
intubation	導管插入	插管法
ionizing radiation	電離輻射; 電離放射	电离辐射
jaundice	黃疸	黃疸
Koplik's spots	柯氏斑點	科氏斑; 麻疹粘膜斑
Leukemia/Leukaemia	白血病	白血病
leukocytes	白血球	白血球 (细胞)
lumbar puncture	腰椎穿刺 (抽腦脊液)	腰椎穿刺 (术)
measles	麻疹	麻疹
meconium aspiration syndrome	胎糞吸入綜合症	胎便吸入综合症
membranes	膜	膜
meningitis	腦膜炎	脑膜炎
mumps	腮腺炎 (俗稱「炸腮」)	腮腺炎
myeloid leukemia/leukaemia	骨髓性白血病	骨髓性白血病; 髓细胞白血病
myocarditis	心肌炎	心肌炎
nasogastric tube	鼻胃管	经鼻胃管; 鼻饲管
necrotized	壞死	坏死
necrotizing enterocolitis (NEC)	壞死性小腸結腸炎	坏死性小肠结肠炎
neonatal care	初生嬰兒護理	新生儿护理
Neonatal Intensive Care Unit (NICU)	初生嬰兒深切治療部	新生儿重症监护病房
orchitis	睪丸炎	睾丸炎
ottitis/otitis media	中耳炎	中耳炎
pancreatitis	胰腺炎	胰腺炎
passive immunization	被動防疫	被动免疫
patent ductus arteriosus (PDA)	動脈導管未閉; 開放性動脈導管	开放性动脉导管; 动脉导管未闭
Pediatrician/Paediatrician	兒科醫生	(小) 儿科医生
Pediatrics/paediatrics	兒科	(小) 儿科
persistent fetal/foetal circulation	胎血循環持續	胎血循环持续
Persistent pulmonary hypertension	持續性肺高血壓循環	持续肺动脉高压
phenylketonuria (PKU)	苯酮酸尿症	苯丙酮尿症
phototherapy	光線療法; 光療	光线疗法; 光照疗法; 光疗
physiotherapy	物理治療	理疗; 物理治疗
Platelets	血小板	血小板
pleural layers	胸 (肋) 膜層	胸膜层

(Continued)

English	Hong Kong & Taiwan	Mainland China
pneumonia	肺炎	肺炎
pneumothorax	胸 (肋) 膜腔積氣; 氣胸	气胸
Preeclampsia/Pre-eclampsia	先兆子癇; 子癇前期	先兆子癇; 子癇前期
prematurity	早產	早产
pulmonary hemorrhage/ haemorrhage	肺出血	肺出血
pyloric stenosis	幽門狹窄	幽门狭窄
radiotherapy	放射治療 (又稱電療)	放射治疗
remission	緩解	缓解
renal ultrasound	腎臟超聲波掃描	肾超声
rheumatic fever	風濕熱	风湿热
rubella	風疹	风疹
scarlet fever	猩紅熱	猩红热
school sores; impetigo	膿疱瘡	脓疱性皮炎; 脓疱病
serum bilirubin level (SBL)	血清膽紅素濃度	血清胆红素浓度; 血清胆红素水平
spinal tap	脊椎穿刺, 抽脊椎液	腰椎穿刺; 脊椎抽液
staphylococci bacteria	葡萄球菌	葡萄球菌
streptococcus bacteria	鏈球菌	链球菌
sudden infant death syndrome (SIDS)	嬰兒猝死綜合症	婴儿猝死综合症
surfactant deficiency	表面張力素缺乏症	表面活性物质缺乏症
thrombocytes	血小板	血小板
tonsillitis	扁桃腺炎	扁桃体炎
TORCH study to detect congenital infection with TO (toxoplasmosis), R (rubella), C (cytomegalovirus) or H(herpes)	TORCH測試 (檢測先天感染弓型蟲、風疹、巨細胞病毒或疱疹)	TORCH測試 (检测先天感染弓型虫、风疹、巨细胞病毒或疱疹)
thyroid function tests	甲狀腺功能檢驗	甲状腺功能试验
ultrasonography	超聲波圖像掃描	超声波图象检查
urea	尿素	尿素; 脲
urinary tract infection	泌尿道感染	泌尿道感染
vaccination	防疫注射; 疫苗接種	疫苗接种
varicella zoster virus	水痘帶狀疱疹病毒	水痘带状疱疹病毒
ventilation	供氧	供氧; 换气
waters (amniotic fluid)	羊 (胎) 水	羊 (胎) 水

Summary of main points

This chapter has offered a brief overview of:

–   Neonatal intensive care units and common reasons for newborns to be
     admitted to such units
–   Equipment encountered in neonatal intensive care settings
–   A large range of possible childhood health problems, with symptoms, causes,
     diagnostic tests and treatment options

Chapter 14

Speech-language therapy

By Dr. Linda Hand, University of Auckland

Speech-language therapy (SLT) focuses on identifying problems in communication rather than enabling communication. Professionals involved in SLT include neurologists and speech language therapists. Speech language therapists are also known as speech pathologists or speech therapists.

1. Common terminology

aphasia	disorder of ability to speak, read, write or understand language (literally means no speech)
articulation	how speech organs are involved in producing sounds and speech
CVA	cerebrovascular accident (stroke)
dysarthria	motor speech disorder resulting from a neurological injury.
	(dys = difficult; arthr- = articulating)
dysphagia	swallowing problems
dyspraxia	the brain has problems coordinating movement of the body parts needed for speech (lips, jaws, tongue)
phonology	study of the sound systems of a language
semantics	study of meaning
speech-language pathologist	specialist in communication and swallowing disorders. SLPs are also known as speech-language therapists (SLT) or speech therapists
speech (language) therapist	see SLP above
syntax	study of the sentence structure of a language
TBI	traumatic brain injury, brain damaged as a result of an accident

2. Communication disorders

Communication disorders can occur from birth to old age and may include:

- Speech/phonological (e.g. "dutty" for "cup"; "tie" for "sky"; seen in dysarthrias)
- Voice (quality of the voice)
- Stuttering (also called dysfluency)
- Swallowing
- Augmentative and alternative communication systems

Language disorders are also a form of communication disorder and may arise for a range of reasons and can include many and varied features. Common causes for language disorders include damage to the brain (e.g. TBI, brain injury or CVA), congenital disorders and developmental disorders (including autism). "Symptoms" of language disorders may include speakers:

- getting words around the wrong way (e.g. *"the horse big"* where you would expect *"the big horse"*).
- getting words muddled (*"the trelly smash"* instead of *"the smelly trash"*).
- getting the wrong words, or cannot find words (*"it's the – oh, whaddya call it – the – um – thingy – you know – corner – no no – come- come – oh what is it?"*).
- appearing to understand what is said (nodding, smiling), but being unable to follow instructions.
- giving responses that have nothing to do with the question (this can be because they have not understood, but sometimes they do understand but are unable to formulate a relevant answer). Such answers may be inappropriate (e.g. too loud, too soft, include swearwords and insults); endlessly repetitive; or be giving the wrong emotional response, such as laughing at a sad story (may again be a comprehension problem, but can be at the level of emotional or empathic grasp rather than language comprehension per se).

3. Assessment

Assessment is a dynamic process, which involves the SLP or SLT gathering information about the client from various sources. Interpreters may be asked to interpret during:

- History-taking/discussing the problem
- Formal tests
- Informal assessments/functional tasks
- Conversation (to provide data on the person's language and speech)

– Intervention (speech and language therapy)
– Feedback and discussion (with patient and his/her significant others)

4. Therapy

Therapy (treatment) can be aimed at the level of impairment or at trying to fix the body part, or body function, that is creating the speech or language problem. Therapy often involves repeated practice of discrete tasks in order to develop new/different muscle or neural pathways and may involve:

– How to produce sounds
– Parents taking an active role by talking to their children in certain ways that will help their child's language development. Likewise, spouses and other family members can have an active role to play in therapy for adults.
– Playing games that require speech sounds, language structures, or words.

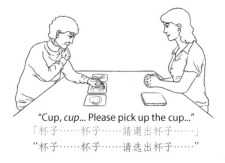

"Cup, *cup*... Please pick up the cup..."
「杯子⋯⋯杯子⋯⋯請選出杯子⋯⋯」
"杯子⋯⋯杯子⋯⋯请选出杯子⋯⋯"

Figure 14.1 Speech language therapy
言語治療
言语治疗

5. Some notes for interpreters and translators

> "Speech Pathologists should be able to assess, diagnose and intervene with communication disorders in a language they do not speak – with the essential help of interpreters".   (Hand 2007)

Interpreting in the area of SLT differs from other types of interpreting in that, rather than conveying *what* the speaker is saying, the interpreter may also need to convey *how* things are being said. In other words, the interpreter may also be expected to provide metalinguistic information, i.e. information about speech and language.

Speech-language therapists work with clients who have language and/or speech disorders, and interpreters need to be able to somehow "reproduce" or comment on the way their clients communicate (Langdon 2002; Langdon & Cheng 2002; Merlini & Favaron 2005, p. 264). This requires a very precise use of vocabulary, starting with the words "language" and "speech," which are used in very specific meanings by speech-language therapists. One interpreter erroneously translated "Tell me about your child's language" as "How well does he speak?", a question with a completely different and much narrower focus.

The speech language therapist will need to know these speech and language 'features,' and it may be important to know how much, and in detail, rather than generally. Langdon (2002, p. 7) stresses the importance of *verbatim translation* of the patients' utterances during assessment sessions by saying: "do not edit what is said, and do not change sounds." In other words, the interpretation should be as close to verbatim as the target language allows. Yet Langdon (2002, p. 7) also urges interpreters to explain to speech pathologists what *is said versus what should have been said*, thereby helping them recognize the extent and causes of the language impairment and provide appropriate feedback. Gentile et al. (1996, pp. 125–135) further clarify that the interpreter's metalinguistic descriptions may refer to *syntax, phonology and semantics.*" (italics added) (Merlini & Favaron 2005, p. 265).

In addition, many formal SLT tests are not appropriate for interpreting, because they are normally very specific to one particular language. This should be accounted for by the SLP or SLT, or else the interpreter should convey why a test is inappropriate or will not work.

When interpreting during formal tests, interpreters need to make sure they avoid:

– Changing the length, structure, kind of vocabulary (e.g. easier for more difficult terms) or references to pictures
– Explaining tasks
– "Helping" the client; for instance by tapping the picture, looking at the picture ("eye pointing"), adding gestures the SLT did not use, repeating words or instructions (where the SLP only gave them once), rephrasing

When interpreting during informal or functional assessment tasks, interpreters should avoid:

– Minimizing or overlooking the significance of what might look like "chat" (but is actually "data collection")
– Reverting to "explaining the meaning"

Likewise when interpreting a client's history or discussing the client's problems, interpreters need to make sure they use the correct terms and reflect the open (non-directive) nature of the SLT's questions and avoid being sidetracked into discussions with the client ("what she meant was …").

During conversation interpreters need to convey what the client says and what is unusual about it.

During feedback and discussion, interpreters should be able to cope with the problem of the meaning of terms and should convey concerns back and forth (i.e. don't try to deal with them yourself).

6. English-Chinese glossary

英漢詞彙表

English	Hong Kong & Taiwan	Mainland China
aphasia	失語	失语 (症)
articulation	發音; 咬字	发音
cerebrovascular accident (CVA)/stroke	腦血管破裂; 腦栓塞; 腦中風; 中風	中风; 脑卒中
dysarthria	發音困難	构音困难; 障碍
dysphagia	吞咽困難	吞咽困难; 噎膈
dyspraxia	運動功能障礙; 動作協調障礙症	动用障碍
Speech (Language) Therapist	言語治療師	言语治疗师
Speech Language Pathologist	言語治療師	言语治疗师
speech language therapy (SLT)	言語治療	言语治疗
stuttering	口吃	口吃
traumatic brain injury (TBI)	腦創傷	外伤性脑损伤

Summary of main points

- Say exactly what the SLT says, with the exact gesture and/or reference to materials.
- Convey back exactly what the client says, letting the SLT adjust what they say if needed.
- Avoid explaining to the client.
- Explain to the SLT if needed.
- If asked questions by parents/family members, convey to SLT to answer.

Chapter 15

Mental health

Mental health interpreting can be a difficult field in which to work. It may be difficult to interpret for clients who suffer from mental health problems which give them a limited or distorted view of what is going on. Clients suffering from episodes of paranoid psychosis may accuse the interpreter of twisting their words or of "being out to get them" and of conspiring against them with the medical staff.

Cultural differences may lead the patient to make references to beliefs or practices which are not shared by mental health professionals in the country in which the patient finds himself. The interpreter may want to obtain clarification from the patient during the interaction. Aside from involving issues of a cross-cultural nature, mental health interpreting for refugees may place an additional load on interpreters due to having to interpret the trauma story in the first person singular (Bot 2005, 2007; Crezee, Jülich & Hayward, 2013; Lai, Heydon & Mulayim, 2015).

In other cases, interpreting assignments may pose a problem due to the fact that the client is depressed to the extent of being totally withdrawn and unwilling or unable to communicate. In some cases, the client may be abusing the interviewer and/or the interpreter. Again, it is important to interpret whatever the client says. The fact that the client is swearing, and even the exact nature of the swear words, may give the mental health professional an important indication of what is going on in the client's mind.

With regard to the terminology used, it should be said that although psychiatric textbooks do not make easy reading due to all the specialized terms, interviews between mental health professionals and clients often involve simple, everyday language, such as: "How are you feeling?" and "I cannot sleep, because they are out to get me". Hence the main aim of this chapter is to ensure the interpreter is familiar with some of the mental health issues with which clients may be struggling, so as to enable them to understand the background of any mental health interviews in which they may be involved.

This chapter will give a very brief overview of some of the most common types of mental illnesses and personality disorders. Please note that these terms will usually not be used in the interviews themselves, i.e. the psychiatrist is not very likely to tell the client "You have a schizoid personality disorder with paranoid components". The overview merely serves to give interpreters some background information as to the disorders, to better understand some of the patient's utterances and responses.

Finally, mental health professionals rely quite heavily on the interview with the client for assessment and diagnosis. They cannot simply order an X-ray or blood test to find out additional information. Therefore, the golden rule is, once again, to interpret whatever the patient says, no matter how odd this may sound to the interpreter.

1.   Terms with Latin and Greek roots

auto	self
bi	two
bipolar	two extremes (two opposite poles)
delude	to make someone/yourself believe something that is not true
delusion	false personal belief
delusional	having false personal beliefs; believing things that are not true
depress	to push down
hallucinate	to feel/hear/see things which are not there
hallucination	feeling/seeing/hearing things which are not there
idio	own; individual
psyche	mind
phrenos	brain
schizo	split
	Please note: schizophrenia does not equal "split personality"; the word schizophrenia is therefore somewhat misleading if taken literally.
therapy	Treatment

2.   Briefing and debriefing

It is important that the mental health professional take the time to (de)brief the interpreter. During the briefing session (also called a pre-session), the professional may talk to the interpreter about the objective of the interview, the client's history/background and any cross-cultural issues. During the debriefing session (also called a post-session), the professional may ask the interpreter if there was anything else the interpreter noted about the client's choice of words, intonation, or pitch that may have carried meaning. It may be appropriate for the interpreter to comment on certain non-verbal aspects of communication, such as gestures, posture, physical space and facial expressions.

The health professional may also ask the interpreter to give him/her some general information on the client's cultural background. The interpreter should emphasize that he or she can only provide some very general cultural background information, and from the interpreter's own point of view. The interpreter should also stress that no two individuals are quite the same and that factors such as personality, age, gender, religion, amount of exposure to other cultures, length of time in the new country and individual life experiences may have shaped the individual to a large extent. Hence the interpreter should phrase his cultural clarification by first stating: "What I am going to say will be objective, a lot will depend on the patient's age, religion, (etc.), however, in general …". (Health Media 1988).

3.   Behaviors and their implications for the interpreter

Some conditions are associated with behaviors and speech patterns which may confuse the interpreter. It may help the interpreter to know that certain behaviors and utterances are commonly observed in certain conditions. The interpreter should interpret everything that is said exactly as it is said.

–   *Psychosis.* Psychotic patients may show signs of paranoia as well; they may also feel that they are receiving special guidance from above. They may say "A voice told me to take the next street, because he wanted to protect me." Again, it is important to interpret this faithfully.

–   *Schizophrenia and psychotic episodes.* Sometimes schizophrenic or psychotic patients hear voices and talk back to them. These clients may seem to listen to "voices" in different corners of the room and reply to those voices, looking in the directions the voices appear to be coming from. The interpreter should simply interpret what they say.

–   *Suicidal patients.* If the patient is thinking about different ways to kill himself or herself, the interpreter should interpret these utterances faithfully. The interpreter should NEVER decide to not interpret these suicidal thoughts simply because the interpreter is against suicide or believes suicide is bad. It is absolutely essential that the professional be aware of these suicidal thoughts, so that the patient can be given all due care and attention.

–   *Disorganized thought patterns.* Sometimes clients can go on and on, expressing seemingly nonsensical thoughts. Such clients may talk non-stop and may not appear to make any sense. They may talk about pigs singing beautiful songs and voting for the conservative party in green underpants on tropical islands, drinking coffee from beer mugs. It is important that the interpreter interpret this stream of consciousness (any seemingly unconnected thoughts that come up) exactly as they are voiced. It may be best to interpret simultaneously, as it is difficult to interpret disorganized thinking consecutively, precisely because it does not make sense and is therefore difficult to remember. Interpreting thoughts accurately may offer the health professional important insights as to what is going on inside the client's mind.

4.   Mental health professionals

Psychiatrist – Medical doctor specializing in mental health, prescribes medication; rarely does therapy.

Psychologist. Not a medical doctor, but someone who has studied the workings of the human mind and completed a Master's or Ph.D. degree in psychology at a university; psychologists are *unable to prescribe medication.*

Psychiatric Nurse Practitioner – An ARNP with specialized training in the diagnosis and treatment of mental illness.

Clinical Psychologist – A Ph.D. psychologist. Psychologists diagnose and do individual/group therapy, and some states allow some very limited degree of prescription of medication as well. There is a specialty in School Psychology as well; these practitioners do a lot of developmental assessments in addition to other tasks.

Clinical Social Worker – A counselor with a masters degree in social work. Diagnoses, does individual/group counseling, provides case management and advocacy, usually in the hospital setting.

Licensed Professional Counselor – A counselor with a masters degree in psychology, counseling or a related field. Diagnoses and does individual/group counseling.

Mental Health Counselor – A counselor with a masters degree and several years of supervised clinical work experience. Diagnoses and does individual/group counseling. *Certified Alcohol and Drug Abuse Counselor* – Counselor with specific clinical training in alcohol/drug abuse. Diagnoses and does individual and group counseling.

Nurse Psychotherapist. RN trained in mental health nursing. Diagnoses and does individual/group counseling.

Marital and Family Therapist – counselor with a masters degree, with special education and training in marital and family therapy. Diagnoses and does individual/group counseling.

Pastoral Counselor – member of the clergy with training in clinical pastoral education. Diagnoses and provides individual/group counseling.

Peer Specialist – counselor with lived experience with mental health or substance use conditions, and with a small amount of training. Assists clients with recovery by recognizing and developing strengths and setting goals.

*Some of these may only be found in the US, not in other English-speaking countries

5.   Some common therapeutic approaches

–   *Classic psychotherapy* also called psychodynamic therapy: the therapist and a client talk about the client's problems, often going back to the client's childhood to find out where problems have come from.

- *Cognitive behavioral therapy (CBT)*: tries to help people understand how (irrational) thoughts can influence the way they behave, and how changing these thoughts can change their behavior. CBT is often used to treat extreme fears (phobias), anxiety, depression and addictions.
- *Dialectal behavioral therapy (DBT)*: aimed at teaching clients skills for coping with stress, managing emotions and improving relationships with others. DBT involves skills training, acknowledging thoughts that are normally avoided, cognitive therapy and amending behavior. Mindfulness (being aware of where you are and what your body is doing without having any particular feelings about this) is an important part of DBT.
- *humanistic therapy* – focuses on the innate goodness of human beings and their ability to overcome a fixed pattern of unhelpful behaviors (based on their past life experience) into a more helpful pattern of behaviors.
- *Mindfulness* – focuses on living in the moment.

6.   Common reasons for counseling

Common reasons for counseling may include grief counseling (following a loss, change or death); relationship counseling (families, marriages, partnerships) and addiction counseling (internet addiction, gambling, sex addiction; substance abuse).

7.   Some commonly used pharmaceutical drugs

Anticonvulsants. These may be given to calm and stabilize the person's moods.

Mood stabilizer. Drugs that act to stabilize mood; these may include tranquilizers and anticonvulsant medication.

Antidepressants. These include selective serotonin reuptake inhibitors (SSRIs), tricyclic anti-depressants (TCAs), serotonin and noradrenaline reuptake inhibitors (SNRIs), monoamine oxidase inhibitors (MAOIs) by tablet or patch, to reduce side-effects.

Antipsychotics. Tranquilizing medication which works against psychotic symptoms such as hallucinations and delusions.

8.   Mental illness

The World Health Organization (WHO) defines mental health as "a state of well-being in which an individual realizes his or her own abilities, can cope with the normal stresses of life, can work productively and is able to make a contribution to his or her community" (WHO, n.d.).

Most mental health professionals follow the American Psychiatric Association's (APA) Diagnostic and Statistical Manual of Mental Disorders or DSM-5 (American Psychiatric Association 2013). The DSM-IV-TR (2000) distinguishes between a large range of mental disorders, including:

1. Anxiety disorders – including: generalized anxiety disorder (GAD); panic attacks; obsessive compulsive disorder (OCD); phobias.
2. Affective disorders – disorders which affect the patient's emotions, including depressive and manic disorders and bipolar (formerly manic depressive) disorder.
3. Personality disorders
4. Psychotic disorders – including psychosis/psychotic episode and schizophrenia
5. Dementias – loss of memory and other mental functions, e.g. in Alzheimer's disease

Interested readers are referred to the DSM-IV-TR (American Psychiatric Association 2000) or the DSM-5 (American Psychiatric Association 2013) which uses a multidimensional approach including clinical syndromes, developmental disorders and personality disorders, physical conditions, severity of psychosocial stressors and highest level of functioning. The categorization into Axis-I and Axis-II disorders in the DSM-5 may be used by health insurance companies as a guideline when deciding whether to provide coverage.

9.   Some mental health disorders

For ease of use, only some of the more common disorders are listed here in alphabetical order, rather than under their APA classification. Developmental disorders such as autism spectrum disorders (ASD) and attention deficit hyperactivity disorder (ADHD) have been included in Chapter 13, because they are often first diagnosed in childhood.

1.   *Acute stress disorder*
Similar to post traumatic stress disorder (PTSD), but symptoms last for less than 30 days.

2.   *Anxiety disorders*
See under *Generalized anxiety disorder* and *Panic disorder* below.

3.   *Bipolar (affective) disorder*
Formerly known as manic depressive disorder.

What happens. This is a major psychological disorder which is characterized by extreme mood swings, ranging from mania (feeling *invincible* and having high energy levels) to depression (feeling *down*, with low energy) to feeling elements of both these moods. Moving from *high* to *low* and back again is known as *cycling*.

People with bipolar disorder may move from one extreme to the other, or feel an element of both extremes at the same time.

Symptoms:

Manic phase. Feeling "on top of the world," showing exaggerated emotions and feelings of extreme happiness; in this phase patients seem to have boundless energy, do not seem to need any sleep and may be agitated, hyperactive and very talkative. They cannot concentrate very well and may have inflated self-esteem and delusions of grandeur ("I am a champion"). Sometimes patients are hypomanic (less severe than manic).

Depressive phase. This phase is the opposite of the manic phase; the patient feels sad, lonely, unworthy, guilty and has very low self-esteem. He or she cannot seem to get anything done and is apathetic and listless.

Causes: Range of environmental, biologic, genetic, psychological and interpersonal factors.

Treatment: Mood stabilizing medication such as lithium, anti-psychotic medication, anti-depressants and sometimes also anticonvulsant drugs.

4.   *Brief psychotic episode* – see under *psychosis*

5.   *Depression* – comes from a word that literally means "pushing down."
Please note: depression is a very general term which can cover a very wide range of moods and situations.

What happens: Clinical depression is an abnormal emotional state with exaggerated feelings of sadness, worthlessness, emptiness and hopelessness. Depression can be a normal response of sadness and despair following a loss.

Causes of major depression: Depression can be triggered by a wide range of factors, including traumatic life experiences, genetic disorders, nutritional disorders (e.g. a Vitamin B deficiency), medication, disorders of the central nervous system (e.g. Parkinson's disease), disorders of the endocrine system (e.g. hypothyroidism), obesity, infections, cancer.

Symptoms: Depressed people may be apathetic (literally: no feelings) and withdrawn; they may either overeat or lose all interest in food.

Types of depression

As with many other mental illnesses, clients may show a mixture of symptoms.

In *neurotic depression*, the individual is being very hard on himself. This can be an exaggerated response to a stressful situation, such as being left by a loved one.

In *psychotic depression*, the individual may not be able to separate the "real" from the "unreal" and have hallucinations, delusions and confusion.

Postnatal depression – some researchers suggest this is triggered by a rapid drop in the female hormone progesterone after childbirth. Postnatal depression is treated with antidepressants, talk therapy, support or natural progesterone. In serious cases, the woman may develop puerperal psychosis, which means she may lose all sense of reality and be at risk of harming herself or her child.

6. *Eating disorders What happens:*

In *anorexia nervosa*, patients starve or purge themselves (using laxatives or inducing vomiting) out of an untrue belief that they are overweight; weight may drop to dangerously low levels.

In *bulimia*, patients binge-eat followed by purging; otherwise similar to anorexia.

Treatment: Therapy (e.g. CBT), closely monitored food intake.

7. *Generalized anxiety disorder (GAD)*

What happens: Ongoing and sometimes disabling anxiety about life in general.

Cause: Unknown, although this disorder tends to run in families. *Symptoms*: Constant worrying; mild heart palpitations; dizziness. *Treatment*: Talk therapy (revisiting childhood), CBT.

8. *Obsessive compulsive disorder (OCD)*

What happens: This is a disorder of checking and doubting. Patients are constantly troubled by obsessions and carrying out repetitive acts to reduce their anxiety (e.g. constant handwashing or cleaning).

Cause: Unknown; tends to run in families.

Symptoms: Performing the same repetitive acts over and over again, thereby wasting a lot of time.

9. *Phobias*

What happens: Intense and paralyzing fear of situations, e.g. an intense fear of mice, spiders, dogs. Some phobias include:

Agoraphobia. An intense fear of leaving the safety of one's house, unless accompanied by a "safe person"

Social phobia. An intense fear of not being able to cope in social situations

Body dysmorphia. Untrue beliefs about the shape of one's own body

10.   *Panic attacks*
What happens: People worry that if they face a particular situation they will panic and lose control. They may avoid driving across bridges, going up escalators, walking past dogs.

Symptoms: Heart palpitations, disordered breathing, tingling around mouth and fingers, chest pain.

Treatment: CBT or DBT, breathing exercises (short breath in, long breath out, so carbon dioxide cannot accumulate and make symptoms worse).

11.   *Post traumatic stress disorder (PTSD)*
What happens: This anxiety disorder may affect people who have seen or experienced a traumatic event involving (the threat of) injury or death; it is very common in war veterans, and in survivors of rape and assault.

Symptoms: (i) Reliving the traumatic event: recurrent intrusive thoughts, nightmares, flashbacks; (ii) Avoiding any possible reminders of the traumatic event: feeling numb, flat, detached, not interested in normal activities; (iii) Hyper-arousal: startling easily, concentration problems, irritability, sleeping problems, hyper-alertness. Depression, alcohol and drug abuse are common.

Treatment: Talk therapy, support groups.

12.   *Psychosis*
What happens: During a psychotic episode, the person is unable to distinguish the "real" from the "unreal" and unable to separate normal thoughts from abnormal thoughts; delusions and hallucinations (e.g. hearing voices) may occur.

Factors: Stress, childhood trauma, (early) cannabis use, changes to brain and brain chemicals (especially dopamine).

Treatment: Antipsychotic drugs.

13.   *Schizophrenia*
What happens: Frequent psychotic episodes, but symptoms last longer than 6 months. Men are often first diagnosed between the ages of 15 and 25, while women are usually affected in their twenties or thirties.

Symptoms include: ·

Disorganized thinking. Thoughts may come and go so quickly that the patient is unable to get "a grip on them." Patients may be easily distracted and "jump" from one topic to the next; others may find it totally impossible to follow these thought processes.

Delusions. False and illogical beliefs; feelings that "people are out to get me" OR feelings of grandeur ("I am a champion")

Hallucinations. Hearing voices, seeing people or things, feeling fingers touching the body.

Treatment: Medication such as anti-psychotic drugs, individual psychotherapy, learning social skills, problem solving, learning independent life skills, family therapy (stable family environment is important).

10. English-Chinese glossary

英漢詞彙表

English	Hong Kong & Taiwan	Mainland China
acute stress disorder	急性壓力症	急性压力症
affective disorders	情緒失調	情绪失调
agoraphobia	空曠恐懼; 恐曠症	恐旷症; 畏旷症
anorexia nervosa	神經性厭食症	神经性厌食症; 神经性食欲不振
anticonvulsants	抗痙攣劑; 抗痙攣藥物; 抗抽搐劑	抗惊厥药
antidepressants	抗抑鬱藥	抗抑郁药
antipsychotics	抗精神病藥物	抗精神病药
anxiety disorders	焦慮症	焦虑症
attention deficit hyperactiviy disorder (ADHD)	注意力失調過度活躍症; 專注不足多動症	注意力缺陷多动障碍; 注意力不足过动症
autism spectrum disorders (ASD)	自閉症譜系障礙; 自閉症	孤独症
Behavior Analyst	行為分析師; 行為分析員	行为分析员
bipolar disorder	躁鬱症	躁郁症
body dysmorphia	身體畸形恐懼症	身体畸形恐惧症
brief psychotic episode	短暫性精神錯亂	短暂性精神错乱
bulimia	貪食症; 暴食症	贪食症
cognitive behavioral therapy (CBT)	認知行為治療 (法)	认知行为疗法
counselling	輔導	辅导
Counselor	輔導員	辅导员

(Continued)

English	Hong Kong & Taiwan	Mainland China
delusions	妄想	妄想
dementia	腦退化症; 失智症; 癡呆症	痴呆症
depression	憂鬱症; 抑鬱症	忧郁症; 抑郁症
depression (clinical)	臨床憂鬱症; 臨床抑鬱症	临床忧郁症; 临床抑郁症
developmental disorders	發展性心理障礙; 精神發育障礙	(精神) 发育障碍
dialectical behavioral therapy (DBT)	辨證行為治療法	辨证行为疗法
disorganized thought patterns	思想模式混亂	思维模式紊乱
eating disorders	進食失調	进食障碍
generalized anxiety disorder (GAD)	廣泛焦慮症	泛化性焦虑症; 广泛性焦虑症
hallucinations	幻覺	幻觉
humanistic therapy	人本主義治療	人本主义疗法; 人文疗法
Licensed Counselor	持牌輔導員	持证辅导员
major depressive disorder (MDD)	嚴重憂 (抑) 鬱症	重症抑郁
MAO inhibitors (MAOIs)	單胺氧化酶抑制藥	单胺氧化酶抑制药
mindfulness	正念	正念
mood stabilizer	情緒穩定劑	情绪稳定剂
neurotic depression	神經官能性憂鬱症	(神经) 官能性抑郁症
serotonin-noradrenaline reuptake inhibitors (SNRIs)	血清素與去甲腎上腺素再攝取抑制劑	血清胺和去甲肾上腺素再吸收抑制剂
obsessive compulsive disorder (OCD)	強迫症	强迫症
panic attacks	恐慌發作	恐慌发作
personality disorders	人格異常; 人格障礙	人格异常; 人格障碍
phobia	恐懼症	恐惧症; 恐怖症
post traumatic stress disorder (PTSD)	創傷後壓力症	创伤后压力症
postnatal depression	產後抑鬱	产后抑郁
Psychiatric Nurse; Mental Health Nurse	精神科護士	精神科护士
Psychiatrist	精神科醫生	精神病学家; 精神科医师
Psychologist	心理學家	心理学家
psychodynamic therapy	心理動力學治療	心理动力疗法
Psychosis	思覺失調	思觉失调
Psychotherapist	心理治療師	心理治疗师
psychotic disorders	精神失常	精神失调症
psychotic episode	精神病發作	精神病发作
Schizophrenia	精神分裂症	精神分裂症

(Continued)

English	Hong Kong & Taiwan	Mainland China
Serotine/Serotonin selective reuptake inhibitors (SSRIs)	選擇性血清素再攝取抑制劑	选择性血清素再吸收抑制剂
social phobia	社交恐懼症; 社交焦慮症	社交恐惧症; 社交焦虑症
tricyclic antidepressants (TCAs)	三環抗抑鬱劑	三环抗忧郁药

Summary of main points

This chapter has given a brief overview of interpreting in mental health, including:

- the importance of briefing and debriefing
- health professionals involved
- commonly used therapies
- some common mental health disorders

Chapter 16

Oncology

With thanks to Dr J. Crezee, Academic Medical Center,
University of Amsterdam

Oncology is the branch of medicine that deals with various types of cancer. Oncologists are doctors who specialize in the treatment of cancer.

The word *cancer* still has a lot of negative connotations. The fact that people still, rightly or wrongly, associate cancer with impending death can make interpreting in this area very difficult. In fact, there are many different types of cancer, and both treatment and outlook can vary enormously. It is important to understand these differences and the variations in outlook.

This chapter will attempt to give some general background information on cancer, related diagnostic procedures, typing and staging as well as treatment options.

1. Cancer

Throughout our body the cells in different organs are designed to do a particular job, e.g. lung cells are different from skin cells. The center of each cell contains a blueprint for new cells: vital information as to exactly what new cells should look like and on how they should behave.

Sometimes, and for reasons unknown, something goes wrong and different new cells start to grow. These cells do not look like the normal cells and do not function like normal cells. They can be benign (not cancerous) or malignant (cancerous).

Cancerous cells usually grow and multiply very fast (compared to normal cells). This is a problem because they spread and take over the organ affected, pushing the normal cells out of the way and interfering with their normal functioning.

By way of analogy, cancer cells may be compared to weeds, because like weeds, they grow very fast and are not useful. If weeds are not removed or destroyed, they can take over the whole garden and choke the normal plants. Similarly, if cancer cells are not destroyed, they can take over the body and 'choke' the normal cells.

Cancer cells can spread in two ways, by:

– *Invasion*, where cancerous cells grow into neighboring tissues and organs. This may be compared to someone having some weeds in his garden, close to the boundary line, and these weeds invading or growing into the weed-free neighboring property, or:

– *Secondaries, in which* new 'colonies' start up. Cancer cells can spread through the blood or lymph system. This may be compared to 'a river carrying weeds downstream', where they then starting growing in a previously weed-free place. It may also be compared to birds carrying seeds over to another area. These new growths are known as *metastases*.

2. Diagnosis

– *History* – The diagnostic process will usually start with a thorough history. The health professional will ask the patient about symptoms including pain, appetite, weight loss, bleeding, vomiting, coughing, history of employment, social background and family history, etc.
– *Physical examination* – Doctors may feel for lumps, size of organs, fluid retention and swelling of lymph nodes. They will judge the patient's appearance and listen to the patient's heart and lungs.
– *Diagnostic tests* – A number of tests may be ordered, including blood tests.
Blood tests: In recent years cancer-specific blood tests (tumor markers) have been developed which can give the doctor an indication of whether the patient might have a specific form of cancer. Some better known tumor markers include prostate specific antigen (PSA) and Ca-125 (which indicates whether the patient may have ovarian cancer). Other tumor markers have been patented for other types of cancer.
– *Imaging* – The patient may be referred on to a specialist for further tests, including X-rays and contrast X-rays. Contrast X-rays may include IVU's (for imaging of the urinary system) or ERCP's (for imaging of the gall-duct system).
A number of increasingly sophisticated scanning methods can be used for precise imaging. These include PET scans, total body scans, VQ Scans, CT scans, ultrasounds, Doppler tests, mammograms, thermograms and so on. Magnetic resonance imaging (MRI scans) can also produce very detailed images of the body, including the soft tissues.
– *Endoscopies* – Endoscopies are procedures in which the doctor has a look inside an organ(s) by inserting a fiber optic tube. Tubes may be inserted through existing body openings. Types of endoscopies include:
Bronchoscopy. Tube inserted through the windpipe into the bronchi.
Colonoscopy. Tube inserted through the rectum into the large intestine (colon).
Colposcopy. Tube inserted through the vagina to look at the birth canal and cervix.
Cystoscopy. Tube inserted through the urethra into the bladder.
Esophagoscopy. Tube inserted into the esophagus.

Gastroscopy. Tube inserted through the esophagus, to look at the inside of the stomach.

Hysteroscopy. Tube inserted through vagina and cervix into the womb.

- *Laparoscopy* – In other cases, the surgeon may need to create a small hole not unlike a key hole and insert the tube through this to gain access to the abdominal cavity. This called a laparoscopy. Many procedures that used to require large incisions (cuts) are today done laparoscopically.

- *Open surgery* – Sometimes open surgery is performed to confirm a suspicion of cancer. The surgeon makes an incision to open the body and have a look inside.

- *Biopsy* – Act of taking a tissue sample. Biopsies can be done by way of fine needle biopsy, hook wire biopsy, during endoscopy or laparoscopy, or by a smear test in which some cells are scraped away from a surface (e.g. the surface of the cervix).

3. Typing and staging

The diagnosis of cancer is usually reached on the basis of history (what the patient tells the doctor) and on the results of a number of tests. Tests are primarily aimed at typing (finding out what type of cancer cell is involved) and staging (finding out what stage the cancer is at, how far it has spread).

Typing involves obtaining a sample of the cancer cells, typically by means of biopsies (removing some living cells, refer above). An operation or endoscopy may be needed to remove some living cells. Examples of endoscopy (looking inside) are listed under Diagnosis above.

Once the sample of cells has been removed, it is sent to a pathologist: (either a histologist (a tissue specialist) or a cytologist (a cell specialist). These specialists look at the cell under the microscope to see if there are any cancer cells and, if so, what type of cells they are. Typing of the cells is important, because it influences the approach/treatment as different types of cancer respond to different types of treatment.

Different types of staging or classification apply to different types of cancer; however, a commonly-used staging system is the 'TNM' classification. In this staging classification system, 'T' describes the size of the tumor and whether it has invaded nearby tissue on a scale of 1 to 4, 'N' describes the degree of regional lymph node involvement on a scale of 0 to 3, and 'M' describes whether the tumor has metastasized (spread) ("0" = no and "1" is yes). For instance, T4N0M0 stands for a size 4 tumor that has invaded neighboring organs but without regional lymph node involvement and without metastases.

For some tumor types specific or earlier staging scales are used, and this may be confusing. Bowel cancer, for example, is usually staged according to the Dukes classification (Dukes A, B, C, D, with A meaning that the cancer is confined to the lining of the bowel and D indicating that there are metastases elsewhere, for example in the liver). Lymphomas may be classified as Stage I, II, III or IV, depending on the spread of the cancer.

The classification of cervical cancer can be confusing, as two different stages are also distinguished. The earliest pre-cancerous cell changes are described as CIN-1, CIN-2 and CIN-3, while developments beyond these very early stages are described as cervical cancer stage I to IV.

It is very difficult to take a general approach to staging, as a lot depends on the condition of the patient, the type of cell involved, the success of previous treatment, and so on.

4. Treatment

Cancer treatment may be *curative* (aimed at achieving a cure) or *palliative* (aimed at lessening the patient's suffering only), and these terms can be very difficult to interpret. When the patient is terminally ill (when death seems inevitable), health professionals will decide on the best palliative approach, which may involve radiation therapy to shrink the tumor, or sustained-release morphine to control the pain.

While researchers around the world are still working on new approaches to cancer, some of the most common treatment options to date include:

- *Surgery* – To surgically remove cancer cells. Surgery is often no longer an option when the tumor has invaded neighboring organs.
- *Radiation therapy* – Concentrated dose of radiation is applied to a specific area. Radiationtherapy may also be used to shrink benign tumors. Radiation therapy may cause side-effects like nausea and irritated skin.
- *Chemotherapy* – Treatment of cancer by chemicals which are intended to 'search out and destroy' predominantly cancer cells. Chemotherapy may have certain side-effects such as hair loss and gastrointestinal complaints such as vomiting and diarrhea.
- *Hormone therapy* – Some cancers are very sensitive to hormones and shrink when treated with appropriate hormones (e.g. prostate cancer is sometimes treated with estrogen). In other cases doctors may withhold hormones, e.g. estrogen may be withheld if the patient is suspected of having breast cancer.
- *Brachytherapy* – Radioactive sources may be temporarily or permanently implanted near the tumor order to destroy the cancer from close by. In order to prevent radiation from affecting health professionals and visitors, these patients are often kept in isolation.
- *Hyperthermia* – Overheating cancer cells can destroy them and also help maintain the effects of radiation therapy. Hyperthermia is now also combined with chemotherapy, where chemotherapy is inside little balls of fat which are placed

near the cancer. Hyperthermia is then used to melt the fat so the chemotherapy medicine can work directly on the cancer.

- *Immunotherapy* – The use of agents to boost the immune response of the body against the cancer cells.
- *Laser treatment* – Using a laser to burn away cancer cells, allowing new cells to grow up from the basal membrane.
- *Cryotherapy* – To freeze off cancer cells, e.g. liquid nitrogen treatment for superficial skin cancers.
- *Proton therapy* – Using a beam of protons to destroy cancer cells, without damaging nearby tissue.

5. Common forms of cancer

1. *Bowel cancer* (*colon cancer*) – Cancer of the large intestine (colon) or rectum.

Cause: Unknown. Risk factors may include age, dietary factors, alcohol intake and family history.

Symptoms: Bowel cancer is usually staged according to the Dukes classification.

Early signs include blood in the stool, changes in bowel habits (diarrhea or constipation) and slight rectal bleeding. Later signs include a feeling of discomfort or fullness in the abdomen, pain, anemia, and weight loss.

Diagnostic tests: barium enema using barium as a radio opaque contrast, colonoscopy, biopsy.

Treatment: Surgery; radiation therapy; chemotherapy.

2. *Breast cancer* – Cancer cells in breast tissue form a lump, cause discharge from a nipple, or cause puckering of the skin (making it look like the skin of an orange), sometimes seen in Paget's disease of the breast.

Cause: Unknown, genetic factors may play a role (especially in HER2 positive cancers, – often found in close relatives of patients with breast cancer, i.e. mother, sister, maternal aunt or grandmother). In other types, alcohol intake may play a role.

Symptoms: Painless lump found during self-examination of the breast, dimpled skin, inward turning nipple, discharge (fluid) from the nipple.

Diagnostic tests: Mammogram; CT scan; breast ultrasound (recommended if breast tissue is dense), MRI, breast biopsy (needle biopsy, hook wire biopsy).

Treatment: Lumpectomy, mastectomy plus reconstruction (breast removed leaving skin and inserting artificial breast) followed by radiation therapy, chemotherapy, hormone treatment (often Tamoxifen®) or treatment with Herceptin. Follow-up including regular mammograms, chest X-rays, bone scans, total body scans.

3.   *Cervical cancer* – Abnormal cells growing on the cervix or mouth of the womb.

Cause: Risk factors include *human papilloma virus* (*HPV*) (wart virus strains) infection; starting sexual intercourse before body's immune system is mature (before age 18); smoking.

Symptoms: Spotting in between menstrual periods; bleeding after intercourse.

Diagnostic tests: Pap smear, colposcopy, cone biopsy.

Treatment: Laser surgery, loop electrosurgical excision procedure (LEEP) or diathermy loop treatment, cryosurgery, cone biopsy, hysterectomy, radiation therapy, chemotherapy, all depending on the stage.

Please see page 186 of this chapter for the classification of cervical cancer. It is important that the interpreter understand these classifications.

4.   *Colon cancer* (refer to Bowel cancer above)

5.   *Lung cancer* – Abnormal cells growing in lung tissue. Differing types include small cell (also called oat cell) and squamous cell carcinoma (often seen in former or current heavy smokers), adenocarcinoma or broncho-alveolar carcinoma (seen in non-smokers). and epithelioma (often seen after asbestos exposure).

Cause: Often related to smoking (active or passive) or inhalation of irritant gases such as asbestos.

Symptoms: Dry cough, coughing up blood, chest pain, wheeze, breathlessness, frequent chest infections or asthma attacks, weight loss. If the cancer has spread, the patient may have headaches or bone pain.

Diagnostic tests: Chest X-ray, needle biopsy or bronchoscopy and biopsy, tomogram of chest, ventilation-perfusion (VQ) scan, perfusion lung scan, CT scan of body (to check for spread), ventilation lung scan (inhaling gas as a contrast medium); blood test; sputum test.

Treatment: Surgery, radiation therapy, chemotherapy.

6.   *Leukemia* – Refer to Chapter 20, page 252.

7.   *Lymphoma* – Any cancer which starts in the lymph glands. Includes non-Hodgkin's lymphoma (including Burkitt's lymphoma) or Hodgkin's lymphoma. There are any different types depending on the type of cell involved (mantle cell, T-cell, B-cell).

Cause: Damage to the DNA of the lymph cells. Exposure to chemicals may play a role.

Symptoms: Painless lumps on lymph glands.

Diagnostic tests: Biopsy, CT scan MRI scan.

Treatment: Radiation therapy, chemotherapy, prednisone. Treatment depends on the stage and the type of cell involved. See Chapter 24 for more information.

8.   *Melanoma* – A cancer which starts from the pigment cells (melanocytes) in the outer layer of the skin.

Cause: Unknown, but risk factors include exposure to UV light, fair skin, moles, family history, and previous skin cancer.

Symptoms: A change in existing freckles or moles, including irregular edges, change of color (including black, blue and red or light grey); also moles or freckles which itch, bleed, are tender or form a crust.

Diagnostic tests: Surgical excision and biopsy, measuring the depth, body scanning; radiotherapy after excision to reduce rate of recurrence.

Treatment: Wide surgical excision and biopsy depending on the depth of the melanoma (measured in millimeters; the thinner the melanoma, the better the outlook), radiation therapy, chemotherapy.

9.   *Myeloma* – cancer starting from the bone-marrow cells.

Symptoms: Severe bone pain and spontaneous fractures; often occurs in ribs, vertebrae, pelvic bone and flat bones of the skull.

Treatment: Radiation therapy. See Chapter 20 for more information.

10.   *Nasopharyngeal Carcinoma (NPC)* – It is a squamous cell carcinoma found in the nose-throat area. It accounts for 18% of all cancers in Mainland China, but is not common in other parts of the world. NPC is sometimes referred to as Cantonese cancer (25 cases per 100,000 people in South China, particularly in Guandong Province. It is also quite common in Taiwan, but not in other areas of the world. There are two peaks, occurring in early adulthood (15–24 years) and later in life (65–79 years).

Diagnostic tests: Biopsy of lymph nodes

Cause: Viral infections, environmental factors (including dietary factors), hereditary.

Symptoms: Swollen lymph nodes in the neck, pain, food or liquid coming back up out of the nose (nasal regurgitation), nasal obstruction, bleeding from the nose, middle ear infection, hearing loss, cranial nerve paralysis, nasal twang when speaking

Treatment: surgery, chemotherapy, radiotherapy, immunotherapy

Prognosis: depends on stage of cancer (4 stages)

11.   *Ovarian Cancer* – Cancer of the ovary/ovaries.

Cause: The exact cause is unknown, but risk factors include: gene mutations; family history of particular types of cancer; and hormonal factors including early start of menstrual periods, late menopause, never having had children, never having used a contraceptive pill.

Symptoms: Symptoms are typically late and include discomfort in abdomen, lump or swelling on ovary*, abnormal vaginal blood loss;, sometimes ascites (fluid collection in the abdomen) or swelling of the legs.

Diagnostic tests: CT scan, Pap smear, laparoscopy or laparotomy, biopsies, Ca125 tumor marker test.

Treatment: Total abdominal hysterectomy with removal of both ovaries (bilateral oophorectomy), irradiation of the pelvis, chemotherapy, iridium treatment (localized radiation through implanted iridium rod).
**different from an ovarian cyst*

12.   *Pancreatic cancer* – Cancer of the pancreas

Cause: Smoking, diabetes, exposure to polychlorinated biphenyl compounds (PCBs), or unknown.

Symptoms: Loss of appetite, weight loss, flatulence, pain around mid-stomach or in the back, jaundice, sudden onset of diabetes.

Diagnostic tests: Laparoscopy, imaging.

Treatment: Partial pancreatectomy (surgical removal of part of the pancreas) plus surgical removal of part of small intestine and stomach, chemotherapy, radiation therapy.

13.   *Prostate cancer* – Abnormal cells in the prostate;

Cause: Unknown. Risk factors may include age, dietary factors and family history.

Symptoms: Prostate cancer may be classified as stage A, B, C, D, where A means that the cancer is confined to the 'capsule' of the prostate and D indicates that there are metastases. Symptoms include a lump in the prostate, and problems with urination (urge, slow start, slow stop, weak stream or trickle).

Diagnostic tests: (Prostate specific antigen (PSA) blood test, rectal examination, biopsy, body scanning.

Treatment: Depends largely on the stage of the cancer, the patient's age and general condition. Treatment may include transurethral resection of prostate (TURP), radical prostatectomy, radiation, chemotherapy, brachytherapy, hormone treatment.

14.   *Sarcoma* – Type of cancer that develops in bone, muscle, fat or softtissue. There are over 50 different types of sarcoma.

15.   *Stomach cancer – gastric carcinoma* – Cancer cells in the lining of the stomach. For more information refer to Chapter 26.

Cause: Unknown, but helicobacter pylori bacteria are thought to play a role, as do genetic mutations in some families.

Symptoms: Aversion to meat, nausea, swallowing problems, lack of appetite.

Diagnostic tests: Barium swallow (contrast X-ray where patient swallows barium), gastroscopy and biopsy, CT scan, PET scan.

Treatment: Surgery (gastrectomy).

16.   *Skin cancer* – Uncontrolled growth of abnormal cells on the skin. There are various types, including basal cell carcinoma (BCC), squamous cell carcinoma (SCC), and melanoma (see page 189).

Cause: Often the result of sun exposure; often seen in farmers, outdoor workers and vehicle drivers (left or right arm).

Symptoms: Sores or changes in the skin that do not heal, crater-like lesions, change in color, bleeding, itching, pain. Sometimes people get patches of *actinic keratosis*, (rough grey-pink scaly patches) as a forewarning that they may be at risk for skin cancer. This cancer can recur or spread.

Diagnostic tests: Regular 'spot checks', biopsy, total body scan (to check for spread).

Treatment: Removal by burning off the patches (*cauterizing*), freezing off the patches with liquid nitrogen (*cryo-surgery*), or removing or cutting out the patches (*radiation* or *excision*). This may be followed by chemotherapy or radiation therapy.

17.   *Testicular cancer* – Abnormal cells in the testicles (balls), usually in men between 15 and 45 years of age.

Cause: Unknown, but risk factors include undescended testicle (see Chapter 27).

Symptoms: Swelling or lump in the testicles, heavy feeling in the testicles, nipples may feel large and tender.

Diagnostic tests: Biopsy.

Treatment: Chemotherapy. Prognosis very good if detected early.

18.   *Uterine cancer – also known as endometrial cancer or cancer of the womb –* Abnormal cells in the uterus (womb) in women, most commonly after menopause.

Cause: Unknown, but risk factors involve hormonal factors, especially unopposed estrogen (estrogen that is not balanced out by natural progesterone). As an example, overweight women may produce more estrogen in their fat tissue (even after menopause) without producing progesterone.

Symptoms: Vaginal bleeding (after menopause).

Diagnostic tests: Hysteroscopy; biopsy.

Treatment: Hysterectomy (surgical removal of the womb); radiation therapy.

6.   Some notes for interpreters and translators

As mentioned in Chapter 2, interpreters need to be aware of the need to convey all information accurately and not censor or leave out information. Interpreters must tell the health professional if they feel unable to convey all information accurately due to cultural or personal restraints or pressure from family members to 'keep the bad news' from their relatives. Interpreters need to be aware that they may themselves feel negatively impacted by any bad news interviews (Lai, Heydon & Mulayim 2015; Crezee, Jülich & Hayward 2013) and practice self-care (Crezee, Atkinson, Pask, Au & Wong, 2015).

Interpreters need to be aware of the various ways in which patients may respond to bad news. Patients may deny that the doctor (or interpreter) has ever given them 'the bad news'; they may get angry and abusive, or they may get depressed and withdrawn. All of these responses are natural and the health professional understands this. Most importantly, perhaps, the interpreter needs to realize that it is the health professional, not the interpreter, who needs to deal with these responses and who is in control of the interview. Occasionally interpreters may feel obliged to admonish the patient for his aggressive responses or withdrawn behavior. Sometimes, the health professional, ignorant of interpreting ethics, may even ask the interpreter to 'get the patient to talk', or to comfort the patient. Neither is appropriate. In some cultures it is not acceptable for patients to be told their real diagnosis, and families may exert pressure on the interpreter to not interpret accurately. In this situation, the interpreter needs to remind a patient's relatives that he needs to adhere to the interpreter code of ethics. The interpreter may want to add: "Please tell the doctor how you feel about this and I will be happy to interpret between you and the doctor. However, please do not ask me to breach my professional code of ethics, which requires me to maintain accuracy and impartiality."

7. English-Chinese glossary

英漢詞彙表

English	Hong Kong & Taiwan	Mainland China
adenocarcinoma	腺癌	腺癌
B-cell	B型細胞	B细胞
barium enema	鋇灌腸	钡 (剂)灌肠
barium swallow	吞鋇	吞钡 (检查)
basal cell carcinoma (BCC)	基底細胞癌	基底细胞癌
bilateral oophorectomy	雙側卵巢切除術	双侧卵巢切除术
biopsy	活組織檢驗	活 (体) 组织检查; 活检
bone marrow	骨髓	骨髓
bowel cancer; colon cancer	腸道癌; 結腸癌	肠癌
brachytherapy	近距療法	短距 (放射) 疗法
breast cancer	乳癌	乳 (腺) 癌
broncho-alveolar carcinoma	支氣管肺泡癌	支气管肺泡癌
bronchoscopy	支氣管內視鏡檢查	支气管镜检查
cauterizing	灸療法	灸疗法
cervical cancer	(子) 宮頸癌	子宫颈癌
cervix	(子) 宮頸	(子) 宫颈
chemotherapy	化學療法; 化療	化学疗法; 化疗
chest X-ray	X光胸肺檢查; 胸肺X-光攝影	胸部X射线检查; 胸透检查
colonoscopy	結腸內視鏡檢查	结肠镜检查
colposcopy	陰道窺鏡檢查	阴道镜检查
computer aided tomography scan; CAT scan; CT scan	電腦斷層掃描; 電腦軸向斷層掃描; 電腦掃描	CT扫描
cone biopsy	錐細胞活組織檢驗; 錐體活組織檢驗	锥体活检
contrast X-ray	造影劑X光檢查	造影剂X光检查
cryosurgery	冷凍外科術	冷冻手术; 低温外科
cryotherapy	冷凍療法	冷冻疗法
cystoscopy	膀胱內窺鏡檢查	膀胱镜检查
loop electrosurgical excision procedure (LEEP)	(宮頸) 環形電切術	(宫颈) 环形电切除术
Doppler test	多普勒測試	多普勒试验
endometrial cancer	子宮內膜癌	子宫内膜癌
endoscopy	內窺鏡檢查; 內視鏡檢查	內窥镜检查; 内腔镜检查

(Continued)

English	Hong Kong & Taiwan	Mainland China
epithelioma	上皮瘤	上皮瘤; 上皮细胞瘤
ERCP; endoscopic retrograde cholangiopancreatography	內窺鏡逆行性膽胰管造影術 (簡稱: 膽管鏡檢查)	内镜逆行胰胆管造影
Esophagoscopy	食道內窺鏡檢查	食管镜检查
Excision	切除 (術)	切除 (术)
Gastrectomy	胃切除術	胃切除术
gastroscopy	胃內窺鏡檢查; 胃鏡檢查	胃镜检查
helicobacter pylori bacteria	幽門螺旋 (桿) 菌	幽门螺旋杆菌
hook wire biopsy	鈎針活組織檢驗	线钩活检
hormone therapy	激素治療	激素疗法
human papilloma virus (HPV)	人類乳突病毒; 人類乳頭狀瘤病毒	人类乳突病毒; 人乳头状瘤病毒
hyperthermia	高溫症; 體溫過高	高热
hysteroscopy	子宮內窺鏡檢查	官腔镜检查; 子宫镜检查
imaging	成像; 造影	显像; 成像
immunotherapy	免疫療法	免疫疗法
iridium treatment	銥療法	铱疗法
IVU	靜脈注射尿道造影檢查	静脉尿道造影检查
jaundice	黃疸	黄疸
laparoscopy	腹腔 (內窺) 鏡檢查	腹腔镜检查
laparotomy	剖腹術	剖腹术
Leukemia/Leukaemia	白血病	白血病
lumpectomy	腫塊切除術	肿块切除术
lung cancer	肺癌	肺癌
lymph node	淋巴結	淋巴结
lymphoma	淋巴瘤	淋巴瘤
magnetic resonance imaging (MRI)	磁力共振掃描 (或直接稱MRI)	磁 (性) 共振成像; 磁振造影扫描
Mammogram/Mammography	乳房X光攝影術	乳房造影; 乳房X线摄影术
mantle cells	套細胞	外膜细胞
mastectomy	乳房切除術	乳房切除术
melanoma	黑素瘤	黑素瘤
Metastases/Metastasis	轉移; 擴散	转移; 扩散
myeloma	骨髓瘤	骨髓瘤
needle (aspiration) biopsy	針吸式活組織檢驗 (俗稱「抽針」)	细针抽吸活检; 针吸活组织检查; 穿刺活检

(Continued)

English	Hong Kong & Taiwan	Mainland China
ovarian cancer	卵巢癌	卵巢癌
pancreatectomy	胰臟切除術	胰切除术; 胰脏切除
pancreatic cancer	胰臟癌	胰腺癌
Pap smear	柏氏抹片	巴氏涂片
perfusion lung scan	肺灌注掃描	肺 (血流) 灌注扫描
PET scan	正電子掃描	PET扫描; 正电子发射断层扫描
prednisone	潑尼松	强的松; 泼尼松
prostate cancer	前列腺癌	前列腺癌
prostate specific antigen (PSA)	前列腺特異抗原	前列腺特异 (性) 抗原
prostatectomy	前列腺切除術	前列腺切除术
radiation therapy/radiotherapy	放射治療 (又稱電療)	放射治疗
sarcoma	肉瘤	肉瘤
skin cancer	皮膚癌	皮肤癌
sputum test	痰液測試	痰测试
squamous cell carcinoma (SCC)	鱗狀細胞癌	鳞状 (上皮) 细胞癌
staging	分期	分期
stomach cancer; gastric carcinoma	胃癌	胃癌
T-cell	T 細胞	T (淋巴) 细胞
testicular cancer	睪 (亦作「睾」) 丸癌	睾丸癌
thermogram	溫度記錄圖	热象图; 热解曲线
TNM classification(Tumor-Node-Metastasis)	TNM (腫瘤) 分期法	TNM分类; 恶性肿瘤国际临床病期分类
Tomogram/Tomography	斷層造影術	体 (断) 层摄影
transurethral resection of prostate (TRP)	經尿道前列腺切除術	经尿道前列腺切除术
tumor/tumour marker	腫瘤標記	肿瘤标记
typing; type and cross match	分 (血) 型; 血型與交叉配型	分型; 血型和交叉配型
ultrasound scan	超聲波掃描	超声扫描
undescended testicle	睪丸未降 (隱睪症)	睾丸未降; 隐睾
uterine cancer	子宮癌	子宫癌
ventilation lung scan	換氣式肺掃描	肺通气扫描
VQ scan	通氣灌注掃描	(肺)通气灌注扫描
womb	子宮	子宫

Summary of main points

This chapter has given a brief overview of oncology, including:

–   common tests used for diagnosis (determining type and stage of cancer)
–   health professionals involved
–   commonly used treatment methods
–   some commonly encountered forms of cancer

PART III

Healthcare specialties

Chapter 17

Neurology

Nerves and the nervous system

The central nervous system (CNS) is literally the control center of the body. The workings of the CNS are very complicated, but to enable interpreters to have a good general understanding of what the neurosurgeon or neurologist is talking about when explaining the patient's condition, the CNS is broadly explained in this chapter.

Some patients require rehabilitative services after suffering neurological events such as strokes. Please refer to Chapter 7 for health professionals involved in rehabilitative services. First, let us look at the Latin and Greek roots that come up frequently in terminology to do with the CNS.

1.　Terms with Latin and Greek roots

cerebellum	part of the brain behind the brain stem (Latin: *small brain*)
cerebrovascular	to do with the blood vessels in the brain
cerebrum	brain
cervix	neck (*cervical* region – C1 – C8)
dura	one of the outer linings of the brain and spinal cord
encephala	brain (tissue)
epi	on top of
epidural	on top of the dura
lumbar puncture	spinal tap (taking a sample of cerebrospinal fluid for testing)
lumbar	lower back (*lumbar* region: L1–L5)
meninges	membranes covering the brain and spinal cord
neuro(n)	nerve cell
para	alongside, beyond
paraplegia	paralysis affecting lower half of the body
paresis	weakness

peripheral nerves	nerves outside of the central nervous system (i.e. **not** in brain and spinal cord)
plegia	paralysis
quadri	four (4)
quadriplegia	paralysis affecting four limbs
sacrum	tailbone (sacral region: S1–S5)
spina	backbone, spine
sub	under
subdural	under the dura
tetra	four (4)
thorax	chest (thoracic region: T1–T12)
vertebra	(plural: vertebrae) one of many bones forming the backbone

2.   Anatomy of the CNS

The CNS consists of the brain and the spinal cord.

2.1   The brain

Structures inside the brain include the cerebrum, cerebellum and ventricles.

Ventricles are chambers filled with cerebrospinal fluid inside the brain, which circulates through these ventricles and down the spinal cord.

Spaces and membranes around the brain include:

–   subarachnoid space
–   subdural space (*sub* being under the dura)
–   dura mater (*dura mater* being hard mother; where the word mother here refers to a thick membrane)
–   epidural space (*epi* being on top of)
–   meninges (outer coverings)
–   inner meninges (*pia mater* or soft mother, where the word mother refers to a thick membrane)
–   middle meninges

2.2   The spinal cord

The function of the spinal cord is to transmit messages from the body to the CNS and vice versa, including reflexes. The spinal cord is enclosed by the vertebral canal or spinal canal (behind the vertebral column).

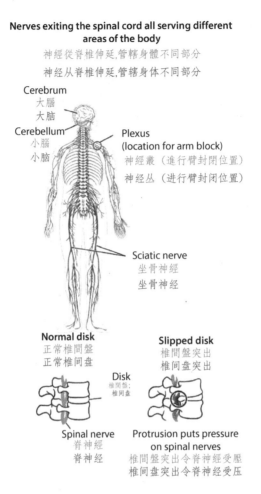

Nerves exiting the spinal cord all serving different areas of the body

神經從脊椎伸延,管轄身體不同部分

神经从脊椎伸延,管辖身体不同部分

Cerebrum
大腦
大脑

Cerebellum
小腦
小脑

Plexus
(location for arm block)
神經叢（進行臂封閉位置）
神经丛（进行臂封闭位置）

Sciatic nerve
坐骨神經
坐骨神经

Normal disk
正常椎間盤
正常椎间盘

Slipped disk
椎間盤突出
椎间盘突出

Disk
椎間盤;
椎间盘

Spinal nerve
脊神經
脊神经

Protrusion puts pressure
on spinal nerves
椎間盤突出令脊神經受壓
椎间盘突出令脊神经受压

Figure 17.1 Spinal nerves
脊神經
脊神经

3. Function of the CNS

The CNS has two main functions: firstly it stimulates movement, and secondly it maintains normal body balance and health (e.g. breathing, digestion, blood pressure, temperature).

These two functions are achieved through the millions of nerve cells that make up the CNS. These nerve cells pass signals (information) to each other in two directions, from the CNS to the body (down the spinal cord and along the "peripheral nerves") and from the body to the CNS (along the peripheral nerves and up the spinal cord).

The CNS also involves hormonal messengers, which are covered in Chapter 25 (endocrinology).

A number of things can go wrong in the transmission of signals from one nerve cell to the other. Most nerve cells have very long arms called *axons*. The axons are protected by myelin, a sort of rolled-up pancake-like sheath. If the myelin gets inflamed (as in multiple sclerosis) and/or damaged, nerve signals cannot be transmitted.

In other illnesses (e.g. Parkinson's disease), there is something wrong with the "transmission fluid" in the space between the nerve cells which stops signals from being properly transmitted.

When people break their neck or back (backbone) and the spinal cord (the bundles of nerves going down the backbone) is damaged, they may be paralyzed as a result, because signals from the brain to the muscles can no longer be transmitted. Likewise, signals to do with sensation and pain can no longer be transmitted to the brain.

4. Health professionals

Neurologist – physician specializing in disorders of the nervous system.
Neurosurgeon – surgeon specializing in surgery involving the nervous system.

5. Disorders of the nervous system

Some common disorders affecting the central and peripheral nervous systems are:

1. *Alzheimer's disease* – see dementia below.

2. *Brain tumor* – Any growth in the brain. Tumors can cause pressure and interfere with normal brain activity. A brain tumor can be benign (not cancerous) or malignant (consisting of cancer cells).

Causes: 20–40% of brain tumors are secondary to cancers elsewhere in the body (e.g. breast, lung, stomach, bowel, kidney or melanoma). Associated factors may include exposure to vinyl chloride and immunosuppressant drugs.

Symptoms: Headaches, nausea, vomiting, seizures, loss of movement or sensation, changes to eyesight, sometimes personality changes.

Diagnostic tests: Brain scan (i.e. CAT/MRI/PET scan) and/or biopsy through craniotomy (making an opening in the skull).

Treatment: Surgery and/or radiation therapy. Note: chemotherapy is not an option due to the blood-brain barrier (the barrier between the blood circulation and the circulation of cerebrospinal fluid), which inhibits treatment effects.

3. *Cerebral palsy* – A group of disorders affecting the CNS, creating mild to severe problems with motor control.

Causes: Damage to motor areas in the developing brain occur during pregnancy, at birth or not long after birth, due to a lack of (or low levels of) oxygen or infection (e.g. rubella).

Symptoms: Floppy muscles, young babies sitting and walking late, *scissors gait* when walking, involuntary movements of face and hands, slurred speech spastic finger Movements, problems seeing/hearing.

Treatment: Physical therapy; braces, crutches or wheelchairs; speech therapy; surgery; muscle relaxants; anti-convulsants.

4. *Coma* – A state of deep unconsciousness making a patient unable to communicate/respond to any stimuli.

Causes: Brain injury, stroke, poisoning, bleeding into the brain, brain tumor, and many other possible reasons.

5. *Cerebrovascular accident (CVA) or stroke* – A incident affecting the blood vessels in the brain.

Causes: A CVA can be caused by either a bleed (brain *hemorrhage*) or a lage blood clot (*embolism*) in the arteries which bring oxygen to the brain.

Symptoms: This depends on which part of the brain is affected by not receiving enough oxygen. The CVA can affect the motor center (which sends signals to the muscles), which can result in hemiparesis (weakness down one side of the body) or hemiparalysis (paralysis down one side of the body). In other cases, the speech center may be affected, which affects the person's ability to speak and understand language (aphasia). The CVA is often preceded by a TIA (transient ischemic attack) or warning stroke.

Treatment: Physical therapy; occupational therapy; speech therapy; drugs to dissolve clots or to prevent further clotting (if the CVA was caused by a blood clot); sometimes *endarterectomy* surgery to open up the carotid arteries, if these are narrowed/blocked.

6. *Dementia* – This involves parts of the brain associated with memory, learning and decision-making which no longer function properly. There are different forms of dementia, including Alzheimer's disease (large percentage of cases), Lewy body dementia and multi-infarct dementia.

Causes: Dementia can be due to conditions like Parkinson's or Huntington's, which cause a loss of brain cells, but can also be due to multiple small infarcts in the brain; alcohol or drug abuse; head injury; lack of certain B Vitamins; anemia; brain tumors; or infections (e.g. AIDS, Creutzfeldt-Jakob's disease).

Symptoms: Memory loss (especially short term memory), confusion, disorientation, personality changes, loss of social skills.

Treatment: Some types of dementia can be treated by treating the cause (e.g. benign brain tumor, lack of Vitamin B12); other forms cannot currently be treated, but research on prevention continues.

7.   *Epilepsy* – Sudden bursts of electrical activity in the brain.
Epilepsy involves sudden and recurrent seizures and is thought to affect 1–2% of the population.

There are many different subtypes of epilepsy, all characterized by a lack of control on the part of the person having the episode. Some subtypes are broadly classified as focal seizures or partial seizures, which affect just one part of the brain. The person may experience strange sensations or movements, and partial seizures may become generalized. Generalized seizures, in comparison, affect both halves of the brain. The person may lose consciousness (sometimes only very briefly).

Patients may get an aura or a feeling that they are going to have an episode.

Causes: Too much electric activity in the brain, causing brain messages to become muddled up. This can be caused by severe head injuries, CVA, a brain tumor, chemical imbalances, infection in the brain, genetic conditions and drug abuse. If the cause of the epilepsy is known, we talk about symptomatic epilepsy, if there is no known cause we talk about idiopathic epilepsy.

Symptoms: These can vary from person to person, depending on the type of episode. Symptoms may include seizures (formerly called fits), loss of consciousness and incontinence, clenching teeth, being mentally *absent* for a very short while, picking at clothes, staring into space, clenching fists, smacking lips.

Diagnostic tests: An EEG, which records the electrical activity of the brain.

Treatment: Anti-epileptic drugs; some patients have a support dog (seizure-alert dog), which can sense an oncoming episode and can warn the person so they are able to get themselves into a safe place before an episode.

8.   *Guillain Barré syndrome* – see Chapter 22.

9.   *Hemorrhage* – Blood "bursting forth"
This is bleeding from a ruptured blood vessel into the brain, or into the space surrounding the brain. The bleeding leads to increased pressure on the brain, and the patient may lose consciousness or go into a coma. Sometimes premature babies also bleed into the brain, which may cause brain damage or cerebral palsy.

Sites of bleeding can include: *subdural* (often slow, signs may occur days after the accident; subdural bleeds are very dangerous for this reason, as some may die unexpectedly); *epidural* (often arterial, signs will develop very quickly); *arachnoid* (congenital malformation of blood vessels in the brain), and *cerebral* (in the brain itself).

Causes: Brain injury, high blood pressure, aneurysm (weakening in blood vessel), blood vessel abnormality, bleeding disorder, brain tumor, liver problem (affecting the blood's ability to clot).

Symptoms: Severe headache, loss of consciousness.

Diagnostic tests: CT scan, cranial ultrasound.

Treatment: Often neurosurgical to relieve pressure on the brain.

10.   *Headache* – Pain in the head

Causes: Headaches can have many different causes. Some of the more common causes are muscle tension (tension headache), migraines (see below) or cluster headaches (these come in clusters followed by long headache-free periods). Hangover headaches are caused by dehydration when a person has drunk too much alcohol. Some causes may be extra-cranial (such as infection of the eyes/ears/sinuses, influenza or tension), or intra-cranial (such as tumors, meningitis or damage (e.g. swelling) to the brain).

Diagnostic tests: History, imaging.

Symptoms: Throbbing, pounding or dull pain in the head, depending on the cause.

Treatment: Muscle relaxants, painkillers.

11.   *Meningitis* – An infection/inflammation of the membranes protecting the brain and spinal cord. Meningitis can cause deafness, brain damage, and life-threatening septic shock if caused by bacteria which multiply rapidly.

Causes: Bacterial or viral infection (e.g. through cup sharing).

Symptoms: Headache, neck stiffness, fever, chills, rash (small spots of bleeding under the skin), drowsiness, nausea, vomiting, child screams when legs are lifted for diaper change (pulling on meninges).

Diagnostic tests: Lumbar puncture to test cerebrospinal fluid.

Treatment: Immediate high-dose antibiotics for bacterial meningitis to prevent septic shock.

12.   *Migraine* – A throbbing headache, usually on only one side of the head.

Causes: Migraines are the end result of a chain of events in the brain and may be triggered by certain foods (e.g. wine, chocolate, coffee), hormones, or stress, though the root cause of migraines is still unknown.

Symptoms: Sensitivity to light, nausea, vomiting. Patients may feel a migraine coming on (aura).

Treatment: Anti-migraine drugs.

13.   *Motor neuron disease* – see Chapter 22.

14.   *Multiple sclerosis (MS)* – A destruction of the protective *myelin sheaths* around the *axons* (long arms) of nerve cells, which results in nerve messages not being passed on.

Causes: Unknown, perhaps genetic predisposition and/or a virus or environmental factors. Autoimmune (the body's own immune cells attack the nervous system).

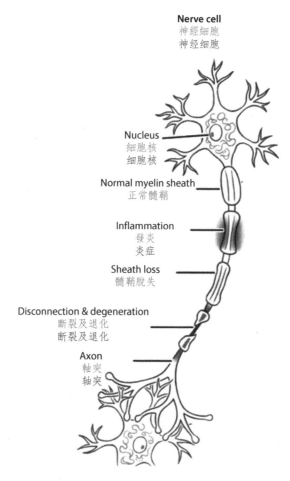

Figure 17.2 Myelin sheath
髓鞘

Symptoms: In MS, attacks alternate with remissions. The disease may lead to a progressive loss of function, which may become fatal if breathing muscles become paralyzed.

Treatment: Medication to control symptoms. Vitamin D.

15.   *Myasthenia gravis* – see Chapter 22.

16.   *Poliomyelitis* – see Chapter 22.

17.   *Parkinson's disease* – A degeneration of the *substantia nigra,* the part of the brain which controls levels of *dopamine* (a neurotransmitter), which consequently means that nerve signals cannot be transmitted properly.

Causes: Unknown.

Symptoms: Mask-like facial expression; wide-eyed, unblinking stare; drooling, open mouth; difficult to start movement; tremor (trembling hands); depression.

Treatment: Physical therapy, anti-Parkinson drugs (to encourage production of dopamine).

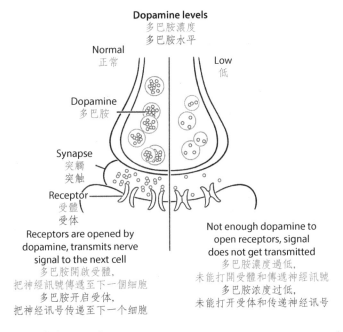

Figure 17.3 Parkinson's disease schematic
帕金森氏病圖示；柏金遜病圖示
帕金森病图示

18.   *Persistent vegetative state* – A situation in which a patient who was previously in a coma, now seems to be awake, but is not able to respond or to communicate. The patient needs to be fed and toileted.

19.   *Sciatica* – Severe pain along the sciatic nerve.

Causes: Slipped disk (see below), irritation due to osteoarthritis (wear and tear) of the vertebrae (see under bone disorders), back injuries/exertion.

Symptoms: Severe pain (sometimes also weakness) down the lower back and leg.

Diagnostic tests: X-ray, CT scan, MRI scan.

Treatment: This is dependent on cause but can include anti-inflammatory drugs, physical therapy, and surgery.

20.   *Shingles* – Inflammation of the nerves caused by the herpes zoster virus. This virus lies dormant in the body of those who have had chickenpox in the past, and is mostly seen in people over 50 years of age, those in a weakened condition due to illness, stress or poor nutrition, or in people who are immunosuppressed (have low immunity) e.g. those who are *HIV positive*.

Causes: Reawakening of the herpes zoster virus.

Symptoms: Pain, blisters and redness along the path of the nerve.

Treatment: Sometimes medication (e.g. acyclovir).

21.   *Slipped disk* – Also known as a *herniated disk, protruding disk, ruptured disk* or *prolapsed disk*. Occurs when the nucleus of an intervertebral disk pops out and presses on the spinal nerves. Can happen in the neck and lower back.

Causes: Incorrect lifting or other sudden injury.

Symptoms: Nerve pain (e.g. sciatica), pins and needles, weakness.

Diagnostic tests: MRI scan; CT scan.

Treatment: Strengthening exercises, surgery (e.g. percutaneous transforaminal endoscopic discectomy).

22.   *Spinal cord injury* – A fractured spine or broken back(bone) in which various nerves are injured and result in a loss of movement/function of parts of the body.

Causes: Typically due to an accident (e.g. being thrown clear of a car, contact sports like American football or rugby, diving into shallow water, falling from a height).

Symptoms: Loss of movement/function in the body; the degree of this loss depends on the level of the injury.

Quadriplegia – Injury to nerves which serve the body from the neck down. The patient may suffer loss of feeling/sensation and paralysis from the neck downwards; this may also affect the patient's breathing muscles.

Paraplegia – Injury to the nerves which serve the lower half of the body. The patient may suffer loss of feeling/sensation and paralysis from the middle of the body down.

Treatment: Wheelchair with/without neck brace, physical therapy for passive movements to prevent contractures; may need in-dwelling catheter; pressure area care to prevent pressure sores.

23.   *Syphilis* – A venereal disease (sexually transmitted disease) which eventually attacks the central nervous system.

Causes: Sex with an infected person.

Symptoms: There are three stages and related signs: (1) chancre, open sore (2) joint aches, rash (latent stage, positive Wassermann blood test), and (3) organ deterioration. We speak of neurosyphilis when the illness has affected the central nervous system, with symptoms possibly including meningitis, memory loss, loss of coordination, personality changes.

Treatment: Antibiotics (also given to all (former) sexual partners).

24.   *Whiplash* – Also referred to as *cervical acceleration deceleration (CAD)*, is an injury of the neck which occurs when the head snaps forwards and then back very fast, such as in a car accident.

Causes: A very sudden snapping movement of the head.

Symptoms: Headaches, pain in shoulders, pins and needles in arms.

Treatment: Depending on severity may include NSAIDS, muscle relaxants, cervical collar, physical therapy, cervical traction.

6.   Some common medications

analgesics	pain killers
anticonvulsants or anti-epileptic drugs	sometimes used as tranquilizers
hypnotics	sleeping medications
muscle relaxants	reduce pain by relaxing tense muscles
psychotropics	have an effect on the mind
sedatives	calming medications

7. Some common tests

- *CT scan* – Computed tomography scan using radiation to produce clear "sliced"
- images of a certain part of the body.
- *EEG* – Electroencephalography, in which leads are attached to the head to test the electrical activity of the brain.
- *Lumbar puncture* – Procedure in which CSF (cerebrospinal fluid) is collected for testing from the lumbar region under local anesthetic using a hollow needle and syringe.
- *Spinal tap* – See lumbar puncture.
- *MRI scan* – Type of scan which uses magnetic fields to produce very clear images

8. English-Chinese glossary

英漢詞彙表

English	Hong Kong & Taiwan	Mainland China
AIDS	後天免疫力缺乏症; 愛滋病	后天免疫缺乏综合症; 艾滋病
Alzheimer's disease	認知障礙症; 腦退化症	阿尔茨海默氏病
analgesic	止痛劑	止痛药; 镇痛药
aneurysm	動脈瘤	动脉瘤
anticonvulsants; antiepileptic drugs	抗抽搐劑; 抗痙攣劑; 抗癲癇藥	抗惊厥药; 抗癫痫药
aphasia	失語	失语 (症)
axon	軸突	轴突
benign tumor	良性腫瘤	良性瘤
blood clot; embolism	血凝塊; 栓塞	血 (凝) 块; 栓塞
blood vessels	血管	血管
braces	支架	支架
brain injury	腦損傷	脑损伤
brain scan	腦掃描	脑扫描
brain tumor	腦腫瘤	脑肿瘤
carotid arteries	頸動脈	颈动脉
CAT	電腦軸向斷層掃描	CAT扫描; 计算机轴位体层摄影术
central nervous system (CNS)	中樞神經系統	中枢神经系统
cerebellum	小腦	小脑
cerebral palsy	大腦麻痹	脑性麻痹
cerebrovascular accident (CVA); stroke	腦血管破裂; 腦栓塞; 腦中風; 中風	中风; 脑卒中

(Continued)

English	Hong Kong & Taiwan	Mainland China
cerebrospinal/Cerebral spinal fluid (CSF)	腦脊髓液	脑脊髓液
cerebrum	大腦	大脑
cervical traction	頸椎牽引	(头) 颈牵引
chancre; open sore	下疳	下疳
chemotherapy	化學療法; 化療	化学疗法; 化学治疗; 化疗
chickenpox	水痘	水痘
clenching teeth	磨牙	磨牙
clots	(血) 凝塊	血块
cluster headache	叢集性頭痛; 群發性頭痛	丛集性头痛; 群发性头痛
coma	昏迷	昏迷
contracture	攣縮	挛缩
craniotomy	顱骨切開術	开颅术; 颅骨切开术
crutches	拐杖	(支撑) 拐
dementia	腦退化症; 失智症; 癡呆症	痴呆症
disk	椎間盤	椎间盘
dopamine	多巴胺	多巴胺
dura mater	腦硬膜	硬 (脑) 膜
electroencephalography (EEG)	腦電圖	脑电图
endarterectomy	動脈內膜切除術	动脉内膜剥除术
endoscopic discectomy	內窺鏡椎間盤切除術	经皮椎间盘切除术
epidural space	硬膜外隙	硬膜外腔; 硬膜外隙
epilepsy	癲癇症	癫痫症; 羊癫疯; 羊角风
hemiparalysis	偏癱; 半身不遂; 半身癱瘓	偏瘫; 半身不遂
hemiparesis	輕偏癱	轻偏瘫
herniated disk (slipped disk, ruptured disk, prolapsed disk)	椎間盤脫出 (椎間盤滑出); 椎間盤破裂; 椎間盤突出)	椎间盘脱出 (椎间盘滑出; 椎间盘破裂; 椎间盘突出)
HIV (human immunodeficiency virus)	人類免疫力缺乏病毒; 愛滋病病毒	人类免疫缺陷病毒; 艾滋病病毒
Huntington's disease	舞蹈症	亨延顿 (氏) 舞蹈病
hypnotics	安 (催) 眠藥	安眠药; 催眠药
idiopathic epilepsy	原發性癲 (羊) 癇	特发性癫痫; 原发性癫痫
immunity	免疫力	免疫; 免疫力
immunosuppressed	免疫抑制	免疫抑制
indwelling catheter	保留性導管	留置导管
incontinence	失禁	失禁

(Continued)

English	Hong Kong & Taiwan	Mainland China
inner meninges (pia mater)	內腦脊膜 (軟腦膜)	内脑膜 (软脑膜)
level of consciousness (LOC)	清醒程度	意识水平; 神志清醒程度
Lewy body dementia	利維體認知障礙症	路维小体痴呆症
lumbar puncture	腰椎穿刺 (抽腦脊液)	腰椎穿刺 (术)
malignant tumor	惡性腫瘤	恶性肿瘤
meninges	腦脊髓膜	脑脊 (髓) 膜
middle meninges	中腦脊髓膜	中脑脊 (髓) 膜
migraines	偏頭痛	偏头痛
MRI	磁力共振掃描	磁 (性) 共振成像; 磁振造影扫描
multi-infarct dementia	多發梗塞性腦退化症	多 (发) 梗塞性痴呆
multiple sclerosis	多發性硬化症	多发性 (脑脊髓) 硬化 (症)
muscle relaxants	肌肉鬆馳劑	肌松药; 肌肉松弛药
myasthenia gravis	重症肌無力	重症肌无力 (症)
myelin	髓鞘質; 髓磷脂	髓磷脂; 髓鞘; 髓脂质
Neurologist	神經科醫生; 腦科醫生	神经科医生
Neurosurgeon	神經外科醫生; 腦外科醫生	神经外科医师
neurosyphilis	神經梅毒	神经梅毒
neurotransmitter	神經遞質	神经递质; 神经介质
nonsteroidal antiinflammatory drug (NSAID)	非類固醇類消炎止痛藥	非甾体抗炎药物; 非类固醇抗炎药物
osteoarthritis	骨關節炎	骨关节炎
paraplegia	截癱; 下肢癱瘓	截瘫; 下身麻痹
Parkinson's disease	柏金遜症; 帕金森氏症	帕金森 (氏) 病
percutaneous	穿皮的; 經皮的	经皮肤的; 透皮肤的
peripheral nerves	週邊神經	周边神经
peripheral nervous system	週邊神經系統	周边神经系统; 末梢神经系统; 外周神经系统
persistent vegetative state	持續陷於植物狀態; 植物人	持续性植物状态; 植物人
PET scan	正電子掃描	PET扫描; 正电子发射断层扫描
physiotherapy	物理治療	理疗; 物理治疗
plexus	神經叢	神经丛
poliomyelitis	脊髓灰質炎; 小兒麻痺症	脊髓灰质炎; 小儿麻痹 (症)
psychotropics	精神藥物	精神药物
quadriplegia	四肢癱瘓; 四癱 (又稱全癱)	四肢瘫痪
radiotherapy	放射治療	放射治疗
reflexes	神經反射	神经反射

(Continued)

English	Hong Kong & Taiwan	Mainland China
rubella	風疹	风疹
sciatic nerve	坐骨神經	坐骨神经
sciatica	坐骨神經痛	坐骨神经痛
scissors gait	剪刀步	剪刀步态
sedatives	鎮靜藥; 鎮靜劑	镇静药; 镇静剂
seizures	抽筋; 癲癇發作	抽搐; 癫痫发作
sexually transmitted disease	性 (接觸) 傳染病; 性病	性传染疾病; 性传播疾病
shingles (Herpes zoster)	帶狀疱疹 (俗稱「生蛇」)	带状疱疹
slipped disk	椎間盤突出	椎间盘突出
slurred speech	言語不清	言语不清
spastic finger movements	手指抽搐	手指抽搐
speech therapy	言語治療	言语治疗
spinal cord	脊髓	脊髓
spinal cord injury	脊髓創傷	脊髓损伤
spinal nerves	脊椎神經	脊椎神经
spinal tap	脊椎穿刺; 抽脊椎液	脊椎穿刺; 脊椎抽液
stroke	中風	中风; 脑卒中
subarachnoid space	蜘蛛膜下腔	蛛网膜下腔
subdural space	硬膜下腔	硬膜下腔; 硬膜下隙
symptomatic epilepsy	症狀性癲癇 (症)	症状性癫痫
synapse	突觸 (兩個神經原的相接處)	突触
syphilis	梅毒	梅毒
tension headache	緊張頭痛	紧张性头痛
transforaminal	經椎間孔	经椎间孔
transient ischemic attack (TIA)	短暫性腦缺血	短暂性缺血发作
venereal disease	性病; 花柳病	性病; 花柳病
ventricles	腦室	脑室
vertebral column	脊柱	脊柱
vertebral canal	椎管	椎管
wheelchair	輪椅	轮椅
whiplash; cervical acceleration decelaration (CAD)	揮鞭式頸部創傷 (由於突然加速或減速的活動, 令頸部有如鞭子般抽動造成的傷害)	急性颈扭伤; 颈加速伸展性损伤

Summary of main points

This chapter has given a brief overview of neurology, including:

- a brief overview of anatomy
- terms with Latin and Greek roots
- health professionals involved
- some commonly encountered conditions relating to the nervous system, together with common diagnostic tests and treatment methods

Conditions affecting the nervous systems can affect level of consciousness (LOC), speech, perception, sensation and movement among others.

Chapter 18

Cardiology

Heart and the circulatory system

The heart is one of the most vital organs in the body (the other two being the brain and the lungs). When the heart stops, circulation stops, and the body's tissues do not receive any more oxygen. Tissue death will start after 5 minutes.

People who suffer a cardiac arrest (when the heart stops beating) are increasingly at risk of brain damage if their heart does not start pumping again within 5 minutes. For this reason cardiopulmonary resuscitation (CPR), which is a combination of artificial respiration and heart massage, is very important.

In order to gain a better understanding of the heart and how it works, it is good to have a look at the heart's structure and function. Firstly, though, let us look at the Latin and Greek roots for related terminology.

1. Terms with Latin and Greek roots

angiography	X-ray examination of the blood vessels, using a radio-opaque fluid which is injected into the blood stream
angioplasty	blood vessel repair, using a thin cardiac catheter with a balloon (and a stent) on it
arrhythmia	irregular heart beat (literally: no-rhythm)
card/cardio	heart
cardiac catheterization	examination of the heart by introducing a thin catheter into an artery and passing it into the coronary arteries
cardiac surgeon	heart surgeon
cardiologist	doctor specializing in the heart
cardiology	special branch of medicine dealing with the heart
cardiomegaly	enlargement of the heart (megalos: big)
cardioversion	an electric shock delivered to the heart to stop abnormal heart rhythms, in the hope that the heart's own pacemaker (the sinus node, see below) will become the pacemaker again and the heart will get back to "sinus rhythm."
carditis	inflammation of the heart (*itis*: inflammation)
chemical cardioversion	attempts to restore normal heart rhythm by administering medication

coronary	like a crown (corona: crown)
coronary artery	artery which takes blood rich in oxygen to the heart muscle itself
Coronary Care Unit or CCU	special care unit for patients with heart problems
cyanosis	looking blue due to lack of oxygen (cyan: blue)
defibrillator	machine for applying electrical shocks to the heart to stop fibrillations (abnormal heart rhythms) or to "jump start" the heart again
EKG or ECG	electrocardiogram, a procedure used to measure the electrical activity of the heart muscle
endocarditis	inflammation of the inner lining of the heart (endo: inside)
fibrillations	irregular heart rhythm where the heart is not contracting properly (a bit like quivering)
infarction	death/damage due to lack of oxygen
ischemic	no blood (i.e. no oxygen)
myocardial	heart muscle (myo: muscle)
myocarditis	inflammation of the heart muscle
palpitations	fluttering of the heart, abnormal heart rate or abnormal heart rhythm
radio-opaque	chemical compound that resists radiation and becomes highly visible in X-rays (so blood vessels filled with the dye show up on X-rays)
sinus rhythm	heart rhythm originating in the sinus node, the natural pacemaker of the heart
thoracic surgeon	surgeon who operates on the thorax (chest)

2. Anatomy of the heart

The heart consists of four compartments or chambers. The top two chambers are called the *atria*, atrium being the Latin word for the vestibule or ante-chamber where people used to wait before being admitted to the main room. The lower two chambers are called the *ventricles*.

There are valves between the atria and the ventricles. The valve between the right atrium and the right ventricle is called the *tricuspid* valve, because it has three (*tri*) leaves. The valve between the left atrium and the left ventricle is called the *mitral* valve, because it has two leaves and looks like a bishop's hat (*miter*).

The heart has two other valves: one valve between the left ventricle and the aorta (called the *aortic* valve), and the other between the right ventricle and the pulmonary artery (called the *pulmonary* valve). Memory aid: mitraL – Left; tRicuspid – Right.

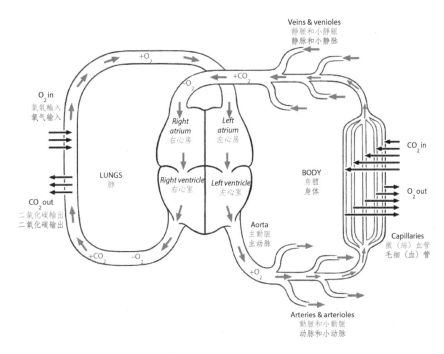

Figure 18.1 Schematic representation of the heart
心臟圖示
心脏图示

Note: Figure 18.1 is a schematic diagram only and not a picture of what the heart really looks like.

3.   Function of the heart

The heart's function is to supply the body with oxygenated blood full of nutrients, and to remove de-oxygenated blood full of waste products from cell metabolism.

The heart pumps blood full of oxygen into the aorta. The aorta branches off into arteries which supply various organs and areas of the body. Arteries are strong, elastic, muscular blood vessels, as they have to withstand high pressure.

Arteries branch off into *arterioles* and finally into *capillaries*, the smallest blood vessels in the body. Oxygen is supplied to the tissues, and the tissues in turn dump their "waste" into the bloodstream.

The capillaries change into small veins, which drain into venioles. Veins contain blood which is low in oxygen (*de-oxygenated*) and which contains various waste products. Veins direct this blood to the right atrium of the heart. This blood goes through the lungs to pick up new oxygen for delivery around the body.

The blood passes from the right atrium through the first valve (tricuspid valve) into the right ventricle. From there it passes through the pulmonary valve into the pulmonary artery into the lungs.

Blood rich in oxygen (*oxygenated*) leaves the lungs and flows into the left atrium. From the left atrium it goes through the mitral valve, into the left ventricle. From the left ventricle, the blood is pumped through the aortic valve into the aorta, for delivery around the body.

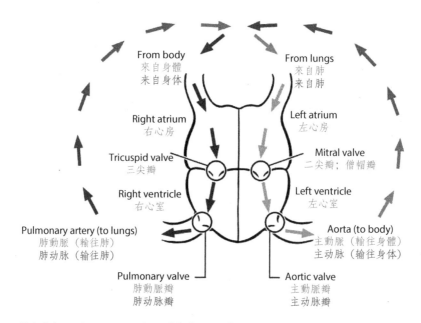

Figure 18.2 Schematic representation of the heart valves
心瓣圖示
心瓣图示

The heart = pump, pumps blood around the body and around the lungs:
right atrium → (tricuspid) valve → right ventricle → (pulmonary) valve →
pulmonary artery/lung →artery → blood to lungs →
→ oxygen in/CO_2 out → to left atrium → (mitral) valve → left ventricle →
→ aortic valve → aorta → arteries → small arteries → capillaries →

oxygen out and CO_2 in, nutrients and wastes exchanged – *you may compare this to a truck doing deliveries to individual houses and picking up their waste for taking to the dump.*
→ small veins → large veins (venioles) → large vein → right
atrium of heart → right ventricle → lungs → heart → body → heart →
lungs → heart → body → heart → and so on…

In addition to the various organs and body tissues that require oxygen to function, the heart muscle itself also needs oxygen to function properly. The very first arteries to branch off the aorta are called the *coronary* arteries because they run around the heart, as if forming a crown (*corona* means crown). It is these coronary arteries that bring blood that is rich in oxygen to the heart muscle itself.

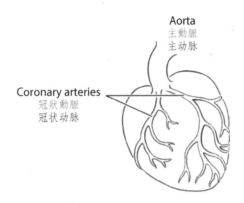

Figure 18.3 Heart and coronary arteries
心臟與冠狀動脈
心脏与冠状动脉

4. Health professionals

Cardiologist – physician specializing in heart disorders
Cardiac surgeon – surgeon specializing in heart surgery
Cardiothoracic surgeon – surgeon specializing in heart and lung surgery

5. Disorders of the heart

Broadly speaking, heart problems can be classified into four main types:

1. *Problems with the coronary arteries*
This affects oxygen supply to the heart muscle and is often referred to as coronary artery disease (CAD) (formerly known as ischemic heart disease; *ischemic* literally means no blood). Obviously a lack of blood equals a lack of oxygen supply, and without oxygen the heart muscle cannot do its job.

In people with CAD there is damage to, or narrowing of, the coronary arteries which supply the heart muscle with blood. As a result, the heart muscle does not get enough oxygen, resulting in chest pain. This chest pain is known as *angina pectoris*, literally meaning a "tightening of the chest."

Patients may have chronic and ongoing CAD, but they may also present with acute coronary syndrome (ACS), i.e. with acute coronary artery problems such as heart attacks (myocardial infarctions),unstable angina, or even sudden cardiac death (SCD), due to sudden cardiac arrest (SCA). This is discussed further below.

2.   *Problems with the heart valves*
People may be born with valve defects or may develop problems with their heart valves following infections somewhere else in the body. When heart valves start to leak, doctors will hear an abnormal heart sound called a murmur, which may be a sign that blood is leaking back (*regurgitation*). Leaky valves may lead to an enlarged heart and heart failure, depending on the valves involved and on what caused the leaky valve. Heart valves can now be replaced through non-invasive procedures, (balloon valvuloplasty) although some surgeons still prefer open heart surgery.

3.   *Problems with the heart's role as a pump*
People may develop problems with their heart not being able to pump blood efficiently anymore. This is known as heart failure. Patients often experience shortness of breath and swelling of the ankles. See page 223 for more information.

4.   *Problems with conduction of electrical activity in the heart*
So, how does the heart muscle know when to contract? The heart is self-sufficient. The *sinoatrial* node (SA node), the heart's own pacemaker found at the top of the right atrium, gives the signal. The SA node sends an electrical impulse directly to the *atrioventricular node* (or AV node), which sends a message to the atria to contract. The signal then passes through the *septum*, the central heart wall dividing the heart into left and right. The two branches branching off into the left and the right side of the heart then spread the message into the ventricle muscle, which synchronizes a ventricular contraction, making both ventricles contract simultaneously.

6.   Some common disorders of the heart

1.   *Acute Coronary Syndrome (ACS)* – ACS can relate to either unstable angina (see angina below) or a heart attack.

Causes: See angina and myocardial infarction.

Symptoms: See angina and heart attack.

Diagnostic tests: Blood test to look for elevated levels of cardiac enzymes, which signal major damage to the heart muscle (these would not be present in unstable angina or non-STEMI heart attacks).

Treatment: Doctors will diagnose whether ACS patients are experiencing unstable angina or a heart attack, and if a heart attack, what kind of heart attack they are having i.e. STEMI or non-STEMI. Please see heart attack below.

2.   *Angina* – From *angina pectoris,* meaning "tightening of the chest." Angina occurs when there is narrowing of the coronary arteries. As a result, the arteries cannot supply the heart muscle with enough oxygen, especially during exertion. This results in chest pain.

Doctors distinguish between stable angina and unstable angina. In unstable angina there are unstable plaques in the walls of the arteries which may break off and cause a blockage of the artery without warning, e.g. at rest or at night. In stable angina, there are partial blockages of the arteries, but they are stable. Stable angina is more common and is also (as the name suggests) more predictable in that the pain usually comes on with physical exertion or emotional stress.

Unstable angina is less common, less predictable and more dangerous, as platelets can suddenly collect on existing plaques in the walls of the arteries. Unstable angina can be the cause of sudden death through a heart attack.

Causes: Being overweight or obese, diabetes, high blood cholesterol, smoking, lack of exercise, "predisposition" through family history.

Symptoms: Stable angina: Pain or tightness in the chest, especially on exertion or following a heavy meal, or when stepping out into the cold. *Unstable angina:* Pain or tightness in the chest at rest or at night.

Diagnostic tests: ECG (EKG), exercise tolerance test (ETT) or stress test, blood tests, angiography; Cardiac CT.

Treatment: Medication (sprayed under the tongue, it helps to open up the coronary arteries so more oxygen can be supplied to the heart), oxygen, coronary artery by-pass surgery, angioplasty using either a balloon or a stent (which is a small mesh tube used to keep the artery open), medications to stabilize the plaques in the walls of the coronary arteries, cholesterol control (by diet or medication or both).

3.   *Conduction problems* – Occurs when the heart's electrical signal is not conducted properly.

Causes: This may be caused by an:

–   *Incomplete heart block*
–   *Complete heart block*
–   *Heart flutter*

There are different types of heart flutter:

1.   *Atrial flutter:* Heart beats at 240–360 beats per minute. Caused by damaged heart muscle.

2.   *Atrial fibrillation (AF)* involves very fast atrial contractions resulting in the heart being unable to pump properly. AF patients are at risk of complications associated with clots which can form in the atrium and travel around the body, causing embolisms, thrombosis or a stroke.

3.   *Ventricular fibrillation* is where the heart is not pumping, only quivering, so there is no circulation, and this leads to death. Ventricular fibrillation is very dangerous because it usually leads to cardiac arrest, in which the heart stops completely.

Treatment: Atrial flutter and atrial fibrillation treatment includes cardioversion, medications (e.g. amiodarone, digoxin), and anti-clotting treatments. For ventricular fibrillation, CPR is performed (a combination of artificial respiration, either mouth to mouth or with an ambu bag, and heart massage), and a defibrillator may be used (two *paddles* are placed on the chest and a shock is delivered) to try and get the heart's own pacemaker (the SA node) working again and the heart pumping in normal sinus rhythm again.

4.   *Congenital heart defects* – Heart disorders that children are born with. Septal defects or a "hole in the heart" are probably the most common, being caused by an opening in the wall (septum) between the heart chambers. An atrial septal defect (ASD[1]) is a hole between the atria. A ventricular septal defect (VSD) is a hole between the ventricles. In ASD, blood which is high in oxygen flows through the hole in the wall between the atria from left to right atrium. As a result, blood which is high in oxygen is mixed with blood which is low in oxygen and this mixing of blood increases the blood flow back to the lungs. The increased blood flow causes a swishing sound, which can be heard as a heart murmur. In VSD, blood which is high in oxygen keeps passing through the hole in the wall from the left ventricle back into the right ventricle. As in ASD, blood which is high in oxygen is mixed with blood which is low in oxygen and this mixing of blood increases the blood flow back to the lungs. The increased blood flow causes a swishing sound, which doctors refer to as a heart murmur.

Causes: There are a number of congenital heart defects, ranging from single conditions such as patent ductus arteriosus (PDA – see Chapter 13), ASD and VSD, to complex heart defects such as transposition of the great arteries (TGA), and tetralogy of Fallot (TOF) (which includes a narrow pulmonary valve, a hole in the wall, an overriding aorta as well as hypertrophy of the right ventricle), double outlet right ventricle or DORV (where the aorta comes out of the right ventricle), valve atresia

---

1.   not to be confused with Autism Spectrum Disorder(ASD).

(valve narrowing or blockage), AV canal defects (combination of septum defects and valve problems).

Symptoms: Very often one of the first things that nurses and parents notice is that the baby looks "dusky" and seems out of breath when feeding. In ASD the baby will be tired and not feeding well, and as a result will not be growing well either. The baby may also have frequent chest colds. In VSD the baby may have fast, shallow breathing, frequent chest colds and sweating; may not be feeding well and/or growing normally, and may be irritable.

Treatments: There is a lot of excellent material (including animations) on congenital heart defects available on the internet. Surgical techniques are continually being improved and updated.

*Please note the abbreviation ASD may also be used to refer to autism spectrum disorder, so please double check before interpreting or translating this abbreviation.

5.   *Congestive heart failure,* also called *heart failure* – Occurs as a result of faulty pump action in which the heart cannot pump sufficient blood and oxygen around the body to meet the body's needs.

Causes: Previous heart attack or CAD, or heart valve problems.

Symptoms: Due to this faulty pump action, some body parts do not get enough oxygen and/or retain fluid. This fluid retention may show in swollen ankles and shortness of breath (fluid retained in blood vessels in the lungs). Some patients may have to sleep sitting up, to avoid shortness of breath at night; some are short of breath when speaking.

Treatment: Medication including anti-arrhythmic drugs to help maintain normal heart rhythm, diuretics to get rid of excess fluid, and drugs to strengthen the heart muscle. Low-salt and low-fat diets are also prescribed, as well as fluid restriction to avoid overloading the heart. Exercise will maintain fitness and health.

6.   *Myocardial infarction (MI) or heart attack* – Occurs when there is a partial or complete blockage of a coronary artery, which can lead to part of the heart muscle being starved of oxygen and dying. Doctors currently distinguish between two types of MIs, the more "common" ST segment elevation myocardial infarction (STEMI) and the less common non-STEMI. In a STEMI, the coronary artery is completely blocked by a blood clot, and a large part of the heart muscle will start to die. This means the heart cannot pump anymore and the patient may die quite suddenly. In a non-STEMI there are unstable plaques in the walls of the coronary artery, and platelets are collecting and sticking to this plaque. As a result, the coronary artery becomes partly blocked.

Because there is less damage to the heart muscle, the heart can continue to pump adequately, which means there is less risk of sudden death.

Causes: Blockage of an already narrowed coronary artery by a *thrombus* (clot) or by a plaque which has broken off from the wall of the artery. Damage to the arteries can

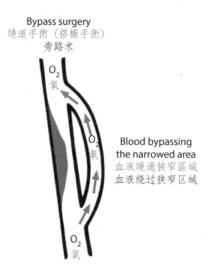

Figure 18.4 Coronary Artery Bypass Graft (CABG)
冠狀動脈繞道手術（搭橋手術）
冠状动脉旁路（搭桥）手术

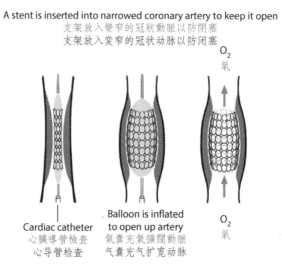

Figure 18.5 Stent in coronary artery
冠狀動脈內支架
冠状动脉内支架

be caused by high blood cholesterol levels (blood fats), smoking, diabetes, high blood pressure, predisposition through family history, gum disease (*gingivitis*). lack of physical activity, stress and obesity.

Symptoms: Shortness of breath, a crushing feeling in the chest which *radiates* to arms and/or jaw. Note: some people only have pain in their arms, either left or right.
Diagnostic tests: 12-lead-EKG or ECG, 5-lead EKG or ECG, angiography. An elevated CPK (creatine phosphokinase) in a blood test may indicate damage to the heart muscle. Other enzyme values may also go up after a heart attack.

Treatment: Depends on the type of heart attack. If the EKG shows ST elevation, there is a big blood clot that needs to be dissolved because it is completely blocking a coronary artery. If there is no ST elevation, there are plaques in the wall of the coronary artery that need to be stabilized to prevent them from causing further blockages. Treatment also includes managing several possible complications, including cardiac arrest (heart stops because heart muscle is so damaged that it cannot contract anymore), systemic embolism, pulmonary edema (swelling in the lung circulation) and shock.

For STEMIs, treatment includes urgent angioplasty, clot-dissolving medications such as Streptokinase® and fibrinolytics (drugs which help to dissolve fibrinogen). Other medications include aspirin, clopidogrel, betablockers and statins (drugs that lower blood cholesterol levels). The patient may also require oxygen, cardiotonic medications (to strengthen the heart muscle), medications to stop irregular heartbeat, pain killers, sedatives, laxatives (to prevent extra strain on the heart), or a coronary artery by-pass graft (CABG). See Figure 18.4. In a CABG, a vein from the patient's legs may be used to create a bypass from the top of the aorta "downstream" past a narrowed area of the coronary artery. Implanting a stent has become a very popular procedure; stents are implanted using a heart catheter. See Figure 18.5. After discharge treatment includes a rehabilitation program involving physical therapy, gentle exercise, limiting caffeine, stopping smoking.

7. *Valve defects* – Occurs when one of the heart valves is not working properly or is damaged/narrowed so that blood leaks back (regurgitation). Valve defects can affect the mitral valve (between the left atrium and the left ventricle), the tricuspid valve (between right atrium and right ventricle), the aortic valve or the pulmonary valve. ·

Causes: Rheumatic fever, valves damaged by strep bacteria, other infections, e.g. gingivitis, high blood pressure, congenital malformation.

Symptoms: Heart murmur, sometimes same symptoms as in heart failure.

Treatment: Medication to control symptoms of heart failure, valve repair or valve replacement.

7. Some common medications

anginine	medication against angina (tablet placed under the tongue, so it can be absorbed directly into the bloodstream)
vasodilator	widens the blood vessels/arteries
antiplatelets	aspirin andclopidogrel stop platelets from sticking together
antifibrinolytics	heparin
betablockers	medication used to slow the heart so it does not have to work too hard
digoxin	drug used to strengthen the pump action of the heart (in heart failure or in problems with irregular heart beat)
diltiazem	used against angina and high blood pressure
nitrolingual spray *glyceryl trinitrate (GTN)* *spray or tablets*	medication sprayed under the tongue, where it is directly absorbed into the bloodstream; used for relief of *angina*. This is a vasodilator, making the arteries widen, resulting in more oxygen to the heart (and hence less pain)
amiodarone®	medication used to correct irregular heartbeat
diuretics	medication used to help reduce fluid retention (e.g. in patients with heart failure)
angiotensin-converting- enzyme inhibitors/ ACE inhibitors	medications used to correct hypertension. ACE inhibitors reduce the body's supply of angiotensin II. Angiotensin makes blood vessels contract and narrow.
calcium channel blockers (CCBs)	slow the movement of calcium into the cells of the heart and blood vessels. Calcium causes stronger heart contractions, so CCBs ease the heart's contraction and relax the blood vessels.
angiotensin receptor blockers (ARBs)	relax the blood vessels by blocking receptors for angiotensin

8. Some common tests

- *Blood pressure* – Blood pressure can tell the health professional a lot about the pump action of the heart. Blood pressure can be taken while the patient is sitting, lying or standing.

Blood pressure can be taken manually with a sphygmomanometer (blood pressure cuff) and stethoscope. Some departments use a cuff attached to a machine which inflates the cuff automatically every 15 or 30 minutes. The reading will show up on a screen.

- *Arterial blood pressure monitoring* – In intensive care units, blood pressure is often monitored through a line in the patient's artery (arterial line) which is connected to equipment which shows the reading up on a monitor screen.
- *Central venous pressure* – Doctors may want to monitor the central venous pressure, by inserting a special line into the neck vein or into the upper hollow vein which drains blood from the body back into the right atrium of the heart.
- *Swan Ganz catheter* – If the doctors are interested in measuring pressures in different areas in the heart, they may insert a Swan Ganz catheter in the large sub-clavian vein just above the heart to monitor these pressures and to measure cardiac output.
- *Cardiac catheter for angiography or angioplasty* – The patient is taken to the *cath lab (special area for cardiac catheterization procedures)* and *EKG* leads are attached. Then a catheter (a long narrow tube) is inserted either through the patient's artery in the left groin (if the doctors want to examine the coronary arteries) or through a vein in the left groin (if the doctors want to examine the right side of the heart and the pulmonary artery).
- The long tube is then slowly pushed up the aorta and then into the coronary arteries. The patient stays awake.
- The doctor will want to do an *angiogram* (a special X-ray of the blood-vessels) and inject some contrast dye so that he will be able to get a good picture of the blood vessels on the screen. The angiogram will show any narrowing or blockages of the arteries.

The angiogram is filmed for later study by the heart surgeon prior to surgery.

If there is narrowing in one or two arteries due to fatty deposits on the walls of the arteries, the patient may be asked to come back to the cath lab for a PTCA or angioplasty. In some cases the angioplasty is done immediately following the angiogram, but this is always discussed with the patient first.

- *PTCA* – Percutaneous (through the skin) transluminal (across the diameter of the bloodvessel) coronary (in the coronary artery) angioplasty (repairing the blood vessel).

The coronary arteries are approached with a catheter (see under cardiac catheter), which is pushed into that part of the coronary artery which is narrowed. The balloon around the catheter is then inflated to squash the fatty plaque in the artery, thus opening that part of the artery again. The EKG is watched all the time for signs that the heart muscle is suffering from a lack of oxygen.

- The stent method often helps to open up arteries for longer periods. Sometimes stents are put in areas where there is severe narrowing to open up the artery at that point. Stents are like little "mesh" tubes.
- *EKG or ECG or Electrocardiogram* – The electrical activity of the heart can be monitored by means of an EKG (a recording of the electrical activity of the heart). In a 12-lead EKG, ten electrodes are placed on the skin (six around the heart and four on arms and legs). For monitoring in a coronary care unit or for telemetry (monitoring from a distance), three or four electrodes are placed on the skin around the heart. Experienced professionals can read ECGs and tell whether everything is normal, or whether the person is suffering from certain disorders.
- *Exercise tolerance test – also called stress test or treadmill test* – ETTs are done to see how the heart copes with exercise. The patient walks on a treadmill, while the EKG leads are attached to their chest. The ETT may help the doctor to diagnose whether the patient has ischemic heart disease. As the patient continues to exert himself, the EKG may start to show signs that the patient's heart is not getting enough oxygen (so-called ischemic changes).
- *Cardiac Computerized tomography or Cardiac CT* – A scan used to create detailed images of heart and blood vessels are created, so physicians can look for calcium buildup, plaques in arterial walls, heart valve defects or other problems.

9. English-Chinese glossary

英漢詞彙表

English	Hong Kong & Taiwan	Mainland China
5-lead ECC; 5-lead EKG	五導聯心電圖	五导联心电图
ACE inhibitors	血管緊張素轉換酶抑制劑	血管紧张素转化酶抑制剂
acute coronary syndrome (ACS)	急性冠狀動脈綜合症	急性冠脉综合症
Ambu bag	安寶膠囊 (復蘇器)	安宝胶囊 (复苏器)
angina pectoris	心絞痛	心绞痛
Anginine; glyceryl trinitrate; GTN	硝酸甘油	硝酸甘油; 三硝酸甘油酯 (抗心绞痛药)
angiography	血管造影術	血管造影 (术)
angioplasty	血管成形術	血管成形术
angiotensin receptor blockers (ARBs)	血管緊張素受體對抗劑	血管紧张素受体拮抗剂
antiarrhythmic drugs	抗心律不齊藥物	抗心律失常药

(Continued)

English	Hong Kong & Taiwan	Mainland China
antifibrinolytics	抗纖維蛋白溶酶藥; 抗血栓溶解劑	抗纤维蛋白溶解药
antiplatelets	抗血小板藥	抗血小板药
aorta	主動脈	主动脉
aortic valve	主動脈瓣	主动脉瓣
arrhythmia	心律不齊	心律不齐; 心律失常
arterioles	小動脈	小动脉
atria	心房	心房
atrial fibrillation (AF)	心房纖維性顫動	心房纤颤; 心房颤动
atrial flutter	心房搏動	心房扑动
atrial septal defect (ASD)	房間隔缺損	房间隔缺损
atrioventricular node (AV node)	房室結	房室结
atrium	心房	心房
AV canal defects	房室傳導缺陷	房室传导缺陷
balloon	氣囊	气囊
betablockers	β-阻斷劑	β-阻断剂
blood clot	血塊; 血凝塊	血块; 血凝块
blood stream	血 (液) 流	血流
calcium channel blockers (CCBs)	鈣通道阻遲劑	钙通道阻断剂; 钙通道阻滞剂
capillary	微 (絲) 血管; 毛細血管	毛细血管
cardiac arrest	心動停止; 心跳驟停	心跳停止; 心搏停止
cardiac catheter for angiography	血管造影術專用心臟導管	血管造影专用心导管
cardiac catheterization	心臟導管檢查	心导管检查; 心导管 (插入) 术
Cardiac CT	心臟電腦掃描; 心臟電腦斷層掃描	心脏CT成像
Cardiac Surgeon	心臟外科醫生	心外科医生
Cardiologist	心臟科醫生	心脏病学家
cardiology	心臟科	心脏病学
cardiomegaly	心臟肥大	心肥大
cardiopulmonary resuscitation (CPR)	心肺復蘇法	心肺复苏
Cardiothoracic Surgeon	心胸外科醫生	胸心外科医生
cardiotonic drugs	強心劑	强心剂
cardioversion	心臟電復律	心脏复律
carditis	心臟炎; 心肌炎	心脏炎; 心肌炎
cath lab	導管化驗室	导管实验室

(Continued)

English	Hong Kong & Taiwan	Mainland China
central venous pressure	中央靜脈壓	中心静脉压; 中央静脉压
cholesterol	膽固醇	胆固醇; 胆甾醇
clopidogrel	氯格雷 (抗血小板藥物)	氯吡格雷 (抑制血小板药物)
clot-dissolving drugs	血凝塊溶解藥	血凝块溶解药
clotting	凝結	凝固
conduction problems	傳導障礙	传导障碍
congenital heart defects	先天性心臟病	先天性心脏缺损
congestive heart failure; heart failure	充血性心臟衰竭; 心臟衰竭	充血性心衰竭; 心衰竭
coronary artery	冠狀動脈	冠状动脉
coronary artery bypass surgery (CABG)	冠狀動脈繞道術 (俗稱「心臟搭橋」)	冠状动脉旁路 (搭桥) 手术
coronary artery disease (CAD); ischemic heart disease	冠狀動脈病; 缺血性心臟病	冠状动脉疾病; 冠心病; 缺血性心脏病
coronary care unit (CCU)	冠心病加護病房	冠心病监护室
creatine kinase (CPK) test	活素測試; 激動酶測試; 肌酸激酶測試	肌酸磷酸激酶试验
cyanosis	(因缺氧而面色) 發紫; 紫紺	发紫; 紫紺
defibrillator	電擊去顫器	除颤器
digoxin	狄各新 (心臟藥)	狄高辛
diltiazem	地爾硫卓; 硫氮草酮 (心臟藥)	地尔硫卓; 硫氮卓酮 (心脏药)
diuretic	利尿劑	利尿剂
double outlet right ventricle (DORV)	右心室雙出口	右心室双出口
electrocardiogram (ECC; EKG)	心電圖	心电图; 心动电流图
embolism	栓塞	栓塞
endocarditis	心內膜炎	心内膜炎
exercise EKG; treadmill test; stress test	運動心電圖; 跑步機心電圖; (心臟) 壓力測試	运动心电图; 跑步机心电图; 压力试验
fibrillation	纖維性顫動	纤维性颤动
fibrinogen	纖維蛋白原	纤维蛋白原
fibrinolytic	纖維蛋白溶解劑	纤维蛋白溶解剂; 纤溶
gingivitis	齒齦炎	(牙) 龈炎
gum disease	齒齦疾病	龈疾病
plaque	斑塊	斑块
Plaque Scan (Carotid Intima-Media Thickness Testing, or CIMT)	頸動脈內膜中層厚度掃描	颈动脉内膜中层厚度扫描

(Continued)

English	Hong Kong & Taiwan	Mainland China
platelet	血小板	血小板
pulmonary edema/oedema	肺水腫／水腫	肺水肿／水肿
pulmonary valve	肺動脈瓣	肺动脉瓣
radio-opaque	射線透不過的	辐射透不过的
regurgitation	反流	逆流; 反流
rheumatic fever	風濕熱	风湿热
sedative	鎮靜藥; 鎮靜劑	镇静药; 镇静剂
septal wall defect	心房間隔缺損; 心漏症	心房间隔缺损; 心漏症
septum	心室隔	心室隔
sinoatrial/sinu-atrialnode(SAnode)	竇房結	窦房结
sinus rhythm	竇節律	窦性节律; 窦性心律
sphygmomanometer	血壓計	血压计
ST elevation	ST段上升	ST上升
stable angina	穩定型心絞痛	稳定型心绞痛
statin drug	抑制劑藥物; 降膽固醇藥物	抑制剂药物; 降胆固醇药物
STEMI	ST 時段上升心肌梗塞	ST段抬高型心肌梗死
stent	支架	支架
stroke	中風	中风; 脑卒中
Swanz Ganz catheter/ Swan-Ganz catheter	氣囊漂浮心臟導管	气囊漂浮导管
systemic embolism	全身性栓塞	全身性栓塞
tetrology/Tetralogy of Fallot (TOF)	法樂氏四聯症	法乐 (氏) 四联症
Thoracic Surgeon	胸腔外科醫生	胸外科医生
thrombosis	血栓	血栓
thrombus; clot	栓塞; 凝塊	栓塞; 凝块
tightness of the chest	胸部壓迫感; 胸悶; 呼吸困難	胸闷; 胸部紧迫感
transposition of the great arteries (TGA)	大動脈錯位	大动脉转位; 大动脉移位; 大动脉错位
tricuspid valve	三尖瓣	三尖瓣
unstable angina	不穩定型心絞痛	不稳定型心绞痛
valve atresia	瓣閉鎖	瓣闭锁
vasodilator	血管擴張劑	血管扩张剂/舒张药
venule	小靜脈	小静脉
ventricle	心室	心室
ventricular fibrillation	心室纖維性顫動	心室纤颤; 心室颤动
ventricular septal defect (VSD)	心室間隔缺損 (心漏症)	室间隔缺损

Summary of main points

This chapter has given a brief overview of the heart, including:

- anatomy
- health professionals involved
- some commonly encountered conditions relating to the cardiac system, together with common diagnostic tests and treatment methods

In adults, heart problems usually affect one of the following:

- arteries
- heart muscle
- conduction of electrical activity
- heart valves

In babies, heart problems usually affect the anatomical structure of the heart, e.g. a hole in the wall between left and right side of the heart.

Chapter 19

Pulmonology

The respiratory system

The respiratory system controls our breathing. Any problems with this system can threaten our survival in the short term. The respiratory rate (the number of breaths per minute) is one of the vital signs observed by health professionals in the emergency room or in intensive care units.

It is important that interpreters understand terminology used when health professionals discuss common breathing problems such as asthma or the breathing problems experienced by premature babies.

1. Terms with Latin and Greek roots

alveolus	little air sac (plural: *alveoli*)
apnea	no breathing
bronchi (plural)	breathing tubes (*bronchus*: single)
dyspnea	difficulty in breathing/abnormal breathing
e or ex	out
expiration	breathing out (spirare: blow)
inspiration	breathing in
larynx	voice box (containing the vocal cords)
pharynx	throat
pneu/pnea	to blow (Greek)
pneumon	lung (Greek)
pulmon	lung (Latin)
pulmonary artery	blood vessel going from the heart to the lung (to pick up oxygen)
re	repeated; again and again
respiration	breathing (in/out)
spirare	to blow (Latin)
trachea	windpipe

2. Other important terms

gas exchange	breathing in *oxygen* (O_2) and blowing out *carbon dioxide* (CO_2)
mucus	slimy substance on inside of membranes
sputum	
or phlegm	the slimy substance that is coughed up from the lungs; spit

3. Anatomy of the respiratory system

Mouth
pharynx/throat epiglottis
larynx/voice box and vocal
cords trachea/windpipe
bronchi
bronchioli (literally:
"smaller bronchi").
alveoli or air sacs
respiratory center in
the brain

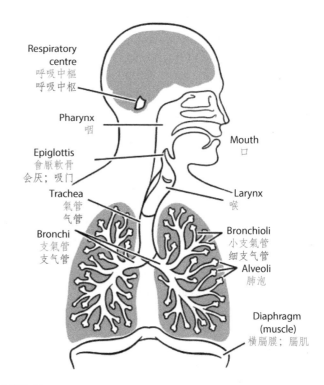

Respiratory
centre
呼吸中樞
呼吸中枢

Pharynx
咽

Mouth
口

Epiglottis
會厭軟骨
会厌；吸门

Larynx
喉

Trachea
氣管
气管

Bronchi
支氣管
支气管

Bronchioli
小支氣管
细支气管

Alveoli
肺泡

Diaphragm
(muscle)
橫膈膜；膈肌

Figure 19.1 Cross-section of the airways
呼吸道橫切面
气道橫截面

4. Function of the respiratory system

The respiratory center in the brain ensures that there is an ongoing exchange of oxygen (O_2) and carbon dioxide (CO_2) between the blood and the lungs. The respiratory center in the brain stem sends a signal to the breathing muscles. The breathing muscles, which run down from the neck to the upper ribs, tighten and pull the chest up and out. At the same time, the large muscle below the lungs (the *diaphragm*) contracts and the chest cavity becomes bigger. As a result of a change in air pressure in the lungs, air is sucked into the chest cavity. This is *inspiration* or breathing in. After inspiration, the breathing muscles relax, the elastic fibers in the lung contract, pressure builds up in the diaphragm below the lungs, and air is pushed out. This is called *expiration* or breathing out.

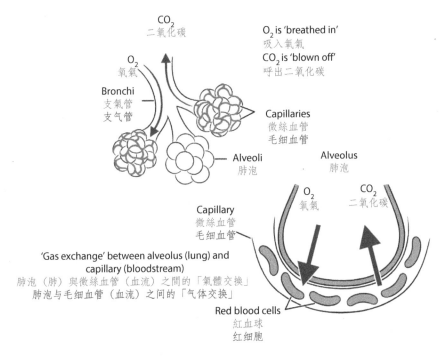

Figure 19.2 Alveoli and gas exchange close-up
肺泡與氣體交換特寫圖
肺泡与气体交换特写

In most people the respiratory center in the brain is stimulated by high levels of CO_2 in the blood, but for those with longstanding lung problems (such as emphysema) it may be stimulated by low levels of O_2 in the blood.

The diagram below may help you understand the mechanism of breathing:

Control: respiratory center in the brain → breathing muscles tighten → inspiration
→ breathing muscles relax → expiration

O_2 inhaled → attached to hemoglobin in the wall of red blood cells → transported around body

CO_2 is blown off

In many cases, patients with breathing difficulties will find it difficult to breathe when they are lying down flat. They will find it easier to breathe when they are sitting up.

Brain injury or drugs which affect the respiratory center in the brain can also adversely affect breathing. In this case, a ventilator or breathing machine may be used to help patients breathe.

5. Health professionals

Respiratory specialists – doctors specializing in disorders of the respiratory system.

Respiratory therapist – health professionals who carry out a wide range of respiratory function tests, including sleep studies.; they may also manage life support for patients in Intensive Care units and EDs, stabilizing patients during transport to hospital; respiratory therapists are often educators in pediatric clinics (e.g. on asthma).

6. Disorders of the respiratory system

1.   *Asthma* – A long term condition in which the airways are inflamed and narrowed (*bronchospasm*), which may lead to attacks of wheezing or coughing, and difficulties in breathing out.

Causes: Many asthma patients are hypersensitive to wheat, dust, airborne pollen or to certain drugs. Sometimes taking deep breaths (when stressed or after exertion) or breathing in cold air may trigger (bring about) an asthma attack. This hypersensitivity causes the muscles in the wall of the bronchi (airways) to tighten so the airways become narrowed. At the same time, the membranes in the lining of the airways swell up and produce a lot of mucus, leading to a clogging of the airways.

Symptoms: The patient finds it very difficult to breathe out and may wheeze when breathing out, producing a sort of whistling sound. Children often cough when they get an asthma attack. Other symptoms include chest tightness, shortness of breath, and use of accessory breathing muscles.

Diagnostic tests: Spirometry (pulmonary function test), using a peakflow meter (to see how much air the patient can still blow out).

Treatment: Preventers (often steroid inhalers) to stop ongoing inflammation and prevent asthma attacks; bronchodilators (given as inhalers or through nebulizers) (see Figures 19.3, 19.4, 19.5) to open up the airways by relaxing the muscles around the bronchi; oxygen; prednisone in tablet form or injected intravenously (into the vein); avoiding triggers; sometimes breathing exercises.

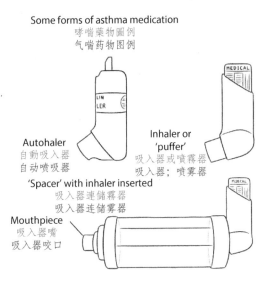

Some forms of asthma medication
哮喘藥物圖例
气喘药物图例

Autohaler
自動吸入器
自动喷吸器

Inhaler or
'puffer'
吸入器或噴霧器
吸入器；喷雾器

'Spacer' with inhaler inserted
吸入器連儲霧器
吸入器连储雾器

Mouthpiece
吸入器嘴
吸入器咬口

Figure 19.3 Some forms of asthma medication
哮喘藥物圖例
气喘药物图例

It should be noted that asthma attacks can become life-threatening within a very short space of time, and an ambulance should be called if a person is having real difficulty breathing and speaking. Children in particular may die if they become exhausted with the effort of pushing the air out.

2.   *Bronchiectasis* – Air passages become dilated (widened) and distorted (misshapen).

Causes: An infection leads to distortion of the airways. Phlegm collects in a pouch-like widening in the walls of damaged bronchi.

Symptoms: Recurrent chest infections, which in turn lead to further damage to the walls of the airways; slightly raised temperature; feeling unwell during an infection.

Treatment: Assistance to help patient to cough up the phlegm (e.g. postural drainage); antibiotics for airway infections.

3.   *Bronchitis* – Inflammation of the bronchi.

Cause: *Acute bronchitis* is caused by a virus in 90% of cases or by bacteria in 10% of cases, while *chronic* (ongoing) *bronchitis* may be due to smoking or working in a dusty, polluted environment.

Symptoms: Coughing up phlegm; raised temperature.

Diagnostic tests: X-ray; sputum specimen sent to lab to test for bacteria.

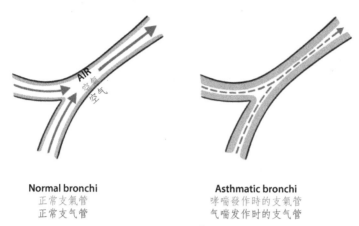

Normal bronchi
正常支氣管
正常支气管

Asthmatic bronchi
哮喘發作時的支氣管
气喘发作时的支气管

Swelling and narrowing of bronchi
resulting in 'wheezing' (a whistling sound)
支氣管壁腫脹,管道收窄,導致呼吸困難（俗稱「扯哮」）
支气管壁肿胀,管道收窄,导致呼吸困难（俗稱「哮鳴」）

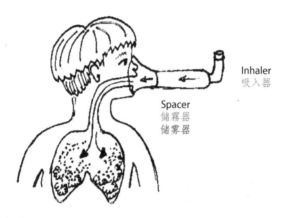

Inhaler
吸入器

Spacer
儲霧器
储雾器

Figure 19.4 Bronchi during an asthma attack
哮喘發作時的支氣管
气喘发作时的支气管

Note: Nebulizers are devices which help patients to inhale medication in spray form. In hospitals, nebulizers are usually connected to oxygen supply to help carry the medication into the lung. The nebulizer may have a mouth piece or a mask to fit around the patient's nose or mouth.

Treatment: Non-steroidal anti-inflammatory drugs; drugs to loosen (and help the patient to cough up) phlegm.

4.   *Cancer of the larynx* – Cancer cells on the vocal cords or on the wall of the voice box.

Causes: Smoking is a risk factor.

Symptoms: Chronic hoarseness; (later) lump on neck; earache; sore throat.

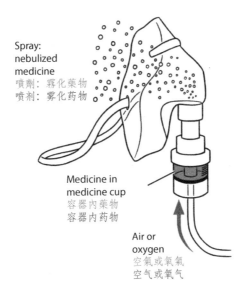

Spray: nebulized medicine
喷剂：雾化药物
喷剂：雾化药物

Medicine in medicine cup
容器内药物
容器内药物

Air or oxygen
空气或氧气
空气或氧气

Figure 19.5 Nebulizer spray
喷雾器；雾化器
喷洒器

Diagnostic tests: Laryngoscopy or micro-laryngoscopy (looking inside the voice box).

Treatment: Laryngectomy (removal of voice box) and creation of a *stoma* (opening in the larynx) radiotherapy; chemotherapy; speech therapy; patient learns to talk again through the stoma.

5.   *Cancer of the lung* (see lung cancer)

6.   *Chronic Obstructive Pulmonary Disease (COPD) or Chronic Obstructive Respiratory Disease (CORD)* – Damage to the alveoli (tiny air sacs).

Causes: Respiratory illness (such as asthma, chronic bronchitis, bronchiectasis or emphysema); smoking.

Symptoms: Wheezing; tight feeling in the chest; constant cough with lots of phlegm; tiredness; weight loss; frequent colds; *cyanosis* (purplish blue color) of fingernails and lips; *edema* (swelling) due to fluid retention.

Diagnostic tests: Pulse oximeter (testing oxygen saturation levels in the blood); spirometry (a type of pulmonary function test); chest X-ray.

Treatment: Oxygen; bronchodilators; corticosteroids; lung training (pursed lip breathing); BiPAP mask (bi-level positive airway pressure mask that helps COPD patients keep their airways open); Pneumococcal vaccine.

7.   *Emphysema* – from the Greek: *blown up, inflated*. Alveoli become permanently enlarged, small bronchi collapse and the lungs lose their elasticity, making chest and lungs appear permanently blown up.

Causes: Long-term exposure to smoking, pollution, industrial dust and fumes.

Symptoms: Severe shortness of breath; lack of oxygen.

Treatment: Oxygen; bronchodilators; corticosteroids; physical therapy: breathing exercises; antibiotics for infection.

8.   *Cor pulmonale* – Sometimes referred to as "fluid on the lungs." Occurs as a result of an increase in pressure in the arteries in the lungs. As a result, the right side of the heart enlarges because it has to work harder to pump the blood through.

Causes: Ongoing lung conditions such as emphysema or COPD.

Symptoms: With increased blood pressure in the lung arteries, breathing becomes increasingly difficult; swollen ankles.

Diagnostic tests: Chest x ray; EKG; echocardiogram.

Treatment: Stop smoking (smoking cessation); oxygen therapy; medication for heart failure.

9.   *Hay fever* – (*Allergic rhinitis*) – An allergic reaction to substances.

Causes: Various substances including plant pollens, dust, dust mites, pets (fur/hair).

Symptoms: Runny, itchy nose, watery eyes, sneezing, stuffy feeling in nose; lack of energy.

Diagnostic tests: Physical examination. Sometimes skin test for allergies.

Treatment: Anti-allergy drugs; nasal sprays.

10.   *Hyaline membrane disease* (see infant respiratory distress syndrome below).

11.   *Infant respiratory distress syndrome (IRDS) or neonatal respiratory distress syndrome* – Occurs in premature babies, with babies of diabetic mothers also at risk (see Chapter 13).

Causes: If a baby is born before 28–32 weeks of pregnancy, its lungs are still premature and not ready for breathing. These babies' lungs lack surfactant and the little air sacs (alveoli) may easily collapse.

Symptoms: The baby's breathing is difficult and labored (grunting.) Other signs may include flared nostrils and in-drawing of the chest.

Treatment: The baby is admitted to the neonatal intensive care unit and given surfactant into the lungs. The baby is put on a ventilator, and positive end-expiratory pressure (PEEP) ventilation or continuous positive airway pressure (CPAP) may be used to help keep the baby's alveoli open. Preventive treatment can also include giving the mother a prenatal course of steroids which helps the baby's lungs mature.

12.   *Lung carcinoma/Cancer of the lung/Lung cancer* – Cancer cells take over normal lung tissue. There are different types of lung cancer (small cell vs. non-small cell) and also different stages (limited – one lung; extensive – spread to both lungs). In lung secondaries or metastases, cancer cells have spread to other parts of the body.

Causes: In most cases lung cancer is caused by smoking. Other causes may include passive smoking or breathing in other irritating substances such as asbestos, coal dust, nickel, petroleum, radon gas.

Symptoms: Chronic coughing or wheezing; blood in phlegm; weight loss; fatigue.

Diagnostic tests: Chest X-ray; spiral CT scanning; angiography or VQ scan (to look at the blood vessels in the lung); bronchoscopy and biopsy; needle biopsy; sputum or phlegm samples. Cancer cells will be checked under the microscope to decide what type of cancer it is (see Chapter 16).

Treatment: The cancer cells may spread to other areas, such as the brain, bone marrow, and liver. Whether the cancer spreads and where it spreads largely depends on the type of cancer. Treatment depends on cell type and spread (stage). This may include surgical treatment such as pneumectomy (removal of entire lung) or lobectomy (removal of one lung lobe). However, surgery is only useful if the cancer has not spread. Non-surgical treatment includes radiation therapy; chemotherapy and targeted therapies.

13. *Pneumonia* – Infection/inflammation of the alveoli (see Figure 19.6).

Causes: Infection (often bacterial), causing the alveoli to swell up, which makes it difficult for oxygen to pass through the wall of the alveoli into the bloodstream.

Symptoms: Tiredness and shortness of breath (due to lack of oxygen); fever.

Diagnostic tests: A chest X-ray may show a *whiteout* (area of no air movement at all); oximetry (percentage of oxygen saturated blood).

Treatment: Bed rest; oxygen; physical therapy; intravenous antibiotics.

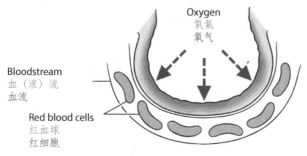

Inflammation and swelling: Difficult for oxygen to enter the bloodstream
發炎與腫脹令氧氣難以進入血（液）流
发炎与肿胀令氧气难以进入血流

Figure 19.6 Swelling and inflammation of the alveoli
肺泡腫脹與發炎
肺泡肿胀与发炎

14.   *Sleep apnea* – The most common form is *obstructive sleep apnea (OSA)*, occurs when a person's throat or windpipe close repeatedly during sleep, obstructing the airway.

Cause: Soft tissue at the top of the airway keeps blocking off the passage of air to the lungs; often in obese individuals.

Symptoms: Snoring; waking up to take a breath (leading to disrupted sleep, lack of deep sleep stages, and waking up feeling very tired).

Diagnostic tests: Sleep study at home (adults only) or in a sleep lab (pediatrics) in sleep lab (with video and continuous pulse oximetry overnight).

Treatment: Continuous positive airway pressure (CPAP) mask/machine to keep airways open; sometimes bi-level positive airway pressure (BiPAP) mask (not continuous).

15.   *Tuberculosis (Tb)* – Infection with Tb bacilli.

Causes: Mycobacterium tuberculosis (bacteria) spread through airborne droplets (coughing, sneezing, laughing). Tuberculosis may be *walled off* and lie dormant in the body for long time (during this time the Tb is called *inactive*). Another infection (including HIV) may reactivate the Tb by allowing it to "break out of the walls." *Active* Tb is infectious to others.

Symptoms: Cough; tiredness; fever; weight loss; night sweats; blood in sputum

Diagnostic tests: Chest X-ray; PPD skin test; the *Ziehl-Neelsen (Zn) AFB stain test*; LED-FM (see page 244) eyesight test (for visual acuity).

Treatment: Depends on whether the patient has inactive tuberculosis or active tuberculosis. Also depends on whether the patient has a drug resistant strain of Tb (common in South East Asia and Africa). *Inactive tuberculosis* can be treated with an antibiotic (INH) to prevent active Tb. *Active tuberculosis* can be treated by INH plus a combination of other drugs. Tb drugs can have side-effects affecting eyesight, liver function and hearing, so visual acuity (eyesight) and audiometry (hearing) tests may be done during treatment. Patients on treatment for Tb should not drink any alcohol. As explained in Chapter 3, for cultural reasons, some interpreters interpret "No alcohol" as "No alcohol – this includes beer," since beer is not considered alcohol in some cultures.

Possible complication: Disseminated tuberculosis: Tb has spread from the lungs to other parts of the body through the blood or lymph system.

NOTE: Interpreters should wear an N-95 face mask or a powered air purifying respirator (PAPR), NOT a simple surgical mask, when interpreting for patients with <u>infectious</u> tuberculosis.

7. Some common medications

cough medicines	prevent too much coughing, by suppressing the inclination to cough (often using codeine)
antihistamines	drugs which prevent allergic reaction by preventing release of histamine
bronchodilators	drugs which open up the bronchi (given as inhalers or through nebulizers)
corticosteroids	may lessen symptoms in life-threatening situations by dampening immune response: they do not address the underlying cause.
expectorants	medications which make it easier to cough up phlegm/sputum from air passages
mucolytics	medications which help dissolve mucus, making it easier to cough up
preventers	medications to prevent asthma attacks; often inhaled corticosteroids

8. Some common diagnostic tests

–   *Arterial blood gases (ABGs)* – Blood is taken from the patient's artery, then sent to the lab for precise measurement of levels of oxygen and carbon dioxide as well as pH and a few other indicators.

–   *Bronchoscopy* – The doctor pushes a flexible fiberoptic tube into the patient's bronchus and examines the lining, taking biopsies if needed. A bronchoscopy may be done if it is difficult to reach a diagnosis in any other way. Sometimes the patient may have washings of the bronchi and alveoli (*lavage*). These washings or biopsies may show up Tb bacilli.

–   *Chest X-ray (CXR)* – An X-ray of the chest area, taken in two directions – one with the patient facing the X-ray machine and one with the patient standing sideways to the X-ray machine. The chest X-ray can give valuable information on the structures in the chest (heart, lungs, windpipe) and any abnormalities such as air, blood or fluid in the chest; thickenings in the lungs; enlarged heart, etc.
–   *CT scan* – Computed tomography imaging.
–   *Light-emitting diode fluorescence microscopy (LED-FM)* – A type of smear microscopy (microscopic examination of sputum specimen), more sensitive and less time-consuming than the standard Ziehl-Neelsen AFB stain.
–   *Pulmonary function test* – Series of tests done in the pulmonary lab, measuring, amongst other things, oxygen uptake on exercise (6-minute walk test) and amount of oxygen inhaled and exhaled.
–   *Mantoux test or PPD (purified protein derivative)* – Skin test whereby a small amount of tuberculin is injected just under the skin. The test is "positive" for tuberculosis if the injection site becomes red and raised two to three days after the test.
–   *Oximetry* – Monitors oxygen saturation of the blood (normally 96–98% on air).
–   *Peakflow meter* – Tube with mouthpiece which measures the amount of air the patient is able to breathe out (or to "shift"). The patient takes a breath in, places the mouth around the mouthpiece (sealing it off), and "huffs" into the peak flow meter.
–   *Pulse oximetry* – Oxygen saturation measured by means of a device placed over the fingertip of the patient (see Figure 11.2, page 120).
–   *Spirometry* – Checking the air capacity of the lung with the aid of a machine
–   *Sputum specimen (sputum spec)* – Patient coughs up some phlegm into a sterile container, which is sent to the laboratory for testing for infection, such as tuberculosis.
–   *Transbronchial biopsies* – Biopsies taken by using bronchoscopy.
–   *Ziehl Nielsen acid-fast bacilli stain test (AFB)* – Traditional test on sputum for tuberculosis bacteria, which will stain (show up) when touched with an acid dye.

9.   English-Chinese glossary

英漢詞彙表

English	Hong Kong & Taiwan	Mainland China
active tuberculosis	活躍性 (肺) 結核病	活跃性结核
air passage	呼吸道	气道
airways	呼吸道; 氣道	气道

(Continued)

English	Hong Kong & Taiwan	Mainland China
alveoli; air sacs	肺泡; 肺泡囊	肺泡
alveolus	肺泡	肺泡
angiography	血管造影術	血管造影 (术)
anti-cough	止咳 (藥)	止咳 (药)
antihistamine	抗組織胺藥; 抗過敏藥	抗组织胺药; 抗过敏药
arterial blood gas (ABG)	動脈血氣	动脉血气
asthma	哮喘	气喘; 哮喘
Autohaler	自動吸入器	自动喷吸器
BiPAP mask	高低式睡眠呼吸機面罩	高低式睡眠呼吸机面罩
bloodstream	血 (液) 流	血流
Bronchi	支氣管	支气管
bronchiectasis	支氣管擴張	支气管扩张
bronchioli	小支氣管	细支气管
bronchodilator	支氣管擴張劑	支气管扩张药
bronchoscopy	支氣管內窺鏡檢查	支气管 (窥) 镜检查
bronchospasm	支氣管痙攣	支气管痉挛
Bronchus	支氣管	支气管
By-Face Positive Airway Pressure (PAP) mask	正氣壓睡眠呼吸機面罩	正气压睡眠呼吸机面罩
cancer of the larynx	喉癌	喉癌
Capillary	微 (絲) 血管; 毛細血管	毛细血管
chemotherapy	化學療法; 化療	化学疗法; 化学治疗; 化疗
chest tightness	胸部壓迫感; 胸悶; 呼吸困難	胸闷; 胸部紧迫感
chest X-ray	X光胸肺檢查	胸部X射线检查
chronic obstructive pulmonary disease (COPD)	慢性阻塞性肺病	慢性阻塞性肺病
Clinical Respiratory Physiologist (CRP)	臨床呼吸生理學家	临床呼吸生理学家
continuous positive airway pressure (CPAP)	持續正氣壓睡眠呼吸機	持续正气压睡眠呼吸机
cor pulmonale	肺原性心臟病; 肺心病	肺 (原) 性心脏病; 肺心病
corticosteroids	類固醇激素; 皮質素	皮质激素; 皮质甾类; 皮质类固醇
chronic hoarseness	慢性聲音嘶啞; 慢性聲嘶	慢性声音嘶哑
cyanosis	(因缺氧而面色) 發紫; 紫紺	发紫; 紫紺
diaphragm	橫膈膜	膈膜
disseminated tuberculosis	傳染性 (肺) 結核病	播散性结核

(Continued)

English	Hong Kong & Taiwan	Mainland China
Dyspnea/Dyspnoea	呼吸困難	呼吸困难
Echocardiogram/ Echocardiography	心臟超音波檢查; 超聲波心動圖	超声心动图
electrocardiogram	心電圖	心电图; 心动电流图
Emergency Room	急症室	急诊室
emphysema	肺氣腫	气肿; 肺气肿
epiglottis	會厭軟骨	会厌; 吸门
expectorant	祛痰劑	祛痰药
expiration	呼氣	呼气; 吐气
gas exchange	換氣	气体交换; 换气
hay fever; allergic rhinitis	花粉症; 花粉熱; 乾草熱; 過敏性鼻炎	干草热; 花粉症; 过敏性鼻炎
Hemoglobin/Haemoglobin	血色素; 血紅素	血红蛋白
HIV	人類免疫力缺乏病毒; 愛滋病病毒	人类免疫缺陷病毒; 艾滋病病毒
hyaline membrane disease; infant respiratory distress syndrome (IRDS); neonatal respiratory disease syndrome	(新生兒) 肺透明膜病; 新生兒呼吸窘迫; 呼吸困難綜合症; 新生兒呼吸疾病綜合症	(新生儿) 肺透明膜病; 新生儿呼吸窘迫综合症; 新生儿呼吸疾病综合症
inactive tuberculosis	非活躍性 (肺) 結核病; 潛復性肺結核	非活动性肺结核; 潜复性肺结核
inhaler; puffer	吸入器; 噴霧器	吸入器; 喷雾器
inspiration	吸氣	吸气; 纳气
Intensive Care Unit	深切治療部	重症监护室
laryngectomy	喉管切除術	喉管切除术
laryngoscopy	喉窺鏡檢查	喉镜检查
light emitting-diode fluorescence microscopy (LED-FM)	發光二極體 (LED) 螢光顯微鏡檢查	发光二极管 (LED) 荧光显微镜检术
lobe	(肺) 葉	(肺) 叶
lobectomy	肺葉切除術	肺叶切除术
lung carcinoma; lung cancer	肺癌	肺癌
Mantoux test	孟都氏試驗 (結核菌素試驗)	曼塔斯试验 (结核菌素皮内试验)
Metastases/Metastasis	轉移; 擴散	转移; 扩散
mucolytics	黏液溶解劑	粘液溶解剂
mucus	黏液	粘液
Mycobacterium tuberculosis	結核桿菌	结核分支杆菌; 鸟型结核杆菌; 结核杆菌
nebulizer	噴霧器; 霧化器	喷雾器; 喷洒器; 雾化器

(Continued)

English	Hong Kong & Taiwan	Mainland China
needle biopsy	針吸式活組織檢驗	针吸活检; 穿刺活检
Neonatal Intensive Care Unit	初生嬰兒深切治療部	新生儿监护病房
oedema; pulmonary edema	水腫; 肺水腫	水肿; 肺水肿
peak flow meter	肺活量計	肺活量计
phlegm	痰	痰; 粘痰
pharynx	咽	咽
pneumectomy	肺切除術	肺切除术
pneumonia	肺炎	肺炎
positive end-expiratory pressure (PEEP)	吐氣末端正壓式	呼气末正压
postural drainage	体位引流; 順位驅痰	体位性引流
prednisone	潑尼松 (屬腎上腺皮質激素)	强的松; 泼尼松
pulse oximeter	(脈搏) 血氧計	脉搏血氧计
radiotherapy	放射治療	放射治疗
red blood cells	紅血球	红细胞,红血球
respiratory rate	呼吸率	呼吸率
sleep apnea/apnoea; obstructive sleep apnea/ apnoea (OSA)	睡眠窒息症; 阻塞性睡眠窒息症	睡眠窒息症; 阻塞性睡眠窒息症
Sleep Physiologist	睡眠生理學家	睡眠生理学家
Sleep Technologist	睡眠技師	睡眠技师
spacer	儲霧器	储雾器
speech therapy	言語治療	言语治疗
Spiral CT scanning	螺旋電腦 (斷層) 掃描	螺旋CT掃描
spirometry	肺活量測定法	肺量测定法; 呼吸量测定法
sputum	痰 (液)	痰 (液)
steroid inhaler	類固醇吸入器	激素吸入器; 类固醇吸入器
steroids	激素; 類固醇	激素; 类固醇
stoma	造口	造口; 小气孔
surfactant	表面張力素	表面活 (性) 剂
trachea; windpipe	氣管	气管
transbronchial biopsy	經支氣管活組織檢查	经支气管 (肺) 活检
tuberculosis (TB)	(肺) 結核	(肺) 結核
ventilator; breathing machine	呼吸器; 人工呼吸機	呼吸器; 呼吸机
VQ scan	通氣灌注掃描	(肺) 通气灌注扫描
Ziehl-Neelsen acid fast bacilli stain test (AFB)	結核菌塗片測試; 抗酸桿菌 (AFB) 測試	抗酸杆菌 (AFB) 測試

Summary of main points

This chapter has given a brief overview of the respiratory system, including:

- a brief overview of anatomy
- terms with Latin and Greek roots
- health professionals involved
- some commonly enountered conditions relating to the respiratory system, together with common diagnotics tests and treatment plans.

Chapter 20

Hematology

Blood and blood disorders

Blood flows through our bodies through a complicated system of blood vessels. This system of blood vessels is described in more detail in the chapter on the circulation. This chapter will deal with the blood itself, with its components and with the various types of blood vessels.

1. Blood

1.1 Terms with Latin and Greek roots

albumin	blood protein
anemia	lack of blood (no blood)
athero	fat(ty)
arterio	arterial; to do with the arteries
arteriosclerosis	hardening of the arteries
atherosclerosis	fatty hardening of the arteries
capillary	to do with the finest (hair-like) blood vessels (capilla: hair)
coagulation	clotting (literally: clumping together)
cyte	cell
embolus	big blood clot
embolism	blockage of a blood vessel by a blood clot (or air bubble)
emia	see: hemia
erythro	red (erythrocyte: red cell)
fuse	to pour (liquids)
-gram/graphy	image; recording (grafein: to write)
haem	see: hem-
hematologist	doctor specializing in the treatment of blood disorders
(h)emia	in the blood (e.g. *leukemia*)
hem-, hemo-, /hemato-	blood (from the greek: *haimos* or *haimatos*)
hemoglobin	protein in red blood cells that allows them to carry oxygen
hemorrhage	bleed (blood bursting forth)
heparin	*anti-clotting agent (hepar: liver)*

infusion	to pour in
leuko	white (*leukocyte:* white cell)
lymphocyte	lymph cell
lymphoma	lymph cancer (*oma:* growth, tumor)
-penia	lack of (e.g. thrombocytopenia: lack of platelets)
plaques	deposit; patch (e.g. *atheromatous plaque:* fatty deposit)
plasma expander	helping to increase the volume of the plasma
thrombo	clot
thrombocyte	platelet (clotting cell)
thrombosis	occurrence of clots (*-osis:* condition, state)
transfuse	to pour (fluid) across

1.2   Anatomy of blood

Blood consists of formed elements and fluid:

–   Formed elements: red blood cells (oxygen; hemoglobin); white blood cells (part of immune system; to fight infections)
–   Platelets (clotting)

Fluid (serum):
–   Salts (electrolytes: Na; Cl; Ca; K, etc.)
–   Oxygen (O_2) and carbon dioxide (CO_2)
–   Food (sugar, fat, proteins), vitamins and minerals
–   Hormones (chemical messengers)
–   Proteins
    –   albumin
    –   globulin
    –   fibrinogen
–   Wastes (removed via kidneys or lungs)

1.3   Function of blood

Red blood cells live for around 90 to 120 days. If a person loses a lot of blood, it will take a few months before they have replaced the lost blood cells.

If a blood-vessel gets cut, blood will start to clot in order to stop the bleeding and start the repair process. Clotting (coagulation or "clumping together") is a very complicated process, involving a chain reaction of many different coagulation factors. Put in a nutshell:

damage → platelets clump together → clots form → bleeding stops

Sometimes, unwanted clotting occurs. This often happens to people who already have damage to the walls of their blood vessels. This damage can be due to fatty deposits, cigarette smoking or many other factors. Unwanted clotting can also be a result of other disorders. Unwanted clotting can be dangerous because it can lead to clots blocking arteries. The medical word for a small clot is thrombus. Thrombosis is a condition where people have clots in their blood vessels. A large clot (consisting of many small clots, sticking together) is called an embolus. When large clots cause a major blockage this is called an embolism.

In short:

plaques in walls of blood vessels may lead to unwanted clotting (thrombosis; embolisms) thrombus → less oxygen to cells

embolism → less or no oxygen to cells   →   lung embolism;

OR   cerebrovascular accident (CVA) (in the brain);

OR   heart attack (in the heart)

1.4   Health professionals

Hematologist – Doctor specializing in blood disorders.

Phlebotomist – Health professional specializing in taking blood samples.

1.5   Disorders of the blood

1.   *Anemia* – There are not enough red blood cells in the blood, or there is not enough hemoglobin, or the volume of red cells is low; often a sign of underlying illness.

Causes: Heavy blood loss (hemorrhagic anemia); heavy menstrual periods; occult (unnoticed) bleeding in stomach or bowels; cancer; sickle cell anemia; inability to absorb iron from food; decreased red blood cell production (e.g. in kidney failure); or *hemolytic anemia* (involving the breakdown of red blood cells), e.g. in malaria, blood transfusion reactions or Rhesus disease.

Symptoms: Feeling cold, weak, tired, irritable; shortness of breath.

Diagnostic tests: Full blood count (FBC); red blood count (RBC); Hb (hemoglobin) Ht (hematocrit); gastroscopy; colonoscopy (to check for blood loss from the digestive tract); CT scan.

2.   *Hemophilia* (bleeder disease) – A hereditary bleeding disorder where either clotting factor VIII (hemophilia A) or clotting factor IX (hemophilia B) are missing, so clotting time is longer than normal.

Causes: Inherited from carrier mother, *mostly* males only are affected.

Symptoms: Bruising very easily; bleeding does not stop.

Diagnostic tests: Clotting test.

Treatment: Transfusion of the missing clotting factors to prevent bleeding. Transfusions can lead to complications such as brain hemorrhage or developing antibodies to transfused Factor VIII.

3.   *Leukemia* (Greek: white blood) – Cancer affecting the white blood cells. Normally stem cells in the bone marrow develop into different types of healthy white cells, red cells and platelets. In leukemia the bone marrow produces lots of immature white cells called *blasts*. The blood is flooded with immature white cells (*white blood*), but there are not enough red cells, platelets or healthy white cells.

There are several types of leukemias: acute myeloid leukemia; acute lymphoid leukemia; chronic myeloid Leukemia (CML); chronic lymphoid leukemia (CLL). Acute leukemia develops very quickly while chronic leukemia develops slowly and symptoms may be less pronounced.

Causes: Exact cause is unknown, but risk factors may include genetic, environmental factors (including infections), all impacting on immune response.

Symptoms: Tiredness; weight loss; looking pale; fever; sweats; repeated infections; enlarged lymph glands; enlarged liver and spleen; abdominal discomfort (large spleen). Patients can also have anemia as well as bleed easily and develop infections, because the *blasts* cannot fight these infections.

Leukemia may also lead to internal hemorrhaging, which may be fatal (lead to death). Likewise, high fever due to uncontrolled infection can also be fatal.

Diagnostic tests: Bone marrow aspiration (sample); blood test (white cell count); biopsy of lymph gland(s).

Treatment: Chemotherapy; radiation; allogeneic bone marrow transplant (transplant using bone marrow from another person). Bone marrow transplants can have complications such as graft-versus-host disease (see Chapter 24), whereby the healthy donor bone marrow attacks the sick body of the person receiving it.

4.   *Malaria* – Parasitic infection of the liver and red blood cells.

Cause: Bite by infected mosquito.

Symptoms: Fever with chills; headache; hemolytic anemia and jaundice. Can result in brain damage leading to coma and death.

Treatment: Preventing mosquito bites in tropical countries; oral medication; recent research suggests a particular type of antiworming medication may work well against malaria.

5. *Myeloma* – Cancer of the blood which develops in the bone marrow.

What happens: Myeloma cancer cells in spine, ribs, pelvic bones; these can destroy the bone.

Causes: Exact cause is unknown.

Symptoms: Severe bone pain; soft spots in the bone; spontaneous fractures (breaks of the bone).

Diagnostic tests: CT scan; MRI scan; bone marrow biopsy; kidney function tests; blood tests for abnormal monoclonal (M) protein (produced by the myeloma cells).

Treatment: Chemotherapy.

6. *Rhesus disease* – See Chapter 28 for specific information on Rh disease.
Please note: Most people are positive for Rhesus factor (Rh+), which means they have this factor on the surface of their red blood cells. Fewer people are Rh negative (Rh-), which means they do not have this factor. If an Rh- person receives Rh+ blood, that person will start to make antibodies against the Rh factor.

7. *Sickle cell disease* – An inherited blood disorder. During an attack of sickle cell anemia, red blood cells take on a rigid "sickle" shape after giving up their oxygen. Sickle shaped cells cannot fit through the narrow capillaries, resulting in a reduced blood supply to that part of the body.

Causes: Genetic/inherited. Sickling attacks are more likely to occur when the patient is in a cold environment or doing exercise.

Symptoms: Sickling attacks are very painful, because parts of the body are deprived of oxygen and therefore send out pain signals. If sickling occurs in the bone, bone may die.

Diagnostic tests: Blood test; if sickling occurs in the lungs, an X-ray may show a complete whiteout, meaning that whole areas of the lungs are no longer involved in oxygen exchange.

Treatment: Treatment of symptoms only. Genetic counseling is advised for carriers of sickle cell anemia wishing to have children.

8. *Thalassemia* – An inherited condition in which the body makes abnormal hemoglobin and many red blood cells are destroyed, resulting in severe anemia. There are several types, including: alpha thalassemia, beta thalassemia and Hb Barts. Common in Southeast Asia, the Pacific Islands and countries around the Mediterranean. The term *thalassemia major* refers to a severe form of the condition, whereas the term *thalassemia minor* refers to a less severe form.

Cause: Genetic

Symptoms: These range from none to mild to severe anemia. Carrier mothers may experience recurrent miscarriages and stillbirths if the unborn baby has inherited a severe form of thalassemia.

Diagnostic tests: Blood tests.

Treatment: Treatment of symptoms only. Genetic counseling is advised for carriers of thalassemia wishing to have children.

9. *Transfusion reaction* – The body's response to receiving non-compatible blood (e.g. wrong blood group, wrong Rhesus factor).

Cause: Non-compatible blood transfusion (e.g. in emergency medicine).

Symptoms: Lower back pain; chills; low blood pressure; sometimes kidney failure (blood in urine); shock; death.

Diagnostic tests: Blood test.

Treatments: Stop transfusion; manage symptoms.

1.6 Some common medications

anticoagulants	medications used to prevent clotting
antifibrinolytics	medications used to break down and dissolve blood clots
heparin	anticoagulant (given by injection or intravenous drip)
vasodilators	drugs used to widen the blood vessels
vitamin K	helps to stop bleeding (given to newborns as they tend to be low on vitamin K)
Warfarin®	anticoagulant; effects are monitored by regular INR blood tests.

1.7 Some common diagnostic tests

- *Bleeding time* – Testing how long it takes before the bleeding stops (earlobe and blotting-paper).

–   *Blood grouping* – Test done to see what blood group a person has: *type A, B, AB* (universal receiver) or *Type O* (universal donor); *Rhesus factor*, Rh+ (rhesus positive) or Rh- (Rhesus negative);
–   *Group and hold* – Checking blood group and keeping blood on standby.
–   *Clotting time* – Test done to see how soon blood clots.

2.   Blood vessels

2.1   Terms with Latin and Greek roots

angio	blood vessel
angiography	process of producing an image of the blood vessels using contrast dye
angioplasty	blood vessel repair (see also Chapter 18)
angiogram	image of the blood vessels following angiography
aorta	largest body artery with smaller arteries branching off to take oxygen to specific areas (comparable to a main road with many side roads branching off)
arterial	relating to arteries
arteries	strong muscular blood vessels transporting blood rich in oxygen
cardiovascular	to do with the heart and blood vessels
claudication	narrowing of leg arteries, causing patients to stop frequently when they are walking due to severe pain in the legs caused by lack of oxygen in leg muscles
cholesterol	blood fats
cyanosis	looking blue (due to lack of oxygen)
endarterectomy	removal of fatty plaque from the wall of the artery (*endo*: inside; *arter*: artery; ec (Greek: *ek*): out: *tomy*: cut)
fem-pop or femoropopliteal	relating to arteries in the upper and lower leg
hematoma	bruise (literally: blood swelling)
hemorrhage	bleed
occlusion	blockage
occluded	blocked
phlebitis	inflammation of the veins
sclerosis	hardening
thrombectomy	procedure to remove a big blood clot from the body either by surgically removing it or by dissolving it and sucking it out through a catheter (thin tube)

thrombophlebitis inflammation of blood vessels with the formation of small clots
vascular   relating to blood vessels
venous   relating to veins

2.2   Anatomy of blood vessels

There are three main types of blood vessels:

–   *Arteries* – Strong, muscular blood vessels which take blood that is rich in oxygen (bright red) around the body, distributing oxygen and nutrients to all the body cells.
–   *Capillaries* – Very fine, hair-like blood vessels, which form the link between the tiniest end arteries and the tiniest little veins.
–   *Veins* – Wide blood vessels which take blood low in oxygen, but high in carbon dioxide (a waste product) back to the heart. This blood looks dark red.

2.3   A word about cholesterol

There are different types of cholesterol, the most well-known types being high density lipoprotein (HDL) or "good cholesterol," which removes cholesterol from the blood vessels, and low density lipoprotein (LDL) or "bad cholesterol," which can build up fatty plaque on the walls of the arteries.

Cholesterol is measured in milligrams per deciliter (mg/dL).

Some people have high cholesterol levels as an inherited condition called *hyperlipidemia* (high fats in the blood). Following are the approximate levels recommended *for healthy people* (at the time of writing) (Mayo Clinic 2014):

Table 20.1 Recommended cholesterol levels

	US	UK, Canada, Australia, NZ
Total cholesterol	< 200 mg/dL	< 5 mmol/L
LDL	< 130 mg/dL	< 1.8 mmol/L
HDL*	> 40 mg/dL	> 1.5 mmol/L
Triglycerides	< 150 mg/dL	< 1.7 mmol/L

*the higher the more protective

2.4   Disorders of the blood vessels

1. *Aneurysm* (Greek: widening) – Local widening of blood vessels, usually in brain, abdomen or chest. There are different types of aneurysms. A dissecting

aneurysm occurs when blood seeps through a lengthwise tear between layers of the wall of the artery. The layers come apart and swell and the artery becomes shaped like a balloon. An abdominal aortic aneurysm (AAA) is a widening in the aorta in the abdomen. Complications can arise as a result of a rupture and bleed which can lead to death.

Causes: Sometimes caused by congenital weakness in blood vessels, but can also be due to injury; smoking; atherosclerosis; ongoing stresses.

Symptoms: Sometimes abdominal discomfort, sometimes no symptoms.

Diagnostic tests: Auscultation (murmur); Doppler; ultrasound.

Treatment: Watchful waiting; repair by vein graft or surgical clipping or by inserting a coil.

2. *Deep vein thrombosiss (DVT)* – A big blood clot in a deep vein, usually the lower leg.

Causes: Being immobile for a long period of time (e.g. bed rest; paralysis); cancer; medications(e.g. birth control pills); injury/damage to veins (e.g. intravenous needle or cannula); varicose veins; old age; previous DVT.

Symptoms: Swelling; pain; warm and tender limb with discolored skin. This condition can lead to a lung embolism (big blood clot stops blood from entering lungs to pick up oxygen), which may be fatal.

Diagnostic tests: Doppler; ultrasound, CT scan.

Treatment: Anticoagulants.

3. *Narrowing of arteries* – When arteries are narrowed or blocked, oxygen cannot get through to the tissue, resulting in pain. If no oxygen gets through at all, cells start to die.

Causes: Artery walls may be damaged due to smoking, high blood pressure, ongoing stresses or high levels of insulin or glucose. Fat may also be deposited on artery walls due to high blood fats (cholesterol).

Symptoms: Narrowed or blocked arteries can lead to a number of conditions, depending on where the blockages are:

   Eyes – Narrowing of the tiny arteries at the back of the eye (in the *retina*) may lead to loss of vision.

   Heart – Coronary artery narrowing may lead to angina or heart attacks (see Chapter 18).

   Neck – Carotid artery narrowing may lead to TIAs or CVAs (see Chapter 17).

Legs – Narrowing of the femoral arteries (in the groin and upper leg) may lead to peripheral vascular disease which may lead to claudication (being able to walk only a small distances before severe pain comes on) or to leg ulcers that do not heal, or to gangrene (tissue dying and going black).

Kidneys – Narrowing of the tiny arteries in the glomeruli, which may lead to kidney failure (see Chapter 27).

Diagnostic tests: angiography; arteriography; Doppler; ultrasound; CT scan.

Treatment: Lifestyle changes such as exercise, cholesterol-lowering diet and stopping smoking; cholesterol-lowering medications; angioplasty with stent; balloon angioplasty (see Chapter 18); endarterectomy (removal of fatty plaque); bypass surgery using vein graft (blood vessel replaced with vein from patient's own leg) or man-made graft. Where there is narrowing of leg arteries treatment may include femoropopliteal (*fem pop*) bypass surgery to bypass narrowed section of leg arteries and improve blood supply to the leg, or amputation of part of the leg.

4.   *Thrombophlebitis* – Inflammation, usually in superficial vein.

Cause: Damage to the vein (e.g. through an intravenous needle or canula); long periods of immobility (e.g. long flight); birth control and *synthetic* progestagens, pills, especially in women who are older or who smoke. Complications can arise if the clot breaks off and causes a blockage elsewhere (e.g. in heart, lungs or brain).

Symptoms: Swelling, redness, tenderness.

Diagnostic tests: Doppler; ultrasound; CT scan.

Treatment: Anti-coagulants; compression stockings; elevating legs; exercise.

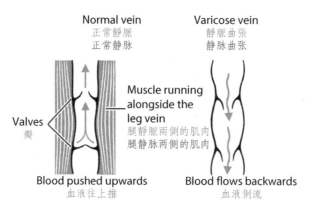

Figure 20.1 Varicose veins
静脉曲张
静脉曲张

5. *Varicose veins* – Bulging, twisted, swollen veins, often in legs.

Causes: Standing for long periods of time; pregnancy; constipation; family history; being overweight. Complications can arise whereby leg circulation can be affected and leg ulcers can occur.

Symptoms: Itching around veins; swelling in legs; aching legs; throbbing pain; muscle cramps; pain behind knee.

Diagnostic tests: Doppler; ultrasound.

Treatment: Exercise; elastic support stockings; sclerotherapy (which entails injecting veins with sclerosing solution to close them down); stripping (surgical removal of veins).

3. English-Chinese glossary

英漢詞彙表

English	Hong Kong & Taiwan	Mainland China
abnormal monoclonal (M) protein	異常單株蛋白 (M蛋白)	异常单克隆蛋白
acute lymphoid leukemia	急性淋巴性白血病	急性淋巴样白血病
acute myeloid leukemia/ leukaemia	急性骨髓性白血病	急性髓性白血病; 髓细胞样白血病
albumin	蛋白	蛋白; 蛋白胚乳
allogeneic bone marrow transplant	異體骨髓移植	异基因骨髓移植
alpha thalassemia/thalassaemia	甲型地中海貧血	甲型地中海贫血
anemia/anaemia	貧血	贫血
aneurysm	動脈瘤	动脉瘤
angiogram	血管造影	血管造影
angiography	血管造影術	血管造影术
angioplasty	血管成形術	血管成形术
anticoagulants	抗凝血劑	抗凝血剂
antifibrinolytics	抗纖維蛋白溶酶藥; 抗血栓溶解劑	抗纤维蛋白溶解药
arteries	動脈	动脉
arteriosclerosis	動脈硬化	动脉硬化
atherosclerosis	動脈粥樣硬化	动脉粥样硬化
auscultation	聽診	听诊

(Continued)

English	Hong Kong & Taiwan	Mainland China
beta thalassemia/thalassaemia	乙型地中海貧血	乙型地中海贫血
blasts	胚細胞	胚细胞
blood clot	血塊; 血凝塊	血 (凝) 块
blood vessel	血管	血管
bone marrow aspirate	抽骨髓	骨髓抽出; 骨髓穿刺
bone marrow	骨髓	骨髓
capillary	微絲血管; 毛細血管	毛细血管
chronic myeloid leukemia/leukaemia (CML)	慢性骨髓性白血病	慢性髓性白血病; 髓细胞样白血病
chronic lymphoid leukemia/leukaemia (CLL)	慢性淋巴性白血病	慢性淋巴性白血病
claudication	跛行	跛行
clotting; coagulation	(血) 凝結	(血) 凝固
Cerebrovascular accident (CVA)	大腦血管意外; 中風	腦血管意外; 卒中綜合症; 中風; 脑卒中
deep vein thrombosis (DVT)	深層靜脈血栓	深部静脉血栓形成
Doppler	多普勒 (檢查)	多普勒 (超声)
embolism	栓塞	栓塞
embolus	栓子	栓子
femoral artery	股動脈	股动脉
femoropopliteal	膝窩動脈 (的) ; 膕動脈	膕动脉
fibrinogen	纖維蛋白原	纤维蛋白原
full blood count (FBC)	血常規; 全血指數; 血細胞數量檢查	全血 (细胞) 计数; 血常规
gangrene	壞疽; 壞死	坏疽; 坏死
globulin	球蛋白	球蛋白
glomeruli	腎小球	肾小球
graft-versus-host disease	移植體對宿主反應; 移植體抗宿主病	移植物抗宿主病
Hb Barts	巴氏血紅素	巴氏血红蛋白
heart attack	心臟病猝發; 心臟病發作	心脏病发作
Hematocrit/Haematocrit (Ht)	血球容積	血细胞比容
Hematologist/Haematologist	血液學專家	血液病学家; 血液病医师
hematoma/haematoma	血腫	血肿
hemoglobin/haemoglobin (Hb)	血色素; 血紅素	血红蛋白
hemolytic anemia/haemolytic anaemia	溶血性貧血	溶血性贫血

(*Continued*)

English	Hong Kong & Taiwan	Mainland China
Hemophilia/haemophilia	血友病	血友病
hemorrhagic anemia/ haemorrhagic anaemia	出血性貧血	出血性贫血
heparin	肝素	肝素
high density lipoprotein (HDL)	高密度脂蛋白	高密度脂蛋白
Leukemia/leukaemia	白血病	白血病
low density lipoprotein (LDL)	低密度脂蛋白	低密度脂蛋白
lymph glands	淋巴腺	淋巴腺; 淋巴结
lymphoma	淋巴瘤	淋巴瘤
malaria	瘧疾	疟疾
myeloma	骨髓瘤	骨髓瘤
occlusion	阻塞; 閉合	阻塞; 闭合
peripheral vascular disease	末梢血管疾病; 周邊血管疾病	末梢血管疾病
phlebitis	靜脈炎	静脉炎
Phlebotomist	抽血員	抽血员
platelet	血小板	血小板
red blood cell	紅血球	红细胞; 红血球
red blood count (RBC)	紅血球數量	红细胞计数
Rhesus disease	溶血性疾病	猕猴 (溶血) 病
sclerosis	硬化	硬化 (症)
sclerotherapy	硬化療法	硬化疗法
sickle cell anemia/anaemia	鐮狀細胞性貧血	镰状细胞性贫血
spleen	脾 (臟)	脾 (脏)
stripping	靜脈剝離術	静脉剥脱术
thalassemia/thalassaemia	地中海貧血	地中海贫血
thrombectomy	血栓清除術	血栓清除
thrombocyte	血小板	血小板
thrombocytopenia	血小板減少症	血小板减少症
thrombophlebitis	血栓性靜脈炎	血栓静脉炎
thrombosis	血栓形成	血栓形成
thrombus	血栓	血栓
transfuse	輸血; 輸液	输血; 输液
transfusion reaction	輸血反應	输血反应
universal donor	全適捐血者	普适供血者; 全适供血者
universal receiver	全適受血者	普适受血者; 全适受血者

(Continued)

English	Hong Kong & Taiwan	Mainland China
varicose veins	靜脈曲張	静脉曲张
vasodilator	血管舒張劑	血管扩张剂
vein	靜脈	静脉
white blood cells	白血球	白细胞; 白血球

Summary of main points

This chapter has given a brief overview of blood and blood vessels, including:

- composition of the blood
- the main blood vessels and their functions
- terms with Latin and Greek roots
- health professionals involved
- some commonly encountered conditions relating to blood and blood vessels, together with common diagnostic tests and treatment methods.

Chapter 21

Orthopedics

The skeletal system

The skeletal system is the supporting framework of the body. It consists of 206 bones in total, including the small bones in the ear. Some of these bones are known only by their Latin names. The list below includes the parts of the skeleton to which medical providers most commonly refer.

1. **Terms with Latin and Greek roots**

ankylo	stiff
arthro	joint
inter	in between
-itis	inflammation
osteoarthritis	inflammation of bone and joint
intervertebral	in between the vertebrae
myelum	bone marrow
osteo	bone
porosis	porous; brittle
sarcoma	cancer of the connective tissue (*sarc* – co tissue; *oma* – tumor or swelling)
spondylos	vertebra
therapy	treatment
vertebrae	33 small bones that make up the spine

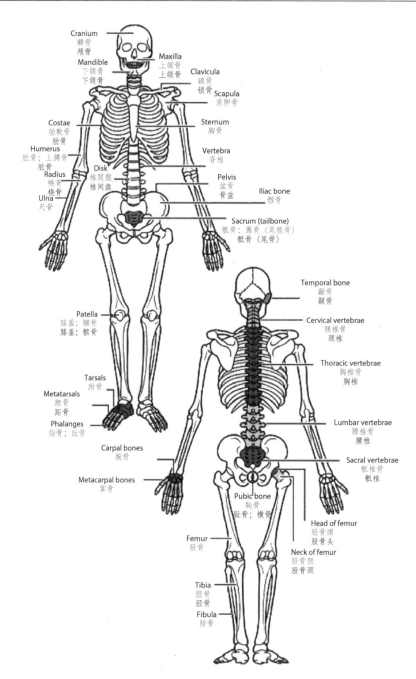

Figure 21.1 Skeleton front and back view

骨骼前後圖示

骨骼前后图示

2.   Anatomy of the skeletal system

2.1   Head

cranium	skull
temporal bone	bone on the side of the skull, above the ear
maxilla	upper jaw
mandible	lower jaw

2.2   Torso

vertebrae	there are 33 vertebrae in the spine, separated by intervertebral disks
cervical	(vertebrae) at neck level
thoracic	(vertebrae) at chest level
lumbar	(vertebrae) at lower back level
sacral	(vertebrae) at the level of the tailbone
clavicle	collarbone
scapula	shoulder blade
costae	ribs
intercostal	between the ribs
sternum	breast bone
pelvis	area between the hip bones
iliac bone	hip bone

2.3   Arms

humerus	upper arm
radius and ulna	two bones of the forearm
metacarpal bones	small bones in the hand

2.4   Legs

femur	thigh bone
neck of femur	neck of the thigh bone
head of femur	head of the thigh bone
patella	kneecap
meniscus	small crescent-shaped piece of cartilage in the knee joint
fibula	one of two long narrow bones in the lower leg
tibia	shin bone
metatarsal bones	small bones in the foot

3.   Function of the bones

The bones have various functions:

-   support of the body
-   protection (e.g. ribs protecting heart and lungs)
-   leverage (movement)
-   production of blood cells (in the bone marrow)
-   storage of minerals (calcium; phosphorus)

Bone has an excellent blood supply and is constantly changing and developing depending on circumstances (e.g. during weight-bearing exercise, bone gets stronger). Bone is made up of minerals and collagen fibers. Healthy bone requires protein, vitamin D3, magnesium, calcium and phosphorus. Excessive consumption of soft drinks containing phosphorus and inadequate intake of calcium may lead to an imbalance in the body, causing bone loss.

The bone marrow (soft center) of some flat bones (hip bones, breast bones) is involved in the production of blood cells.

4.   Health professionals

Chiropractor – health professional who has completed studies in the area of musculoskeletal disorders; often specializing in manipulation of the spinal column.

Orthopedic surgeon – medical doctor specializing in orthopedic surgery.

Orthopedist – physician specializing in orthopedics

Osteopath – health professional specializing in trying to eliminate structural problems of the skeletal system, and especially in manipulation of the spinal column.

Physical therapist – health professional who has completed studies in the treatment of muscular disorders; physical therapists are often involved in treatment of sporting injuries, rehabilitation of patients (e.g. following surgery or strokes) or in helping prevent breathing problems (e.g. patients with chronic lung disorders). See also Chapters 7 and 22.

5.   Disorders of the bones and joints

1.   *Ankylosing spondylitis* (also called *bamboo spine* or *poker spine*) – Ongoing inflammation and stiffness of the spine and pelvic joints. Eyes, heart, lung and bowels may

also be involved. Eventually the joints involved start to fuse together. The spine becomes rigid. Usually occurs in men between 20 and 40 years of age.

Causes: Autoimmune disease.

Symptoms: Worsening pain and stiffness in the lower back.

Diagnostic tests: Blood tests.

Treatment: Nonsteroidal anti-inflammatory drugs (NSAIDs).

2.   *Anterior cruciate ligament rupture* – Rupture of ligament that runs across the front of the knee.

Cause: Twisting force to the knee while foot firmly on the ground, during sports or motor vehicle collision.

Symptoms: Pop and severe pain when injury happens; initial instability, extensive swelling.

Diagnostic tests: Physical examination (patient cannot fully straighten the leg); MRI.

Treatment: Surgery

3.   *Curvature of the spine* – Spine curves to the left or right side – the most common type of curvature is scoliosis (from the Greek, meaning *crooked*).

Causes: Unknown.

Symptoms: Depends on curvature.

Diagnostic tests: X-ray.

Treatment: Back brace; surgery in severe cases.

4.   *Bone cancer* – A fast growing tumor in the bone and/or the connective tissue, in the leg or in the upper arm. There are many different types of primary bone cancer (cancer that starts in the bone); osteosarcoma is one of these. Secondary bone cancer refers to cancer spread (to the bone) from somewhere else. Common in breast, prostate or lung cancers.

Causes: Unknown.

Symptoms: Pain; problems with movement; fracture.

Investigations Diagnostic tests: X-ray, MRI scan, bone scan, bone biopsy. For secondary forms tests include CT scan.

Treatment: Limb-sparing surgery with bone graft or prosthesis; amputation; radiation therapy, chemotherapy, palliative treatment. For secondary forms treatment can include surgery; chemotherapy; radiation therapy.

5. *Fractures* – Broken bones. There are several types of fractures: open fractures (bone sticking out through the skin), closed fractures/simple fractures (skin is not broken) and greenstick fractures (incomplete fractures). Children's bones, in particular, are a bit like young green twigs and often bend rather than break completely. Fractures can also be displaced (bone pieces are out of place), non-displaced (bone pieces are still in place) or comminuted (bone has been broken into more than two pieces).

Some common fractures include: a fractured neck of the femur (abbreviated as #NOF) (especially in older women), dinner fork fracture (when radius and ulna are broken close to the wrist); fracture of the spine (which may cause injury to the spinal cord, see Chapter 17), and fractured tibia and fibula (abbreviated as #tib fib).

Causes: Impact of some kind.

Symptoms: Depends on the fracture, please see above.

Diagnostic tests: X-rays.

Treatments: General treatment methods for fractures include repositioning (putting it back in place) or reducing the fracture (bringing it back into position); collar-and-cuff; sling; plaster cast; sometimes traction (pulling it into alignment using a weight and pulley system) is used for broken thigh bones. Surgical treatment may include total hip replacement for a broken neck of femur (NOF); screw and plate; dynamic hip screw; pin; external fixation (bone supported by metal rods from outside of the body).

For open fractures the skin wound will not be closed so as to not lock in bacteria (anaerobic bacteria thrive if there is no oxygen) that could cause gas gangrene under the skin. Complications such as compartment syndrome can arise when plaster casts become too tight, blocking blood flow or putting pressure on the nerves. Symptoms of compartment syndrome may include pain; tingling; 'pins and needles'; numbness; patient is unable to move toes or fingers (flex, extend). In this case the cast will need to be split to relieve the pressure and restore the blood flow.

6. *Hydrocephalus* (from the Greek meaning: water on the brain) – Cerebrospinal fluid (CSF) is not absorbed, leading to too much fluid in the ventricles (cerebrospinal fluid spaces) in the brain. Hydrocephalus may also result from brain injury (including stroke).

Causes: In infants: not well understood. In older people: brain injury. *Symptoms*: In infants, the skull will grow bigger to accommodate the fluid. *Diagnostic tests*: CT or MRI scan.

Treatment: Shunt (or other surgery) to drain away excess cerebrospinal fluid.

7. *Osteoarthritis* – "Wear and tear" of joins/spine

Causes: Overweight; too much jarring exercise.

Symptoms: Stiffness; tenderness; deformity; difficulty moving.

Diagnostic tests: X-ray; arthroscopy; ESR blood test *to exclude* rheumatoid arthritis and other conditions.

Treatment: Weight loss; corticosteroid injections into joint; NSAIDS; physical therapy; knee brace. Surgical treatment may include total hip/knee replacement; osteotomy (to realign bone).

8. *Osteomalacia* – Referred to as rickets in children and osteomalacia in adults.

Cause: Malabsorption of calcium in the gut (either because there is not enough calcium in diet, or because of a lack of vitamin D) or because of a phosphate deficiency (because phosphate is lost through the kidneys).

Symptoms: In rickets, children's bones may become soft and bowed. In osteomalacia bones in the arms, legs, ribs and/or lower back are painful. Other symptoms include muscle weakness; waddling (duck-like) gait; chronic fatigue; bones lose their shape.

Diagnostic tests: X-ray; bone density (DEXA) scan

Treatment: Exposure to sunlight (vitamin D3); diet with calcium and/or phosphorus; vitamin D supplements.

9. *Osteomyelitis* – Inflammation or infection of bones and bone marrow.

Causes: Usually from infection elsewhere in the body (e.g. pneumonia or a urinary tract infection); open wound over bone (e.g. small heel wound) or open fracture.

Symptoms: Pain; fever; chills.

Diagnostic tests: Erythrocyte sedimentation rate (ESR); CT or MRI scan.

Treatment: Immobilizing affected bone (e.g. brace, splint); high dose of IV antibiotics; surgery.

10. *Osteoporosis* (also *"brittle bone disease"*) – Bones become thinner, lighter, and more brittle, and they break more easily.

Causes: Lack of vitamin D3; lack of weight-bearing exercise; poor diet (not enough calcium, too much soda pop); certain medications (e.g. long-term use of corticosteroids); loss of estrogen protection after menopause or due to prolonged use of certain birth control pills; family history of osteoporosis; smoking; excessive alcohol intake.

Symptoms: Bones break easily.

Diagnostic tests: DEXA scan (bone density scan).

Treatment: Increase calcium intake; weight-bearing exercise; vitamin D; hormone replacement therapy.

11.   *Rheumatic fever* – see Chapter 13.

12.   *Rheumatoid arthritis* (RA) – A connective tissue disorder involving inflammation of the connective tissue in joints, tendons and other parts of the body.

Cause: Not known; auto-immune disease – some link it to gluten intolerance.

Symptoms: Patients often feel ill, painful and stiff; small joints may be swollen or deformed.

Diagnostic tests: Blood tests: ESR (erythrocyte sedimentation rate) and C-reactive protein (CRP) are high, indicating inflammation; rheumatoid factor is positive in the blood; X-rays; family history.

Treatment: Disease modifying anti-rheumatic medication and biologic drugs (such as Humira®); some patients benefit from a diet that is gluten-free and high in fish oil. Surgery: joint replacement may be considered (total hip replacement; total knee replacement; finger bone replacement).

13. *Slipped disk* – See Chapter 17.

14. *Whiplash* – See Chapter 17.

6.   English-Chinese glossary

英漢詞彙表

English	Hong Kong & Taiwan	Mainland China
ankylosing spondylitis	關節僵直性脊椎炎	强直性脊柱炎
anterior cruciate ligament rupture	前十字韌帶撕裂	前十字韧带断裂; 前交叉韧带断裂
arthroscopy	關節內窺鏡檢查	关节 (内窥) 镜检查
autoimmune disease	自體免疫病	自身免疫性疾病
back brace	背部支架; 背封	背支具
bone cancer	骨癌	骨癌

(Continued)

English	Hong Kong & Taiwan	Mainland China
C-reactive protein (CRP)	丙種反應蛋白	C反应性蛋白
Chiropractor	脊椎治療師; 脊醫	脊椎治疗师
closed fracture; simple fracture	閉合性骨折; 無創骨折; 簡單骨折	闭合性骨折; 无创骨折; 简单骨折
comminuted fracture	粉碎性骨折	碎裂性骨折
compartment syndrome	骨筋膜室綜合症	骨筋膜室综合症
CT scan	電腦斷層掃描; 電腦掃描	CT掃描
DEXA scan; bone density scan	骨質密度掃描	骨密度扫描
dinner fork fracture	橈尺骨 (手腕骨) 骨折; 餐叉狀骨折	橈尺骨 (手腕骨) 骨折; 叉状骨折
displaced fracture	移位性骨折	移置性骨折
dynamic hip screw	動力加壓髖螺釘	动力性髋螺钉
ESR (erythrocyte sedimentation rate)	紅血球沉降率	红细胞沉降率; 血沉
external fixation	外固定術	外固定
finger bone replacement	指骨置換術	指骨置换
gas gangrene	氣性壞疽	气性坏疽
greenstick fracture	青枝骨折	青枝骨折
hydrocephalus	腦積水	脑积水
knee brace	護膝	膝关节固定带
MRI scan	磁力共振掃描	磁 (性) 共振成像; 磁振造影扫描
neck of femur	股骨頸	股骨颈
nonsteroidal antiinflammatory drug (NSAID)	非類固醇類消炎止痛藥	非类固醇抗炎药物
numbness	麻木; 麻痹	麻木; 麻痹
open fracture	哆開骨折; 開放性骨折	哆开骨折; 开放性骨折
Orthopedic/Orthopeadic Surgeon	骨科外科醫生	骨科医生; 骨外科医生
osteoarthritis	骨關節炎	骨关节炎
osteomalacia; rickets	軟骨病	软骨病; 骨软化症
osteomyelitis	骨髓炎	骨髓炎
Osteopath	骨療師; 整骨治療師	骨科医师
osteoporosis	骨質疏鬆 (症)	骨质疏松 (症)
osteosarcoma	骨肉瘤	骨肉瘤
osteotomy	截骨術	截骨术
Rheumatic fever	風濕熱	风湿热
rheumatoid arthritis (RA)	類風濕性關節炎	类风湿性关节炎

(Continued)

English	Hong Kong & Taiwan	Mainland China
sarcoma	肉瘤	肉瘤
scoliosis	脊柱側彎	脊柱側弯; 脊柱側凸
screw and plate	骨釘及骨板	骨钉及骨板
skeletal system	骨骼系統	骨骼系统
slipped disk	椎間盤突出	椎间盘突出
spinal column	脊柱	脊柱
total hip replacement	全髖關節置換術	全髋关节置换术
total knee replacement	全膝關節置換術	全膝关节置换术
X-ray	X光; X射線	X(射)線

Summary of main points

This chapter has given a brief overview of the skeletal system, including:

–   anatomy of bones and joints
–   terms with Latin and Greek roots
–   health professionals involved
–   some commonly encountered conditions relating to the bones and joints, together with common diagnostic tests and treatment methods.

Chapter 22

Muscles and the motor system

The motor system involves both nerve cells and muscle cells.

Within the motor system, the brain coordinates and controls movement by sending signals to the muscles; that is, the brain sends signals to the muscles, the muscles then contract and movement results. The cerebellum ensures that movement is smooth and coordinated.

Please note: Alcohol influences the cerebellum, resulting in movement that is less smooth and coordinated.

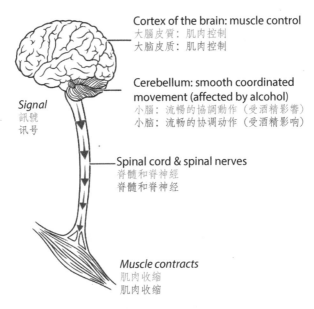

Figure 22.1 Schematic overview of the motor system
運動系統圖示
运动系统图示

1.　Terms with Latin and Greek roots

atrophy	absence of growth (muscle atrophy)
a	not; without
ab	away from

ad	towards (Note: *adc...* often changes into *acc...*)
-algia	pain
anti	against
bi	two (biceps = two headed)
chondro	cartilage-
con	together
contract	pull together
duct	lead
dys	bad; difficult; painful
dystrophy	abnormal growth
fascia	bundle
hernia	broken
-lysis	destruction of; loosening of; freeing of
malacia	softening
myalgia	muscle pain
myo	muscle
neuromuscular	to do with both nerves and muscles
-oid	resembling (e.g. deltoid muscle resembles a river delta)
ortho	straight
para	beside/alongside; beyond; accessory to (e.g. paramedic)
pathos	sick/diseased
ped	child; grow
plasty	repair
sarco	connective tissue
syn	together
tonus	tone (muscle tone)
tract	route; pull
tri	three (triceps = three-headed)
trophy	growth

2.   General terminology in relation to muscles

EMG	electromyography (electrical stimulation of muscle to measure strength of muscle contractions)
lesion	damage; injury; wound
ligament	band of fibrous tissue binding joints together
physical therapy	literally: physical treatment
	– active movement
	– passive movement

posture	The way somebody holds their body (e.g. stooped; hunched shoulder)
RICE	Rest; ice; compression; elevation treatment for injuries
ROM	range of movement exercises
sphincter	circular band of muscle fibers around natural orifices (openings)
sprain	traumatic injury to muscle, tendon, or ligament around joints: creates pain and swelling
strain	damage (usually muscular) due to excessive physical effort (overdoing it)
tendon	strong fibrous cord attaching muscle to bone
torn muscle	tear in muscle fibers

3. Anatomy of the muscles

There are three main types of muscle in the body:

- *cardiac muscle* – muscle in the wall of the heart. The cardiac muscle (myocard) responds to the heart's own pacemaker, the sinus node.
- *skeletal muscle* – role is to provide movement (voluntary, automatic or reflex) of skeleton (e.g. breathing; walking; grasping)
- *smooth muscle* – involuntary muscle in hollow organs and blood vessels that play a role in digestion and circulation.

4. Function of the muscles

In general, muscles provide movement, maintain posture and produce heat, e.g. when someone with a high fever gets the *chills* because the "thermostat" in the brain has been reset and the person feels cold.

5. Health professionals

See Chapter 17, page 202 and Chapter 21, page 266.

6. Disorders of the motor system

1. *Guillain Barré syndrome* – A virus infection leads to an antibody response in which the body's immune system mistakenly attacks part of the nervous system, resulting in nerve damage.

Causes: Viral infection.

Symptoms: Weakness; muscle wasting; paralysis (may need ventilator); tingling; numbness. Mostly affects people between 20 and 50 years of age. Note: Guillain-Barré symptoms can worsen very quickly.

Diagnostic tests: Blood tests; lumbar puncture; MRI scan.

Treatment: Acute stage – rest; pain relief; physical therapy; ventilator/respiratory support. Recovery stage – strengthening exercises.

2.   *Motor neuron disease (MND)* – Degeneration of nerve cells results in progressive muscle wasting; usually affects patients over 50 years of age (this condition is often fatal within 3–10 years). MNDs include amyotrophic lateral sclerosis (ALS), also called Lou Gehrig's disease or classical motor neuron disease.

Causes: Toxins; inherited; viral and environmental causes have also been suggested.

Symptoms: Muscle wasting and weakness; spasticity; difficulty swallowing. Can lead to complications due to respiratory infections.

Diagnostic tests: Electromyography (EMG); MRI scan; muscle biopsy.

Treatment: Physical therapy; occupational therapy; wheelchair.

3.   *Muscular dystrophy (MD)* – Group of inherited disorders of the motor system, which lead to gradually worsening muscle weakness and muscle loss. One form of MD is Duchenne's muscular dystrophy (DMD), which only affects boys.

Causes: Genetic disorder; missing protein (in DMD).

Symptoms: Affected children may develop problems walking by age 6 and may be in a wheelchair by age 12. Breathing may be affected by age 20.

Diagnostic tests: Electromyogram (testing muscle tone and strength); muscle biopsy

Treatment: Braces; walker; wheelchair; ventilator support if necessary.

4.   *Myasthenia gravis* – An autoimmune disorder affecting the motor system. Antibodies attack the junction between nerves and muscles, and the nerve signal is not transferred to the muscles.

Causes: Autoimmune.

Symptoms: Drooping eyelid is often an early sign. Painless muscle weakness can progress to paralysis, which is dangerous if breathing and swallowing are affected.

Diagnostic tests: Repetitive nerve stimulation.

Treatment: Immunosuppressants; immunoglobulins; removing the thymus gland; stem cell treatment is being investigated.

5. *Poliomyelitis* – Infection in which the polio virus destroys the *motor nerves*.

Causes: Polio virus.

Symptoms: Sore throat, malaise; headache; fever (non-paralytic poliomyelitis); in paralytic poliomyelitis, this is followed by muscle pain, muscle weakness, problems urinating, problems breathing, and may lead to paralysis. If breathing muscles are paralyzed, it may result in death.

Diagnostic tests: Lumbar puncture (to distinguish it from meningitis); blood test for polio antibodies.

Treatment: Ventilator support if necessary; physical therapy, leg braces.

6. *Polyneuropathy* – A malfunction of many peripheral nerves at the same time, leading to degeneration of those nerves.

Causes: Many different causes, including diabetes, alcohol abuse or infections such as *herpes zoster* or *Guillain Barré* (see page 275).

Symptoms: Itchiness; "crawling" sensation; "burning" sensation; pain.

Diagnostic tests: Electromyogram; nerve conduction velocity test (NCV).

Treatment: Painkillers; physical therapy.

7. Disorders of the muscles

Disorders to do with the muscles proper are often related to either exercise, overuse, trauma, injury or infection. Patients will often see their primary doctor or physical therapist (see Chapter 7) for advice. Assessment will involve physical examination and history-taking.

1. *Carpal tunnel syndrome* – Increased pressure in the carpal tunnel (a narrow space inside the wrist) causes pressure on the median nerve.

Causes: Occupational overuse; wrist injury; swelling during pregnancy or menopause.

Symptoms: Leads to numbness, pain and tingling or pins and needles in the hand and/ or arm.

Diagnostic tests: Physical examination; history.

Treatment: Wrist supports or splints; avoiding repetitive movements; steroid injections; surgery.

2.   *Groin strain* – Adductor muscle in the inner thigh muscle stretched too far.

Treatment: Rest, stretching, ice, heat.

3.   *Hematoma* – Literally, blood swelling. Blood leaks into the muscle tissue after injury, causing tenderness and bruising.

Treatment: Ice packs.

4.   *Myositis* – Inflammation of muscle tissue.

Treatment: Corticosteroids.

5.   *Occupational overuse syndrome (OOS)* (*also known as repetitive strain injury or RSI*) – Carpal tunnel syndrome and tendonitis may be examples of OOS (although they may also have a different cause).

6.   *Shin splints* – Swelling or inflammation of muscles and tendons over the shin bone due to overuse or increased activity.

Treatment: Rest, ice; stretching, strengthening; orthotics; taping.

7.   *Ruptured Achilles tendon* – Rupture of tendon at the back of the heel, causing pain, swelling, inability to walk.

Treatment: Cast or walking boot; surgery.

8.   *Sprained ligament* – Stretch and/or tear of a ligament.

Treatment: *RICE*; immobilization and surgery if severe.

9.   *Strained muscle* – Injury of a muscle or tendon.

Treatment: *RICE*; immobilization and surgery if severe.

10.   *Tendonitis* – Inflammation of the tendons (fibrous cords connecting muscles to bones) e.g. tennis elbow; Achilles tendonitis; rotator cuff injury.

Treatment: *RICE*; anti-inflammatory medications; physical therapy.

8.   Common treatment methods for muscle injuries

Medications   Anti-inflammatory medications or gels; painkillers

Physical therapy   Physical therapy may include exercises; electrical stimulation; massage; taping (rigid sports tape; stretchy kinesiology tape); applying heat or cold (ice).

9.   English-Chinese glossary

英漢詞彙表

English	Hong Kong & Taiwan	Mainland China
Achilles tendonitis	跟腱炎	跟腱炎
cardiac muscle; myocard/Myocardium	心肌	心肌
carpal tunnel syndrome	腕管綜合症	腕管综合症
cerebellum	小腦	小脑
cortex of the brain	(大) 腦皮質	大脑皮层; 大脑皮质
corticosteroids	類固醇激素; 皮質素	皮质激素; 皮质类固醇
Duchenne's muscular dystrophy (DMD)	杜氏肌肉萎縮症	杜氏肌肉萎缩症
electromyography (EMG)	肌電圖	肌电图
Guillain Barré syndrome	吉巴氏綜合症	巴格二氏综合症
herpes zoster infection	帶狀皰疹感染	带状疱疹感染
Immunoglobin/Immunoglobulin	免疫球蛋白	免疫球蛋白
Immunosupressant drug	免疫抑制劑; 免疫抑制藥物	免疫抑制剂; 免疫抑制药
kinesiology	肌動學; 運動機能學; 人體運動學	运动学
ligament	韌帶	韧带
lumbar puncture	腰椎穿刺 (抽腦脊液)	腰椎穿刺 (术)
motor neurone disease (MND); Amyotrophic lateral sclerosis (ALS)	運動神經元病; 肌萎縮性脊髓側索硬化症 (又稱漸凍人)	运动神经元病 (变) 肌萎缩性 (脊髓) 侧索硬化
motor system	運動系統	运动系统
MRI scan	磁力共振掃描	磁 (性) 共振成像; 磁振造影扫描
muscle cell	肌細胞	肌细胞
muscular dystrophy (MD)	肌肉萎縮症	肌肉萎缩症
myasthenia gravis	重症肌無力	重症肌无力; 假麻痹性重症肌无力
myositis	肌炎	肌炎
nerve cell	神經細胞	神经细胞
nerve conduction velocity (NCV) test	神經傳導速度檢查	神经传导速度试验
occupational overuse syndrome (OOS); repetitive strain injury (RSI)	職業性筋肌勞損綜合症; 重複性肌勞損	作业过度劳损综合症; 重复性肌劳损
poliomyelitis	脊髓灰質炎; 小兒麻痹症	脊髓灰质炎; 小儿麻痹
polyneuropathy	多發性神經炎	多发性神经炎

(Continued)

English	Hong Kong & Taiwan	Mainland China
RICE (rest ice compression elevation treatment)	RICE療法 (休息-冰敷-加壓-抬高)	RICE疗法 (休息-冰敷-加压-提升)
ROM (range of movement exercises)	ROM (活動度訓練運動)	ROM (活动幅度训练运动)
rotator cuff injury	旋轉帶肌肉損傷	回旋肌套损伤; 肩袖损伤
ruptured Achilles tendon	跟腱斷裂	跟腱断裂
shin splints	脛痛; 外脛炎; 外脛夾	胫痛; 外胫炎; 外胫夹
skeletal muscle	骨骼肌	骨骼肌
smooth muscle	平滑肌	平滑肌
sphincter	括約肌	括约肌
spinal cord	脊髓	脊髓
spinal nerves	脊神經	脊神经
sprain	扭傷	扭伤
stem cell treatment	幹細胞療法	干细胞疗法
strain	拉傷	扭伤
tendon	腱	腱; 筋
tendonitis	(肌) 腱炎	腱炎
thymus gland	胸腺	胸腺

Summary of main points

This chapter has given a brief overview of the muscles and motor system, including:

- anatomy of the muscles and the motor system
- terms with Latin and Greek roots
- health professionals involved
- some commonly encountered conditions relating to muscles the motor system and joints, together with common diagnostic tests and treatment methods.

Chapter 23

The sensory system

The sensory system is the system that deals with the five senses:

- Eyesight
- Smell and taste
- Hearing
- Balance
- Touch

Impressions of the outside world (e.g. sights, sounds, smells, tastes and "feels") are picked up by our eyes, nose, taste buds, ears and other receptors, and messages are sent to the brain as to what we are seeing, smelling, tasting, hearing or feeling.

1. Terms with Latin and Greek roots

astigmatism	distorted images cornea is not symmetrical (*a*: no; *stigma*: mark)
cataract	cloudy, opaque lens
cochlea	(Greek: snail shell) hearing organ which looks like a snail shell
corneal implant	artificial cornea
Eustachian tube	tube connecting middle ear with nose/throat cavity
excimer laser	special type of laser used for eye surgery
hyperopia/	
hypermetropia	farsightedness; condition where person has difficulty seeing things close-up
kerato-	cornea; having to do with the cornea
- metrist	someone who measures
myopia	shortsightedness
ophthalmos	eye
opt/optic	relating to the eye
photorefractive	light bending (rays) *photorefractive*
keratectomy	laser surgery to reshape the corneas to improve vision (less or no need for corrective glasses)
nystagmus	quick jittery movements of both eyes related to either loss of vision or loss of muscle control

retinoblastoma   tumor of retina (blast: immature cell; oma: growth)
strabismus   crossed eyes
tympanometry   checking how well the ear drum moves

2. The eye

Light enters the eye through the opening, the *pupil*. It then passes through the *lens* and is received by the nerve cells which are situated on the *retina*, at the back of the eyeball. The nerve cells pass the messages along the *optic nerve* on to the brain, which interprets the light patterns as images. The so-called blind spot is where the optic nerve leaves the retina.

3. Anatomy of the eye

This is a cross-section of the eye.

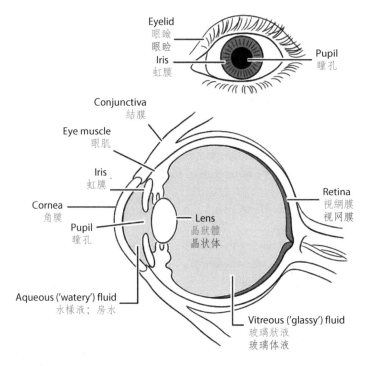

Figure 23.1 Cross-section of the eye
眼球横切面
眼球横截面

4. Different parts of the eye

conjunctiva	the inner lining of the eyelids
cornea	the clear, dome-shaped, outermost layer of the eye
iris	the round colored disk which floats in the watery fluid between the cornea and the lens of the eye
lens	thin but tough see-through membrane in front of the eyeball. The lens focuses by changing its curve. When the curve of the lens changes, the light rays passing through the lens are bent at a different angle so as to all converge at one spot on the retina.
macula	the part of the eye that provides sharp, central vision, helping you see things clearly
optic nerve	takes images from the retina to the brain
pupil	the "black" hole in the middle of the iris. Muscles in the iris can make the pupil opening bigger or smaller. If there is not much light, the pupil opening will enlarge, to let more light in
retina	the nerve cells of the eye are situated on the retina, at the back of the eyeball

5. Health professionals

Ophthalmologist – Doctor specializing in eyes and eye complaints.
Optometrist – Health professional specializing in measuring eyesight.
Optician – Professional specialized in providing people with the right glasses or contact lenses.

6. Disorders of the eye

1. *Cataract* – Lens becomes increasingly cloudy or opaque.

Causes: Age; eye injury; diabetes; X-rays; microwaves; UV light; long-term use of corticosteroids.

Symptoms: Blurry vision; "grey film" covering the eye.

Diagnostic tests: Eye examination.

Treatment: Surgery to remove cloudy lens and insert an artificial lens; phacoemulsification (ultrasound is used to break up lens into small pieces, which are then suctioned out).

2. *Conjunctivitis* – (also called pink eye) – infection or inflammation of the conjunctiva.

Cause: Viral or bacterial infection; irritation; allergy; chemicals.

Symptoms: Painful, swollen, red eyes; bacterial infection may cause yellow discharge.

Diagnostic tests: Swab; culture to see which bacteria has caused the infection.

Treatment: Anti-bacterial ointment; steroid or antihistamine eye drops for allergic conjunctivitis.

3. *Floaters* – Spots, flecks or "cobwebs" in the vision.

Cause: Bits of debris floating in the gel-like fluid (vitreous humor) in front of the retina, due to aging, injury or bleeding into the vitreous humor. Sudden increases in floaters with light flashes may be followed by retinal detachment (see below – medical emergency).

Symptoms: As above

Diagnostic tests: Eye examination

Treatment: None.

4. *Glaucoma* – Too much pressure in the fluid in front of the lens, leading to pressure on lens. This pressure is transferred to the fluid in front of the retina and may

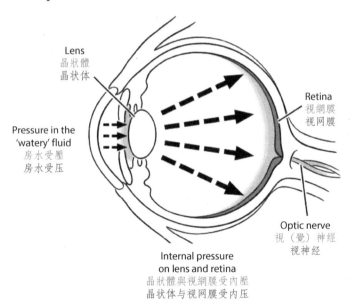

Figure 23.2 Schematic representation of glaucoma
青光眼圖示
青光眼图示

eventually lead to damage of the nerve cells on the retina. There are different types of glaucoma; the two most common are open-angle glaucoma, which develops gradually (slow onset), and angle-closure glaucoma, which can have an acute onset (start suddenly).

Cause: Risk factors include age; family history; myopia; diabetes.

Symptoms: Pain; reduced vision or even blindness; sudden loss of vision in one eye; halos around lights; often acute episodes with severe pain; nausea and vomiting.

Diagnostic tests: Regular eye examinations; pressure test in which a puff of air is blown against the eye (tonometry).

Treatment: Eye drops: surgery aimed at allowing fluid to seep away by enlarging drainage openings, e.g. laser treatment: laser iridotomy; laser trabeculectomy (filtration surgery).

5.   *Macular degeneration, also Age-Related Macular Degeneration (AMD or ARMD) –* a range of conditions affecting the macula, the central part of the retina. AMD is a leading cause of blindness.
There are two types of AMD: dry and wet.

Cause: Deterioration of the retina. Risk factors include age; smoking; light eye color. *What happens*: the macula deteriorates, especially in those aged 55 and older.
Dry (atrophic) form: This type results from the gradual breakdown of cells in the macula, resulting in a gradual blurring of central vision. Single or multiple, small, round, yellow-white spots called *drusen* are the key identifiers of the dry form.
Wet form: Abnormal blood vessels grow under the center of the retina, leaking, bleeding and scarring, leading to a rapid loss of vision.

Symptoms: Dry AMD: gradual blurring of central vision. Wet AMD: rapid loss of vision, usually in one eye first.

Symptoms: Blurry vision; blind spots.

Diagnostic tests: Visual field testing; special eye tests using contrast dye.

Treatment: Low vision aids; stopping smoking.

6.   *Nystagmus* – Rolling or jerking eye movements.

Cause: Some form of brain dysfunction; multiple sclerosis; use of alcohol or barbiturates (drugs causing sleepiness).

Symptoms: As above.

Diagnostic tests: Eye examination.

Treatment: Treating underlying condition.

7. *Retinal detachment* – Retina comes away from the back of the eye.

Cause: Age, myopia.

Symptoms: Shower of sparkling spots and/or floaters, followed by feeling as if a curtain is moving across the eye. Note: this is a medical emergency, as it can lead to blindness.

Diagnostic tests: Eye examination.

Treatment: Immediate laser surgery to reattach the retina.

8. *Trachoma* – Type of conjunctivitis.

Causes: Contagious bacterial infection.

Symptoms: Pain; redness; swelling; scarred eyelids rub on eyeballs, can lead to blindness

Diagnostic tests: Eye examination.

Treatment: Urgent medical attention required, including tetracycline (medication) and surgical repair of scarred eyelids.

7. The ears

Sound waves enter through the outer ear and the ear canal until they hit the ear drum, making it vibrate

The middle ear is situated between the ear drum and the inner ear. In the middle ear, the sound waves are passed from the ear drum to a number of small bones (the hammer, the anvil and the stirrup), until they reach the inner ear.

The inner ear is the part of the ear that contains the cochlea, the hearing organ, which is shaped like a snail shell and lined with nerve cells. The inner ear also contains the balance organ. The nerve cells in the inner ear receive the sound message and send it on to the brain by way of the auditory nerve.

There is a tube called the Eustachian tube which leads from the nose/throat area to the middle ear. This tube is one reason why infections are easily transferred from the nose/throat area to the middle ear.

8. Anatomy of the ear

The ear consists of three sections:

- the outer ear – where sound is received and transferred to the eardrum.
- the middle ear – where sound is transferred from the eardrum to the inner ear.

– the inner ear – which contains the hearing organ and the balance organ. The illustration shows a cross-section of the ear.

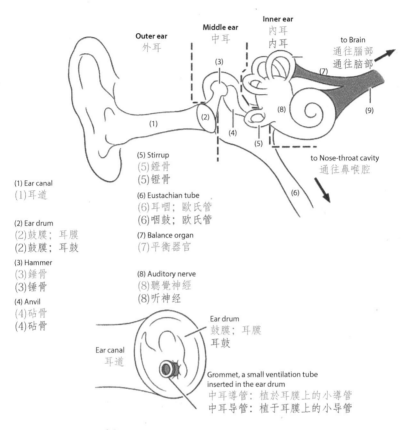

Figure 23.3 Cross-section of the ear
耳蝸橫切面
耳蝸橫截面

9. Health professionals

Audiologist – Health professional who diagnoses hearing or balance problems; may dispense hearing aids or recommend cochlear implants.

Audiometrist – Hearing tester.

Otorhinolaryngologist (ORL), also called an ENT for Ear-Nose-Throat (ENT) specialist – Doctor specializing in disorders of the ear, nose and throat. The ENT also treats patients with disorders of the balance organ, as this is situated near the inner ear.

10. Conditions of the ear and balance organ

1. *Deafness* – Inability to hear (can be nerve deafness or conductive hearing loss).

Causes: Can be congenital; damage to auditory nerve through ongoing noise, drugs or trauma.

Symptoms: Hearing loss.

Diagnostic tests: Otoscopy; audiometry.

Treatment: Cochlear implant, a surgically implanted electronic device that provides a sense of sound. Cochlear implants comprise a microphone, a speech processor, a transmitter (behind the ear), a receiver and stimulator (placed in bone beneath the skin), and electrodes wound through the cochlea, which send nerve messages through to the brain. For this to be successful the patient needs a functioning auditory nerve, profound deafness in both ears, and a desire to become part of the "hearing" world.

Note: Not all deaf individuals view their deafness as a deficit; some consider their deafness as a normal part of who they are and choose to forego treatment.

2. *Ear infection (also otitis media or middle ear infection)* – Bacterial infection of the middle ear whereby the middle ear fills up with fluid, causing pressure against eardrum.

Cause: Cold blocking off the Eustachian tube; bacteria trapped inside middle ear (where they multiply, causing infection). More common in young children as the Eustachian tube is smaller and floppier and becomes more easily blocked.

Symptoms: Hearing loss; pain. Additional complications can arise for children if left untreated. Glue ear (gluey fluid remains in middle ear) leads to hearing loss which can affect (delay) speech development.

Diagnostic tests: Checking ear for fluid with otoscope.

Treatment: Antibiotics; ear tubes if repeated ear infections.

3. *Impacted cerumen (ear wax)* – Ear wax blocks the outer ear so sounds cannot get through.

Cause: Ear wax (often pushed inside when cleaning ear with cotton swabs).

Symptoms: Tinnitus (roaring sound in ear); hearing loss.

Diagnostic tests: History.

Treatment: Syringing or irrigating ear with lukewarm water.

4. *Glue ear* (see ear infection).

5. *Meniere's disease* – Fluid increases in the ear canals in the inner ear, which leads to more pressure in the inner ear, disturbing the sense of balance.

Cause: Unknown; factors may include food allergy (including beans and legumes) or injury to middle ear.

Symptoms: Vertigo (dizziness) with a sense of the room spinning; tinnitus (ringing in the ear); nausea, sweating. The increase in pressure can also damage the *cochlea* (hearing organ), leading to hearing loss.

Diagnostic tests: Audiometry; MRI brain scan.

Treatment: Medication.

6. *Middle ear infection* (see ear infection).

7. *Motion sickness* (also called seasickness or carsickness) – Motion of plane, car or ship makes person sick.

Cause: Very sensitive balance center (inherited) in the inner ear.

Symptoms: Nausea and vomiting.

Diagnostic tests: History.

Treatment: Antihistamines; skin patch, worn close to the ear (and balance organ).

8. *Otitis media* (see ear infection).

9. *Seasickness* (see motion sickness)

11. Medications (for eyes and ears)

antihistamines	used for allergy relief; prevent the allergic reaction by preventing the release of histamine.
blocking agents	lower the pressure in the eye.
miotics	lead to narrowing of the pupil (treatment of glaucoma).
antibiotics	help the body fight bacterial infections.

12. Touch

The skin contains many nerve endings. When we touch something, for example something hot, a message travels back from the nerve receptor, along a long path, back up along the spinal cord to the brain. The brain then realizes that we are touching something hot and sends another message down along nerve paths to a muscle, saying: "Pull that hand back! Quick!" Those of us who have ever touched something very hot and pulled our hand back, will realize that these messages travel to and from the brain incredibly quickly.

13. Disorders of touch

Disorders of touch/sensation will usually be investigated by the *neurologist* (nerve specialist).

1. *Loss of sensation*

Cause: Many different factors may be involved, including nerve damage (please refer to Chapters 17 and 25) due to diabetes; a break in the spinal cord; a nerve having been accidentally cut; swelling and pressure on the nerves (e.g. after having a plaster cast applied). Loss of sensation may also result from nerve cells not getting enough oxygen due to loss of blood supply to a certain area. Blood supply may be lost due to a blood clot blocking circulation, or to a narrowing of arteries, limiting the amount of blood to the area. Compartment syndrome may also be involved.

Symptoms: Loss of sensation.

Diagnostic tests: Neurological studies.

Treatment: Treating the underlying cause.

2. *Unusual sensation or paresthesia*

Causes: There may be pressure on a nerve either at the level of the spine (e.g. whiplash injury or prolapsed disk) or at another level, (e.g. on the nerve in the wrist in carpal tunnel syndrome or due to a cast which is too tight as in compartment syndrome).

Symptoms: Tingling; pins and needles; numbness. *Diagnostic tests*: MRI scan; neurological studies.

Treatment: Treating underlying cause.

14.   English-Chinese glossary

英漢詞彙表

English	Hong Kong & Taiwan	Mainland China
angle-closure glaucoma	閉角青光眼	闭角型青光眼
antihistamine	抗組胺藥; 抗過敏藥	抗组胺药; 抗过敏药
anvil	砧骨	砧骨
aqueous fluid	水樣液; 房水	房水
astigmatism	散光	散光
Audiologist	聽力學家; 聽覺學家	听力学家; 听力师
Audiometrist	聽力測定師	测听师
auditory nerve	聽 (覺) 神經	听神经
balance	平衡	平衡
balance organ	平衡器官	平衡器官
blind spot	盲點	盲点
blocking agent	阻斷劑	阻滞剂; 阻断剂
cataract	白內障	白内障
cochlea	耳蝸	耳蜗
conjunctiva	結膜	结膜
conjunctivitis	結膜炎	结膜炎
cornea	(眼) 角膜	角膜
corneal implant	角膜植入	角膜植入
ear canal	耳道	耳道
ear drum	鼓膜; 耳膜	鼓膜; 耳鼓
Eustachian tube	耳咽管; 歐氏管	咽鼓管; 欧氏管
excimer laser	準分子雷射; 準分子激光	准分子雷射; 准分子激光
eye muscle	眼肌	眼肌
eyesight	視力	视力; 眼力
eyelid	眼瞼	眼睑
floaters	飛蚊症	飞蚊症
glaucoma	青光眼	青光眼
glue ear; otitis media with effusion	積液性中耳炎; 中耳積水	胶耳; 中耳积水
grommet	中耳導管	鼓室通气管
hammer	錘骨	锤骨
hearing	聽覺	听力

(Continued)

English	Hong Kong & Taiwan	Mainland China
hyperopia; hypermetropia; farsightedness	遠視	远视
impacted cerumen; impacted ear wax	耳垢阻塞	耳垢阻塞
inner ear	內耳	内耳
iris	虹膜	虹膜
lens	晶狀體	晶状体
macula	黃斑	黄斑
macular degeneration (AMD)	黃斑退化; 視網膜黃斑病變	黄斑病变
Meniere's disease	美尼爾氏病; 耳病性眩暈; (俗稱「耳水不平衡」)	梅尼埃尔氏病; 耳性眩晕病
middle ear	中耳	中耳
miotics	縮瞳劑	缩瞳剂
motion sickness	暈浪	晕动病
myopia; shortsightedness	近視	近视
numbness	麻木; 麻痺; 無感覺	麻木; 麻痹
nystagmus	眼球震顫; 眼震	眼球震颤
open-angle glaucoma	開角青光眼	开角型青光眼
Ophtalmologist	眼科醫生	眼科医生
optic nerve	視 (覺) 神經	视神经
Optician	配鏡師	眼镜师
Optometrist	視光師; 驗光師	配镜师
otitis media; middle ear infection; ear infection	中耳炎	中耳炎
Otorhinolaryngologist (ORL); Ear-Nose-Throat (ENT) specialist	耳鼻喉專科醫生	耳鼻喉科医师
otoscope	耳窺鏡	耳镜
outer ear	外耳	外耳
photorefractive keratectomy	鐳射屈光角膜切除術	屈光性角膜切除术
pins and needles	發麻	發麻
pressure in the 'watery' fluid	水樣液內壓	房水内压
pupil	瞳孔	瞳孔
retina	視網膜	视网膜
retinal detachment	視網膜脫落	视网膜脱落; 视网膜剥离
retinoblastoma	視網膜胚細胞瘤	视网膜母细胞瘤
smell and taste	嗅覺與味覺	嗅觉与味觉
stirrup	鐙骨	镫骨

(Continued)

English	Hong Kong & Taiwan	Mainland China
Strabismus/strabilismus	斜視	斜視; 斜眼
syringing	沖洗	冲洗
tetracycline	四環素	四环素
tingling	刺痛; 麻刺感	刺痛; 麻刺感
tinnitus	耳鳴	耳鸣
touch	觸碰感覺; 觸覺	触碰感觉; 触觉
trachoma	砂眼	沙眼; 粒性结膜炎; 椒疮
tympanometry	鼓室圖 (聽力) 檢查; 鼓膜測試	鼓室测定法; 鼓室压测量
vertigo	眩暈	眩晕
vitreous fluid	玻璃狀液	玻璃体液; 玻璃狀液

Summary of main points

This chapter has looked at the sensory system, including:

- anatomy and physiology of the ears and eyes
- terms with Latin and Greek roots
- health professionals
- some commonly encountered conditions affecting the sensory system, together with common diagnostic tests and treatment methods.

Chapter 24

Immunology

The immune and lymphatic systems

The immune system is like the body's 'bodyguard'. It involves, amongst other things, the lymphatic system and special white blood cells called lymphocytes. During an infection, the lymph nodes become large and tender, because they are involved in fighting the infection. You may notice the doctor palpating (feeling) the lymph nodes during a physical examination.

1. Terms with Latin and Greek roots

antibodies	proteins produced by the body's lymphocytes to identify and fight particular bacteria or viruses
antigen	from **anti**body **gen**erator, a substance in viruses or bacteria that generates or triggers an antibody response
autoimmune disease	an illness in which the body attacks its own cells (e.g. in *rheumatoid arthritis*)
foreign substances	substances from outside of the body which are alien to the body
immunocompromised	the immune system is not able to fight off infections very well
immunoglobulin	protein produced by the immune system to identify and fight foreign substances such as bacteria and viruses
immune deficiency	the immune system is not able to fight off infections, as in AIDS (acquired immune deficiency syndrome)
immunosuppressant drugs	medications which suppress the immune system, making it less able to fight off infections
immunity	body's ability to overcome illnesses
immunization	*the introduction of an antigen that provokes the* immune system into developing 'weapons' against that particular bacteria or virus
active immunization	body is exposed to foreign substances and develops antibodies. Active immunization is long-lasting.

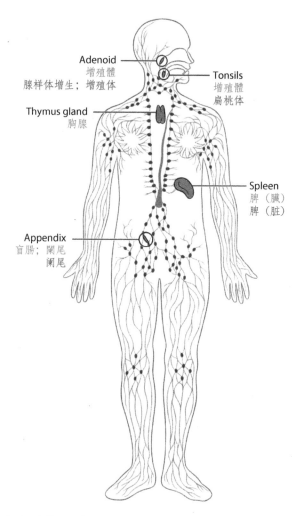

Figure 24.1 Lymph circulation system
淋巴循環系統
淋巴循环系统

passive immunization	mother passes her immunity on to baby during pregnancy or while breastfeeding; passive immunization does not last long.
lymph tissue	lymph cells or lymphocytes (T cells and B cells)
lymphedema	swelling of a part of the body (usually an arm or a leg) due to lymph being 'collected' in that body part that cannot drain away to rejoin the lymph vessels in the rest of the body (e.g. women who have had the lymph nodes in their armpit removed may develop lymphedema of the arm later on).
lymphocyte	special white blood cells that make antibodies against antigens; lymph cells

lymphoma	cancer involving the lymph cells
lymphatic ducts	network of lymph vessels that unite to form larger vessels called ducts
lymph nodes	lymph nodes filter the lymph, trapping foreign substances so the body can fight them
vaccination	artificial active immunization (body is exposed to weakened component of bacteria or virus, so it starts to make antibodies) artificial passive immunization – person is given serum containing antibodies (short-acting immunity)

2. Anatomy of the immune and lymphatic systems

The body has two main circululatory systems: the blood circulation system and the lymph circulation system. Not many people are aware of the second system, and yet it plays a very important role. The lymphatic system consists of a system of lymph vessels and lymph nodes. The lymph nodes are like truck depots or bus stations, where lymph collects *en route*.

3. Lymphatic organs

appendix	Small pouch in the GI tract, containing lymph tissue situated close to where the small intestine joins the large intestine
bone marrow	contains stem cells which develop into specialized blood cells (red and white blood cells and platelets)
gut or intestine	the lining of the gut contains many lymphocytes which scan food to see if an immune response is warranted. Food is thought to play a much more important role in the development of (autoimmune) disease than previously thought
thymus	lymph tissue behind breast bone which generates T-lymphocytes
tonsils and adenoid	lymph tissue in the throat
spleen	lies behind/under the stomach. The spleen breaks down and filters out old red blood cells; gets rid of bacteria and produces lymphocytes. *Sometimes the spleen is ruptured in accidents. This can result in a serious bleed leading to shock. A ruptured spleen is a medical emergency and must be removed immediately by a surgeon as it is too 'spongy' to be sutured.*
	The spleen may also be larger than normal and prone to rupture in viral illnesses such as glandular fever; care needs to be taken in these cases as well and contact sports avoided.

4.   Function of the immune and lymphatic systems

The lymphatic system drains lymph fluid which has collected in tissue and takes it back to the blood circulation system. This fluid contains protein and fats which have escaped from the blood circulation system.

The lymphatic system also produces lymphocytes (big white cells) which play a role in our immune system. Through our immune system our body's defense system develops, i.e. we develop immunities. These include B lymphocytes which may grow into plasma cells (which develop antibodies) and T lymphocytes which destroy infected cells or bacteria and also have an effect on other parts of the immune system.

5.   Health professionals

Immunologist – Physician specializing in the immune system.
Hematologist – Physician specializing in the blood and related body systems.

6.   Disorders of the immune and lymphatic systems

1.   *Acquired immune deficiency syndrome (AIDS)* – condition following infection with human immunodeficiency virus (HIV), which attaches itself to the CD4 helper T-cell lymphocytes so the body can no longer respond to infections. The virus can also stop B-cell lymphocytes from doing their job properly. Slowly, the CD4 cell count goes down and the immune system starts to fail.

AIDS is different to HIV infection. A diagnosis of AIDS requires HIV infection plus one of the following:

-   a CD4+ T-cell count below 200 cells/μL;
-   a CD4+ T-cell percentage of total lymphocytes of less than 15%;
-   diagnosis of one of a list of defining illnesses.

Causes: HIV can only be transmitted through blood, semen, vaginal secretions and breast milk, i.e. through sexual intercourse, sharing of intravenous needles, breast-feeding by an HIV-infected mother; or receiving organs from an infected donor.

Symptoms: Vary over the course of the disease. Those with blood (serum) which is positive for HIV antibodies may not show any symptoms of AIDS (sometimes for a long time). Early symptoms of HIV infection can include brief periods of illness (fever; chills; feeling unwell; headache); tiredness; oral thrush; weight loss; diarrhea. In full-blown AIDS the patient has very low immunity and develops major infections characteristic of AIDS (e.g. cytomegalovirus infection or CMV; tuberculosis; chronic herpes simplex virus infection or one of many others) or one of the secondary cancers characteristic of AIDS (e.g. Kaposi's sarcoma or non-Hodgkin's lymphoma).

Diagnostic tests: CD4 cell count below 350 cells/mm3; over-the-counter saliva testing kit.

Treatment: Highly active antiretroviral rherapy (HAART). *The patient will remain infectious even when on HAART*. Research is ongoing. AIDS can be prevented through practicing safe sex, i.e. use of condoms, and using clean sterilized needles

2.   *Allergic reactions* – An overreaction of the body to foreign substances from out-side the body (e.g. pollen, seafood, peanuts or medication).

What happens: An allergen is any substance which causes an allergic reaction (e.g. nuts, eggs, shellfish, wasp or bee stings, pollen, antibiotics, latex). On first contact, the body makes the antibodies to the allergens. On second contact an antibody-allergen reaction takes place. Body cells are damaged and histamine comes out, causing the body's tissues to swell up. At the same time, blood vessels in the area widen, leading to redness.

If this allergic reaction takes place in the airways, the breathing tubes become narrowed with swelling and the person produces a wheezing sound when trying to breathe out.

Symptoms: See anaphylactic shock below.

Diagnostic tests: Skin test; history.

Treatment: Avoiding triggers; special diet; EpiPen® autoinjector if necessary.

3.   *Anaphylactic shock* – Anaphylaxis is a severe allergic reaction which affects the whole body.

Symptoms: Blood vessels widen all over the body, leading to an enormous drop in blood pressure, which in turns leads to *shock*. There may be redness all over the body (an all-over body rash) as well as itching and swelling all over the body. Breathing is difficult as airways can swell up.

Diagnostic tests: Blood pressure; pulse; history.

Treatment: Epinephrine (adrenaline) injections must be given fast, preferably using an autoinjector such as the EpiPen®.

4. *Elephantiasis* – (also known as *filariasis*) – A parasite infection leading to enlargement of a limb due to blockage of lymph glands.

Causes: Tiny parasitic worm found in tropical countries which is conveyed through the bites of mosquitoes infested with the parasite.

Symptoms: Enlargement of a limb due to obstruction (blockage) of lymph glands.

Diagnostic tests: Finger-prick test followed by checking blood smear under microscope.

Treatment: Medications (diethylcarbamazine, also known as DEC); sometimes plastic surgery; bed rest; tight bandages. Elephantiasis can be prevented through medications (*DEC*) and avoiding mosquito bites.

5. *Graft-versus-host-disease* (*GVHD*) – Occurs when the healthy donor cells attack the weakened body of the host (the person receiving the donor cells or transplant).

Symptoms: Red rash; abdominal pain and cramps; nausea; dry mouth and dry eyes.

Diagnostic tests: Biopsy of skin or mucosa of the mouth.

Treatment: Immunosuppressant medications.

6a. *Hodgkin's lymphoma* – Cancer of the lymphocytes.

Causes: Exact cause is not known.

Symptoms: Painless, enlarged lymph nodes (lumps), usually in the neck first, then spreading to other lymph nodes; tiredness; night sweats; weakness.

Diagnostic tests: Biopsy of lymph nodes; body scan to check for spread.

Treatment: Combination of radiation therapy and chemotherapy; stem cell transplant (using healthy bone marrow from patient); monoclonal antibodies. For young patients, special measures are taken which include sperm storage for men prior to chemotherapy and hormone replacement therapy for young women following chemotherapy, as they may go into early menopause.

6b. *Non-Hodgkin's Lymphoma* – Cancer of the lymphocytes which is not Hodgkin's lymphoma. There are sixteen different types, ranging from very slow growing to very aggressive, but usually B-cells and sometimes T-cells are affected.

Symptoms: Enlarged lymph nodes; tiredness; weight loss; sometimes enlarged spleen.

Diagnostic tests: Bone marrow biopsy; blood counts; CT scan.

Treatment: Chemotherapy; stem cell transplant (using healthy bone marrow from patient); monoclonal antibodies; immunotherapy.

7. *Lymphoma* – There are several types of lymphoma including *Burkitt's lymphoma* (a type of Non-Hodgkins Lymphoma, see above).

8. *Lymphedema* – Swelling (edema) that occurs when lymph cannot drain away as normal, causing the affected body part to swell up.

Causes: Lymph nodes removed from armpit or groin following breast surgery or abdominal surgery; lymph drainage blocked for another reason, e.g. inflammation or blockage of lymph vessels, or patient does not have sufficient lymph vessels.

Symptoms: Arm or leg swells up; feels very 'tight'.

Diagnostic tests: History; physical examination.

Treatment: Sleeping with legs/arm elevated; elastic stockings; low salt diet (to reduce fluid retention); diuretics; sometimes surgery.

9. *Systemic Lupus Erythematosus or (SLE)* – Autoimmune disease affecting connective tissue in any part of the body. SLE most often affects heart, joints, skin, lungs, blood vessels, liver, kidneys, and nervous system.

Causes: Exact cause is not known.

Symptoms: General malaise; fever; joint pains; butterfly rash on face.

Diagnostic tests: Blood tests.

Treatment: Immunosuppressants; disease-modifying antirheumatic drugs.

10. *Tissue rejection* – Occurs when antibodies are formed against the transplanted tissues following a transplant. To prevent tissue rejection, tissue typing takes place before transplantation. The tissue typing is done in order to make sure that the tissues of the receiving person and the donor are very similar, so that, hopefully, the receiving person's immune system will not reject the donor organ. In addition, patients are given special immunosuppressant drugs to prevent rejection.

11. *Tonsillitis* – Painful, red and swollen tonsils.

Causes: Bacterial or viral infection of the throat.

Symptoms: Red, swollen tonsils. Can lead to complications including abscess and strep throat, which may lead to rheumatic fever.

Diagnostic tests: Throat swab to check for bacteria.

Treatment: Antibiotics; chronic and recurrent episodes may require a tonsillectomy (tonsil surgically removed).

7. English-Chinese glossary

英漢詞彙表

English	Hong Kong & Taiwan	Mainland China
Acquired Immune Deficiency Syndrome (AIDS)	後天免疫力缺乏症; 愛滋病	获得性免疫缺乏综合症; 艾滋病
adenoids	腺樣增殖體	腺样体增生; 增殖体
anaphylactic shock	過敏性休克	过敏性休克
antibodies	抗體	抗体
antigen	抗原	抗原
appendix	盲腸; 闌尾	阑尾
autoimmune disease	自體免疫病	自身免疫性疾病
B-cells	B細胞	B細胞
Bone marrow	骨髓	骨髓
Burkitt's lymphoma	伯基特; 伯奇氏淋巴瘤	伯基特淋巴瘤
CD4 helper T-cell lymphocytes	CD4輔助型T淋巴細胞	CD4辅助型T淋巴细胞
chemotherapy	化學療法; 化療	化学疗法; 化学治疗; 化疗
CT scan	電腦斷層掃描; 電腦斷層攝影; 電腦掃描	CT扫描
cytomegalovirus infection (CMV)	巨細胞病毒感染	巨细胞病毒感染
diethylcarbamazine (DEC)	乙胺嗪 (抗絲蟲藥)	乙胺嗪
elephantiasis	象皮病	象皮病; 象皮肿
epinephrine	腎上腺素	肾上腺素
filariasis; lymphatic filariasis	絲蟲病; 淋巴絲蟲病 (俗稱「象皮病」)	丝虫病; 淋巴丝虫病
graft-versus-host disease (GVHD)	移植體對宿主反應; 移植體抗宿主病	移植物抗宿主病
Hematologist/Haematologist	血液學家; 血液病科醫生	血液学家; 血液病学家
highly active antiretroviral therapy (HAART)	高療效抗逆轉錄病毒療法; 效能抗愛滋病毒治療法 (俗稱「雞尾酒療法」)	高活性抗逆转录病毒治疗
Hodgkin's lymphoma	何傑金氏淋巴瘤	霍奇金氏淋巴瘤; 何杰金氏淋巴瘤
human immunodeficiency virus (HIV)	人類免疫力缺乏病毒; 愛滋病病毒	人类免疫缺陷病毒; 艾滋病病毒
immune system	免疫系統	免疫系统
immunoglobulin	免疫球蛋白	免疫球蛋白
Immunologist	免疫學家	免疫学家
Kaposi's sarcoma	卡波西氏肉瘤	卡波济氏肉瘤

(Continued)

English	Hong Kong & Taiwan	Mainland China
lymph	淋巴液	淋巴
lymph node	淋巴結	淋巴结; 淋巴腺
lymph vessel	淋巴管	淋巴管
lymphatic duct	淋巴導管	淋巴导管
lymphedema/lymphoedema	淋巴水腫	淋巴水肿
lymphocite/lymphocyte	淋巴球; 淋巴細胞	淋巴细胞
lymphoma	淋巴瘤	淋巴瘤
lymphatic system	淋巴系統	淋巴系统
monoclonal antibodies	單純系抗體; 單克隆抗體	单克隆抗体
non-Hodgkin's lymphoma	非何傑金氏淋巴瘤	非霍奇金淋巴瘤; 非何杰金淋巴瘤
spleen	脾 (臟)	脾 (脏)
stem cell transplant	幹細胞移植	干细胞移植
systemic lupus erythematosus (SLE)	系統性紅斑狼瘡	全身性红斑狼疮; 系统性红斑狼疮
T-cell lymphocyte	T 細胞淋巴球	T淋巴细胞
thymus gland	胸腺	胸腺
tissue rejection	組織排斥性	组织排斥
tonsillectomy	扁桃腺切除術	扁桃体切除术; 扁桃体摘除
tonsillitis	扁桃腺炎	扁桃体炎
tonsils	扁桃腺 (體)	扁桃体

Summary of main points

This chapter has given a brief overview of the immune system, including:

- anatomy of the immune system
- terms with Latin and Greek roots
- health professionals involved
- some commonly encountered conditions relating to the immune system, together with common diagnostic tests and treatment methods.

Chapter 25

Endocrinology

The endocrine system

The endocrine system manages the body's hormones (chemical messengers). A number of organs and glands are involved in producing these chemical hormones and releasing them into the body. The following Latin and Greek roots form the basis of many medical words that have to do with the endocrine system.

1. Terms with Latin and Greek roots

acro	topmost; extreme
adrenals	hormone producing glands found *alongside the kidneys* (*ad-renal*)
diabetes	running through
ectomy	cut out; surgical removal of
endocrine	releasing internally
endocrinologist	doctor who specializes in the endocrine system
glyco	glucose, sugar
glycemic	sugar in the blood
hyper	too high, too much (compare *super – very high, very much*)
hyperthyroidism	hyperactive thyroid
hypo	too low, not enough (compare *sub – very low, very little*)
hypothyroidism	underactive thyroid
insipidus	tasteless (people with *diabetes insipidus* do not care what their drinks taste like, as long as they have something to drink!)
megaly	largeness (*megalos* – big)
mellitus	sweet as honey – in *diabetes mellitus* – fluid sweet as honey is running through the body (blood, urine)
parathyroid	alongside the thyroid
thyroid	shaped like a shield

2.   Overview of the endocrine system

These glands	Produce these hormones	Which do this:
adrenal glands	corticosteroids	encourage the body to repair after injury
	aldosterone	helps the body retain water and sodium
	adrenaline (also called epinephrine)	helps the body's *flight-fight* response, increases heart rate and breathing rate
hypothalamus (in brain)	stimulating and inhibiting hormones	switch hormone secretion by pituitary gland on or off
ovaries	estrogen and progesterone	female sex hormones
pancreas	– enzymes for digesting food – insulin (produced in cells called the Islets of Langerhans)	lowers blood sugar levels
	– glucagon	raises blood sugar levels
parathyroid gland (in the neck)	parathyroid hormone	regulates calcium levels in the blood and bone metabolism
pineal gland (in brain)	melatonin	manages sleep-wake patterns
pituitary gland (in brain)	thyroid-stimulating hormone (TSH); follicle-stimulating hormone (FSH), luteinizing hormone (LH); human growth hormone (HGH); adrenocorticotropin hormone (ACTH); prolactin and oxytocin	LH and FSH trigger ovulation; ACTH triggers release of corticosteroids; prolactin stimulates production of breast milk; oxytocin causes contractions of the womb
testicles (testes)	testosterone	male sex hormone
thyroid gland	thyroxin (T4)	helps regulate metabolic rate

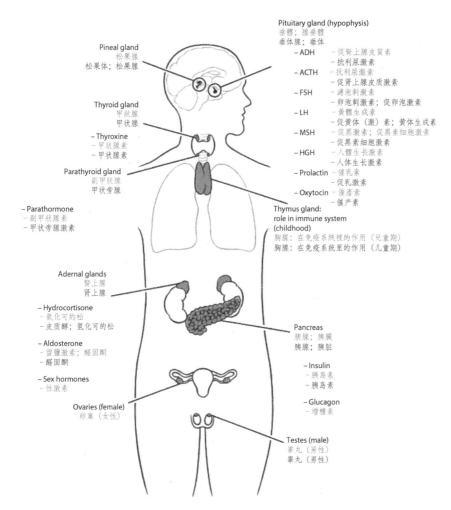

Pineal gland
松果腺
松果体；松果腺

Thyroid gland
甲狀腺
甲状腺
– Thyroxine
– 甲狀腺素
– 甲状腺素

Parathyroid gland
副甲狀腺
甲狀旁腺

– Parathormone
– 副甲狀腺素
– 甲状旁腺激素

Adernal glands
腎上腺
肾上腺

– Hydrocortisone
– 氫化可的松
– 皮质醇；氢化可的松

– Aldosterone
– 留鹽激素；醛固酮
– 醛固酮

– Sex hormones
– 性激素

Ovaries (female)
卵巢（女性）

Pituitary gland (hypophysis)
垂體；腺垂體
垂体腺；垂体
– ADH   – 促腎上腺皮質素
             – 抗利尿激素
– ACTH   – 抗利尿激素
             – 促肾上腺皮质激素
– FSH   – 濾泡刺激素
             – 卵泡刺激素；促卵泡激素
– LH   – 黃體生成素
             – 促黄体（激）素；黄体生成素
– MSH   – 促黑激素；促黑素细胞激素
             – 促黑素细胞激素
– HGH   – 人體生長激素
             – 人体生长激素
– Prolactin – 催乳素
             – 促乳激素
– Oxytocin   – 催產素
             – 催产素

Thymus gland:
role in immune system
(childhood)
胸腺：在免疫系統裡的作用（兒童期）
胸腺：在免疫系统里的作用（儿童期）

Pancreas
胰腺；胰臟
胰腺；胰脏

– Insulin
– 胰島素
– 胰岛素

– Glucagon
– 增糖素

Testes (male)
睾丸（男性）
睾丸（男性）

Figure 25.1 Endocrine system
內分泌系統
内分泌系统

3.   Health professionals

Endocrinologist – Doctor specializing in complaints involving the endocrine (hormone) system.

Diabetes nurse educator – Registered nurse specializing in educating patients with diabetes about managing their symptoms, checking blood sugar levels, administering insulin and so on.

4.   Disorders of the endocrine system

Endocrine disorders are affected by the hormone involved and by whether there is too much or too little of this hormone. Some of the most common disorders are listed below.

5.   Pituitary gland

1.   *Dwarfism* – Adult stature of less than 4 ft 10 in or 147 cm.

Causes: Dwarfism can be due to more than 200 different medical conditions, with achondroplasia the most common, followed by growth hormone deficiency (pituitary dwarfism), in which the pituitary gland does not produce enough growth hormone.

Symptoms: In achondroplasia limbs are proportionately shorter than trunk, head is larger than average.

Diagnostic tests: Physical examination; growth chart; X-rays.

Treatment: Human growth hormone (HGH); sometimes surgery to increase height; shoe lifts.

2.   *Gigantism* – Massive growth before the growth plates have closed.

Causes: Abnormality (often pituitary adenoma) in pituitary gland resulting in over-production of HGH.

Symptoms: Abnormally rapid growth.

Diagnostic tests: Brain scan; blood tests.

Treatment: Removing pituitary adenoma (benign tumor); radiation therapy.

3.   *Acromegaly* – Developing big hands, feet, chin and nose in adulthood.

Causes: Abnormality in pituitary gland (often pituitary adenoma) resulting in over-production of HGH.

Symptoms: Very gradual increase in size of hands, etc.

Diagnostic tests: Brain scan; blood tests.

Treatment: As for gigantism.

4.   *(Central) Diabetes insipidus* – The pituitary gland does not produce enough ADH, so the body cannot retain enough sodium and water.

Causes: Inadequate release of anti-diuretic hormone (ADH).

Symptoms: Excessive urination and thirst.

Diagnostic tests: Blood tests.

Treatment: Synthetic form of ADH.

6. Thyroid gland

1. *Cretinism* – Severe hypothyroidism (see below) in young children, leading to a combination of growth failure and mental retardation. Sometimes symptoms are related to thyroid gland failure due to autoimmune disease.

Causes: Lack of iodine, necessary for the synthesis of thyroid hormone in womb or in infancy.

Symptoms: Growth failure and mental retardation. *Diagnostic tests*: Blood tests.

Treatment: Thyroid hormone. Prevented through the use of iodized salt.

2. *Hypothyroidism (underactive thyroid)* – Thyroid gland does not produce enough thyroxin and the person's metabolic rate slows down. Common in women over 50 and men over 65.

Causes: Lack of thyroid hormone.

Symptoms: *Myxedema,* water retention with puffy, cheesy face; hair loss; brittle nails; memory loss; lack of concentration; fatigue (in spite of sleeping enough); lack of energy; depression.

Diagnostic tests: Check levels of thyroid hormone (T3 and T4) and of TSH. If TSH levels are high, the thyroid may in fact be struggling to maintain (normal) thyroid function.

Treatment: Thyroxine (hormone replacement).

3. *Hyperthyroidism* – An overactive thyroid where the thyroid gland produces too much T3 and T4 and the person's metabolic rate is increased.

Causes: Overproduction of thyroid hormone.

Symptoms: Weight loss; lots of nervous energy; increase in body temperature and sweating; feeling ravenously hungry all the time; sometimes bulging eyes and goiter (swelling around thyroid gland).

Diagnostic tests: Blood tests; scan.

Treatment: Medication; radioactive iodine to destroy thyroid hormone producing cells; subtotal thyroidectomy or hemi-thyroidectomy (partial removal of the thyroid gland).

7. Parathyroid gland

1. *Hypoparathryoidism* – Underactive parathyroid gland.

Causes: Not enough parathyroid hormone (PTH) is released, leading to a drop in blood calcium levels.

Symptoms: Muscle twitches; spasms; convulsions; abdominal pain; cataracts.

Diagnostic tests: Blood tests.

Treatment: Calcium; vitamin D.

2. *Hyperparathyroidism* – Overactive parathyroid gland.

Causes: Too much parathyroid hormone (PTH) is released resulting in a rise in blood calcium levels.

Symptoms: High blood calcium levels; unspecific symptoms.

Diagnostic tests: Blood tests.

Treatment: Remove gland.

8. Adrenal glands

1. *Addison's disease* – Form of adrenal gland failure.

Causes: Adrenal glands do not produce enough steroid hormones.

Symptoms: Low blood sugar; muscle weakness; fatigue; weight loss. Note: people with Addison's disease can go into a 'crisis' during surgery or pregnancy and therefore need to wear Medic Alert bracelets.

Diagnostic tests: Blood tests.

Treatment: Replacing steroid hormones.

2. *Cushing's syndrome* – High levels of cortisol.

Causes: High levels of cortisol produced by adrenal glands; corticosteroid medication; pituitary gland tumor resulting in too much adrenocorticotropin hormone (ACTH).

Symptoms: High blood sugars leading to redistribution of fat, especially a buffalo hump and moon face; easy bruising; poor wound healing.

Diagnostic tests: Blood tests.

Treatment: Depending on the cause, tapering off corticosteroids if necessary.

9. Pancreas

1. *Diabetes* – High levels of sugar (glucose) in the blood. Sugar is unable to enter the body's cells to be used for energy because there is a problem with the hormone insulin, which helps glucose enter the cells. There are two main types of diabetes. Type 1 diabetes (T1DM) is relatively rare (10% of patients) while type 2 diabetes (T2DM) is by far the most common (90% of patients).

Causes: Type 1 diabetes is an autoimmune disease in which the pancreas quite suddenly stops producing insulin. More common in persons under 30 years of age.

In Type 2 diabetes, the pancreas either does not produce enough insulin, or the insulin receptors on the body's cells are no longer 'receptive' to insulin (insulin resistance), meaning cells do not 'open up' to absorb sugar from the blood stream (see Figure 25.2). Traditionally found in persons 45 years plus of age, but with the number of overweight people increasing around the world, a growing number of children and young people are now developing type 2 diabetes.

Symptoms: Sugar is needed in the cells for energy. Without sugar in the cells, the person feels tired and listless. Eventually, the body will start to burn off fat for energy, resulting in *ketones* in the urine (*acetone* smell on breath or skin).

If diabetes is undiagnosed and untreated, sugar will remain in the bloodstream and blood sugar levels will become very high. In type 2 diabetes, insulin levels may also be very high, because the insulin receptors are not responding to it. High insulin levels disturb fat metabolism and make arteries more likely to clog.

In many cases, people with type 2 diabetes may walk around undiagnosed for a long time. They may develop symptoms very gradually and therefore get used to not feeling 'the best'.

Diabetes can lead to complications such as hypoglycemia (note: this can only occur in people who use insulin or other diabetes medication); hyperglycemia and problems with nerves (diabetic neuropathy) and blood vessels (summarized below).

Hypoglycemia occurs when there is not enough sugar in the blood stream because insulin has allowed all sugar to leave the bloodstream and enter the cells. This results in the brain cells not receiving enough sugar, which can lead to aggression, confusion, loss of consciousness and potentially a hypoglycemic coma.

Hyperglycemia happens when the kidneys allow sugar overload into the urine. This very sweet urine attracts more fluid from the body, leading to polyuria (too much

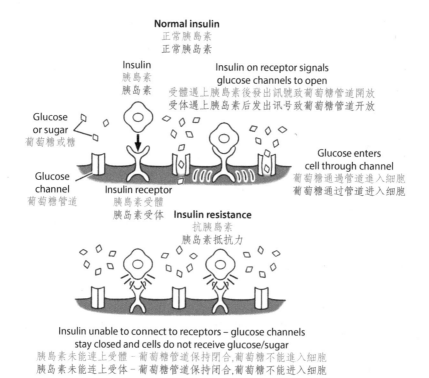

Figure 25.2 Insulin resistance
胰島素抗性
胰岛素抗性

urine produced) and the person becoming very thirsty (polydipsia). A very high blood sugar may lead to a diabetic coma, (as can acidemia, in which the blood is too acidic), dehydration and electrolyte imbalances.

Symptoms of diabetes can include excessive thirst and urination; weight loss; fatigue, weakness (can be extreme); blurred vision; frequent and persistent skin and bacterial infections; slow healing and itching; numbness, pain and tingling in hands or feet and leg cramp.

Diabetes can also lead to nerve and circulation disorders affecting every part of the body, specifically eyes (blindness; eyesight problems); feet (small wounds don't heal, leading to tissue dying off and amputation); legs (chronic leg ulcers); brain (CVAs); heart (heart attacks); kidneys (renal failure or diabetic nephropathy); nerves (loss of sensation in fingertips and toes).

Symptoms of hypoglycemia can include trembling; sweating; ravenous hunger; palpitations of the heart; headache; tingling of fingers and lips; disturbances of concentration; abnormal speech; confusion; aggressive behavior and blurred vision. Note: Hypoglycemic patients have been mistaken for drunks and arrested!

Diagnostic tests: Blood glucose level, which may be tested in different ways, including:

– fasting blood sugar (FBS)
– two-hr postprandial blood sugar test (2-h PPBS) – 2 hours after meal
– oral glucose tolerance test (OGTT) – after drinking sugary drink (also called oral glucose challenge test)
– random blood sugar (RBS)
– Patients monitoring their own blood sugar levels using a small card-like blood glucose meter or a continuous glucose monitor, with a sensor under the skin
– A1c Test (or HbA1c – glycated hemoglobin or glycosylated hemoglobin) – indicates somebody's average blood glucose level over the past few months

A person without diabetes will have a normal blood glucose of between 62 to 125 mg/dL and a HbA1c of 4–6%.

Treatment: Type 1 – Insulin injections; insulin pump (attached to abdomen); low fat diet; careful balance between diet (timing, carbohydrates and amount), insulin (timing and amount) and exercise. Type 2 – Medications to help the pancreas produce more insulin; insulin injections; low fat diet; careful balance between diet (timing, carbohydrates, amount), insulin (timing and amount) and exercise. Some diabetic patients have been able to reduce their medication following gastric bypass (or gastric banding) surgery.

10.   The glycemic index (GI)

Researchers think that a low glycemic index (low GI) diet may help prevent type 2 diabetes. Food containing carbohydrates that break down quickly have a high GI and rapidly increase blood glucose levels. Foods with carbohydrates that break down more slowly have a low GI and release glucose into the bloodstream gradually. Sugar is the standard measure, with a GI of 100. An example of GI can be found in comparing different types of rice, where jasmine rice has a very high GI, while basmati rice has a medium GI; hence a low GI diet should not include jasmine rice.

Another way of describing food is using the glycemic load (GL). Similarly to GI, GL is a number that describes how quickly blood glucose levels go up after consuming certain foods. One unit of GL reflects the effect of consuming one gram of glucose. A low GL is <10, a high GL is >20.

11.   English-Chinese glossary

英漢詞彙表

English	Hong Kong & Taiwan	Mainland China
A1c test; HbA1c; glycated hemoglobin; glycosylated hemoglobin	糖化血色素 (HbA1)	糖化血红蛋白 (HbA1)
acromegaly	肢端肥大症	肢端肥大症; 肢端巨大症
Addison's disease	愛迪生氏病	艾迪生病; 肾上腺皮质功能衰竭症
ADH	抗利尿激素	抗利尿激素
adrenaline; epinephrine	腎上腺素	肾上腺素
adrenocorticotropin hormone/ Adrenal corticotrophic hormone (ACTH)	促腎上腺皮質 (激) 素	促肾上腺皮质 (激) 素; 促皮质素
aldosterone	留鹽激素; 醛固酮	醛固酮; 醛甾酮
autoimmune disease	自體免疫病	自身免疫性疾病
chemical messenger	化學信使; 化學訊息	化学信使
continuous glucose monitor	連續血糖監測	连续血糖监测
corticosteroids	類固醇激素; 皮質素	皮质激素; 皮质类固醇
cortisol	皮質醇	皮质醇; 可的松
cretinism	先天性碘缺乏症候群; 克汀病; 呆小症	先天性碘缺乏症候群; 克汀病; 呆小病
Cushing's syndrome	庫興氏綜合症; 皮質醇增多症	库兴 (氏) 综合症; 皮质醇增多综合症
diabetes	糖尿病	糖尿病
diabetes insipidus	尿崩症	尿崩症
diabetic nephropathy	糖尿引發腎病變	糖尿病性肾病变; 糖尿病肾病
diabetic neuropathy	糖尿病引發神經病變	糖尿病 (性) 神经病变
dwarfism; achondroplasia	侏儒症; 軟骨發育不全症	侏儒症; 软骨发育不全
endocrine system	內分泌系統	内分泌系统
Endocrinologist	內分泌科醫生	内分泌学家
estrogen	雌激素	雌激素; 女性激素
fasting blood sugar (FBS)	空腹血糖	空腹血糖
follicle stimulating hormone (FSH)	濾泡刺激素	促卵胞激素; 促卵胞成熟激素; 卵胞刺激素
gigantism	巨人症	巨人症
glycemic index (GI)	血糖指數; 升糖指數	血糖 (生成) 指数

(Continued)

English	Hong Kong & Taiwan	Mainland China
glycemic load (GL)	血糖負荷; 升糖負荷	血糖 (生成) 負荷
goiter	甲狀腺腫	甲狀腺肿
human growth hormone (HGH)	人體生長激素	人生长激素
hydrocortisone	氫化可體松	氢化可的松
hyperglycemia	高血糖; 血糖過高; 多糖症	高血糖; 高血糖症
hyperparathyroidism	副甲狀腺機能亢進	甲狀旁腺功能亢进 (症)
hyperthyroidism	甲狀腺機能亢進	甲狀腺功能亢进 (症)
hypoglycemia	低血糖 (症) ; 血糖過低	低血糖 (症)
hypoparathyroidism	副甲狀腺機能減退	甲狀旁腺功能减退 (症)
hypophisis	腦下垂體	脑下垂体
hypothalamus	下視丘	下丘脑
hypothyroidism	甲狀腺機能減退	甲狀腺功能减低 (症)
islets of Langerhans	胰島	胰岛
ketone	酮	酮
luteinizing hormone (LH)	黃體生成素	促黄激素; 黄体化激素
melatonin	褪黑激素	褪黑激素
myxedema ; myxoedema	黏液性水腫	粘液性水肿
oral glucose tolerance (test) (OGTT)	口服葡萄糖耐量試驗; 口服耐糖試驗	口服葡萄糖耐量试验
oxytocin	催產素	催产素; 缩宫素
parathormone	副甲狀腺素; 甲狀旁腺激素	甲狀旁腺激素
parathyroid gland	副甲狀腺	甲狀旁腺
pineal gland	松果腺 (體)	松果体; 松果腺
pituitary adenoma	垂體腺瘤	垂体腺瘤
pituitary gland	垂體	垂体; 垂体腺
polydipsia	多渴	烦渴
polyuria	多尿	多尿
progesterone	黃體素; 孕酮	黄体酮
prolactin	催乳素	催乳激素
random blood sugar (RBS)	隨機血糖	随机血糖
sex hormones	性激素	性激素
testosterone	睪丸素; 睪丸酮	睾酮; 睾丸酮; 睾丸素
thyroid stimulating hormone (TSH)	甲狀腺刺激素	促甲狀腺激素
thyroidectomy	甲狀腺切除術	甲狀腺切除术
thyroxin (T4)	甲狀腺素	甲狀腺素

English	Hong Kong & Taiwan	Mainland China
two-hr postprandial blood sugar (2-h PPBS)	飯後兩小時血糖指數	餐后兩小時血糖

Summary of main points

This chapter has given a brief overview of the endocrine system, including:

- various hormones and the role they play
- terms with Latin and Greek roots
- health professionals involved
- some commonly encountered conditions relating to the endocrine system, particularly diabetes, together with common diagnostic tests and treatment methods.

Chapter 26

Gastroenterology

The digestive system

The digestive system is involved in the process of taking in food, breaking it down and processing it for absorption, absorbing it into the blood stream, and eliminating the waste products from the body. Consequently, the digestive system involves a range of different organs.

Different medical words are also used when talking about the digestive system. Some doctors talk about the alimentary canal (the route the food takes through the body) or the gastrointestinal tract or GI tract (the route the food takes through stomach and bowels). The following Latin and Greek roots form the basis of many medical words that have to do with the digestive system.

1. Terms with Latin and Greek roots

absorb	to take in
chole	bile, gall (breaks fat globules down into smaller ones)
cholecystectomy	to cut out the gallbladder (chole: bile; cyst: bladder)
cyst	Literally: bladder; fluid-filled sac (e.g cystitis)
digest	to break down
enter	inside (entrails: bowels)
esophagus	gullet (*phago*: eat; *eso*: going to carry)
gaster/gastro	stomach
gastrointestinal (GI)	relating to stomach and bowels
hepato	Liver
intestino	entrails, bowels
oesophagus	see esophagus
pancreas (pancreatic)	large gland (*pan*: all; *creas*: flesh/meat)
parenteral	by-passing the bowels (*para*: alongside)
peri	around
scopy	looking
sorb	to soak (up)
stoma	mouth; artificial opening

| *tomy* | cut |
| *tract* | route |

2. Anatomy and function of the digestive system

The gastrointestinal tract (GI tract) consists of a range of organs and accessory glands. Figure 26.1 represents the digestive system.

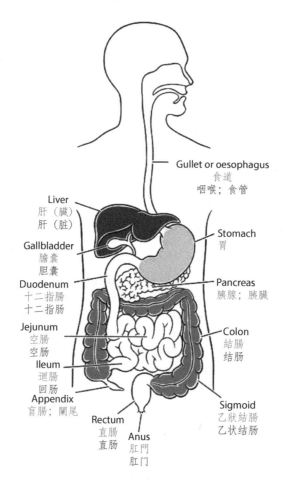

Figure 26.1 Digestive system
消化系統
消化系统

Table 26.1 gives an overview of the main organs and accessory organs of the digestive tract.

Table 26.1 The GI Tract

Organs	Accessory organs/glands	Role
Mouth	tongue	taste buds (papillae)
	salivary glands	saliva is released when food enters; food starts to dissolve (especially white bread; rice)
	teeth	food is broken up into small pieces and can be swallowed more easily
esophagus		tube behind the windpipe, connecting the throat to the stomach: food slides down to stomach
stomach		gastric juices to break down protein and carbohydrates
	liver	enzymes and bile (bile breaks down fat)
	gallbladder	storage place for bile; bile is squeezed into the intestine when fatty foods come along
	pancreas	digestive enzymes; insulin; glucagon
small intestine (duodenum, jejunum, ileum)		20 feet (6.3 meters) long; intestinal juices containing digestive enzymes help break down the food into tiny particles; these are absorbed into the blood stream through the wall of the small intestine and travel to the liver for processing
	appendix	includes lymph tissue
large intestine (ascending colon, transverse colon, descending colon, sigmoid colon, rectum, anus)		5 feet long (1.5 meters); mainly fluid is absorbed here and stools are moved towards exit (the anus)

In short, the process of digestion involves the following:

– eating or taking in food
– moving food along the digestive tract
– digestion (breaking it down into smaller bits)
– absorption
– defecation (elimination from body)

The digestion process starts in the mouth and continues in the stomach. When food is ready, the stomach contracts and pushes the food into the bowels, usually 2–6 hours after eating. Carbohydrates are digested quickly, protein and fats are digested more slowly. Some foods and medicine are readily absorbed in the stomach (i.e. water; Vitamin B12; aspirin; whey protein shakes).

The pyloric valve is the muscular opening between the stomach and the small intestine. The pylorus opens when food is ready to leave the stomach. In some infants the pyloric valve is narrowed and food is pushed out the other way, resulting in forceful projectile vomiting (see Figure 26.2).

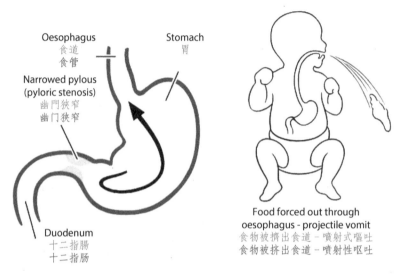

Oesophagus
食道
食管

Stomach
胃

Narrowed pylous
(pyloric stenosis)
幽門狹窄
幽门狭窄

Duodenum
十二指腸
十二指肠

Food forced out through
oesophagus - projectile vomit
食物被擠出食道 – 噴射式嘔吐
食物被挤出食道 – 喷射性呕吐

Figure 26.2 Pyloric stenosis and projectile vomiting
幽門狹窄及噴射式嘔吐
幽门狭窄及喷射性呕吐

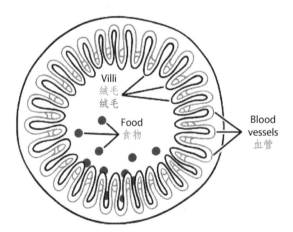

Villi
絨毛
绒毛

Food
食物

Blood
vessels
血管

Figure 26.3 Villi in the lining of the bowel
腸道內壁的絨毛
肠道内壁的绒毛

When food comes out of the stomach, carbohydrates and protein have been partly digested, but fats have not been digested. Glucose, fat and protein are absorbed in the small intestine, where nutrients are trapped between fingerlike protrusions in the lining of the bowel called villi, before passing into the blood which takes them to the liver for processing. Once processed, the nutrients are taken to the cells or stored in the form of glycogen or fat.

The many functions of the liver are represented in Table 26.2.

Table 26.2 The many functions of the liver

Functions of the liver	Examples
makes plasma proteins, also heparin destroys old red blood cells	
liver enzymes break down poisons, making them harmless	includes medication, e.g. paracetamol
collects nutrients	
processes nutrients	can change sugar into: stored sugar (glycogen) stored fat (body fat)
	can change glycogen: back to sugar
	to protein to fat
	as required
stores nutrients	iron, copper, vitamins A, D, E, K
	also stores proteins which cannot be broken down (e.g. DDT) and heavy metals
makes bile (gall)	stored in gallbladder (bile breaks down fat)

3. Peritoneum

The peritoneum is a membrane lining the abdominal wall. It contains a lot of blood vessels and nerve endings, making it very sensitive to pain. The peritoneal cavity, is the space surrounded by the peritoneum. Some of the organs in the abdomen are inside the peritoneal cavity. The peritoneum has a rich blood supply (mesenterium). Mesenterial infarcts are very painful.

4. Health professionals

Gastroenterologist – Physician mainly specializing in disorders affecting all parts of the digestive system i.e. stomach, liver, pancreas, small and large intestine and rectum.

5. Disorders of the digestive system

1. *Appendicitis* – Inflammation of the appendix.

Cause: Bacteria entering the appendix, usually preceded by an obstruction or infection of the gut.

Symptoms: At start: pain around belly button; then: loss of appetite; nausea; vomiting; the pain will then shift to the right lower quadrant (RLQ) of the abdomen, getting worse with coughing, sneezing, or body movements; rebound tenderness (pain gets worse when the doctor removes his hand after pushing down on the abdomen). If the appendix perforates (breaks and contents come out), this can lead to peritonitis and sepsis (bacteria overwhelming organs and the bloodstream).

Diagnostic tests: Ultrasound; CT scan; laparoscopy.

Treatment: Appendectomy (removal of appendix); antibiotics.

2. *Cirrhosis* – Occurs when the liver is infiltrated with fibrous tissue and fat. This 'destroys' liver function, i.e. the liver cannot make glycogen, absorb vitamins, break down bilirubin, process food, or detoxify alcohol and drugs. Blood flow through the liver is also obstructed (like a huge backlog of traffic) and there is back flow into the GI tract resulting in hypertension in the portal vein and in the veins alongside the esophagus.

Cause: Often chronic alcohol abuse; hepatitis (especially B or C).

Symptoms: Anorexia (which literally translates as *no appetite*); nausea; weight loss; more than 5 spider naevi (spiderweb-like blood vessels just below the surface of the skin); fatigue; ascites (fluid in the peritoneal space). Esophageal varices (weak dilated veins along the esophagus) can lead to a massive hemorrhage, hepatic coma, and kidney failure.

Diagnostic tests: Liver biopsies; liver function tests.

Treatment: Depends on cause.

3. *Crohn's disease* – Inflammatory bowel disease which can affect both the small and large intestine.

Causes: Genetic predisposition in which the immune system attacks harmless bowel bacteria.

Symptoms: Ongoing disease with periods of remission and flare-ups (known as *exacerbations*) which can include malabsorption (leading to malnutrition and weight loss);

anal fistulas; anal fissures (small tears); perianal abscesses. Can lead to a bowel blockage (ileus).

Diagnostic tests: Colonoscopy; stool tests; CT scan.

Treatment: Meal replacements; diet (bananas); anti-diarrhea medications, antiinflammatory medications; corticosteroids; immunomodulators; biologicals; antitumor necrosis factor (anti-TNF) medications; occasionally surgery to remove rectum and colon (proctocolectomy); ileostomy or intestinal resection (removing diseased part of the bowel).

4. *Dental caries* – Tooth decay.

Causes: Breakdown of the tooth enamel due to acid-producing bacteria which destroy tooth enamel.

Symptoms: Often no symptoms; sometimes toothache or pain when eating or drinking hot or cold foods; cavities discovered during dental examination

Diagnostic tests: Dental examination; X-ray.

Treatment: Fillings; root canal treatment; crown (cap fitted over remainder of tooth).

Prevention: Good oral/dental hygiene (brushing, flossing); water fluoridation, dental sealants.

5. *Diverticulitis* – Inflammation of small pouches (*diverticula*) in the lining of the colon.

Causes: Pressure on weak places in the wall of the colon, resulting in pouches forming.

Symptoms: Pain lower left abdomen; change in bowel habits. Can lead to complications including infections, tears and blockages.

Diagnostic tests: Colonoscopy.

Treatment: Surgery for blockages; high-fiber diet.

6. *Duodenal ulcer* – see peptic ulcer.

7. *Gallstones* – Solid particles that form from bile in the gallbladder.

Causes: Crystallization of cholesterol (cholesterol stones) or excess bilirubin pigment stones.

Symptoms: Often no symptoms; sometimes pain after a fatty meal; pain if there is blockage and infection of the gallbladder; nausea, vomiting, jaundice, fever.

Diagnostic tests: Ultrasound scan; endoscopic retrograde cholangiopancreatography (ERCP), looking at part of the gall ducts using a flexible scope; cholescintigraphy (HIDA), scan following intravenous injection of a special solution.

Treatment: cholecystectomy, laparoscopic surgery to remove the gallbladder. Extra-corporeal shockwave lithotripsy (ESWL) is only used for patients who cannot have surgery, breaking up stones using sound waves; dissolving the gallstones.

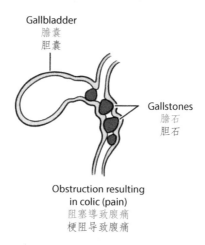

Gallbladder
膽囊
胆囊

Gallstones
膽石
胆石

Obstruction resulting
in colic (pain)
阻塞導致腹痛
梗阻导致腹痛

Figure 26.4 Gallstones
膽石
胆石

8. *Hepatitis* – Inflammation of the liver.

Causes: Infection with the hepatitis virus. The means of transmission depends on the type of hepatitis (see below).

Hepatitis A and E result from infection through contaminated food and water. A complete recovery is possible.

Hepatitis B infections are common in Asian and Pacific Island populations, with infections possibly partly spread by eating food with shared eating utensils.

Hepatitis C and D are common in drug users, infants from infected mothers, people infected through hemodialysis or contaminated transfusions prior to the introduction of screening tests. That is, infection occurs through contact with blood or other body fluids or transferred to infants at birth. Infection with hepatitis B, C or D virus can result in chronic hepatitis; cirrhosis; liver failure and liver cancer.

Symptoms: Tiredness; nausea; loss of appetite; jaundice (skin looks yellow); whites of the eye look yellow.

Diagnostic tests: Blood tests (to check for antibodies).

Treatment: Antiviral drugs; occasionally liver transplant.

9. *Hemorrhoids* (also referred to as *piles*) – Inflammation/enlargement of veins in anus (internal or external).

Causes: Constipation may play a role as it causes pressure on the veins.

Diagnostic tests: Physical examination.

Symptoms: Bright red blood in stools; pain on defecating (passing stools).

Treatment: Local cream; surgery.

10. *Inflammatory bowel disease* – see *Crohn's disease* and *ulcerative colitis*

11. *Irritable bowel syndrome (IBS)* – Not a disease but a set of symptoms resulting from an abnormal functioning of the bowel.

Causes: Combination of factors, including genetics, food sensitivity and mental stress.

Symptoms: Abdominal pain; cramping; bloating; diarrhea alternating with constipation.

Diagnostic tests: Colonoscopy; stool test.

Treatment: Diet (typically avoiding certain foods).

12. *Lactose intolerance* – inability to process lactose.

Causes: A lack of the lactase enzyme used to break down milk sugar (*lactose*).

Symptoms: Abdominal bloating.

Diagnostic tests: Stool acidity test; hydrogen breath test.

Treatments: Avoiding lactose in diet.

13. *Pancreatitis* – Acute or chronic inflammation of the pancreas.

Causes: Alcohol abuse; gallstones, abdominal surgery.

Symptoms: Acute pain; nausea; vomiting; jaundice; diabetes symptoms.

Diagnostic tests: Imaging.

Treatment: Stopping food by mouth; intravenous nutrition or fluids, plus no alcohol and frequent small meals for those with chronic condition.

14. *Peptic ulcer (gastric ulcer or duodenal ulcer)* – Ulcer in the stomach or duodenum.

Causes: Infection with Helicobacter pylori (H. Pylori) bacterium; stress; aspirin, NSAIDS.

Symptoms: Intense and acute pain. Peptic ulcers may lead to perforation (a hole in the wall of the stomach), leading to a hemorrhage (severe bleeding) which can result in shock, board-like stomach and death.

Investigation: Gastroscopy; breath test; stool test.

Treatment: Antibiotics against H. Pylori; medication to stop production of stomach acid.

15.   *Tumors* – Cancers can occur anywhere in the digestive tract.

Causes: Depends on type of cancer.

Symptoms: Loss of appetite; weight loss; ascites (fluid); pain (usually a late symptom); jaundice.

Diagnostic tests: Gastroscopy; sigmoidoscopy; colonoscopy; CT scan.

Treatment: Depends on type of cancer, (see also Chapter 16) e.g. gastrointestinal stromal tumors (GISTs) respond well to drugs other than chemotherapy.

16.   *Peritonitis* – Acute inflammation of the peritoneum (membrane lining the abdominal wall). This is a very serious condition.

Causes: Infection through wounds after childbirth or through CAPD (see Chapter 27); perforation of infected organs; perforation of Fallopian tube after ectopic pregnancy. Can be prevented with antibiotics before abdominal surgery and using sterile procedures.

Symptoms: Rigid washboard abdomen; pain; nausea and/or vomiting; reduced bowel sounds/movement; fever; chills.

Diagnostic tests: Blood tests; sometimes laparotomy.

Treatment: Immediate antibiotics; surgery and lavage (washing infectious fluids out of abdomen).

17.   *Ulcer* – see peptic ulcer

18.   *Ulcerative colitis* – Type of inflammatory bowel disease in which there is ongoing inflammation and sores in the large intestine (colon) and rectum.

Causes: Genetic predisposition (immune system responds abnormally to some of the bacteria in the bowel).

Symptoms: Periods of remission and flare-ups (known *as exacerbations*) involving fever, bloody diarrhea and cramping.

Diagnostic tests: CT scan; stool test; colonoscopy.

Treatment: Special diet; nutritional supplements; anti-inflammatory medications; corticosteroids; immunomodulators or anti-tumor necrosis factor (TNF) medications; occasionally surgery to remove part of the colon and create a pouch by attaching the ileum to the anus; sometimes ileostomy.

6. Some common medications

antacids	neutralize excessive stomach acid
antiemetics	stop vomiting
antispasmodics	calm stomach/intestinal muscles; stop cramping of smooth muscle tissue (given for colic)
digestives	help digestion (breaking down of food)
emetics	induce vomiting
laxatives	induce bowel movements

7. Some common diagnostic tests

- *Endoscopy* – Use of a scope (a flexible or rigid fiber-optic tube) to look inside organs and take biopsies: e.g: gastroscopy; colonoscopy
- *Contrast X-rays*, which may include:
  endoscopic retrograde cholangiopancreatography (ERCP) – Tube inserted into duodenum and dye injected to take X-rays of the bile ducts.
  percutaneous transhepatic cholangiography (PTC) – Dye injected to take X-rays of liver and bile ducts.
  magnetic resonance cholangiopancreatography (MRCP) – MRI used to obtain pictures of the bile ducts.

8. Additional comments

Occasionally people are unable to take in food: for example, a person with cancer in the gastrointestinal tract that prevents food from passing through, or babies who have a heart condition, which means they are unable to feed properly due to a lack of energy. In such instances, different feeding methods have to be used. These may include:

- nasogastric feeding tube (NG tube) (e.g. premature babies)
- percutaneous endoscopic gastrostomy tube (PEG): a tube inserted through the gastrostomy opening

–   intravenous nutrition (IVN) or total parenteral nutrition (TPN) being a mix of glucose, lipids, amino acids, minerals, and electrolytes (Na+, K+, Cl–) given directly into the bloodstream.

Similarly, sometimes people are unable to defecate (pass stools/have bowel movements, poop) due to surgical treatment for bowel cancer or very severe Crohn's disease. In these cases, an artificial outlet called a stoma may be created in the wall of the abdomen. Stoma (which means "mouth") is the general name given to artificial outlets for either the colon, the ileum or the ureters.

A colostomy is an artificial outlet for the colon (large intestine); an ileostomy is an artificial outlet for the ileum (part of the small intestine), a jejunostomy is an artificial outlet for the jejunum (part of the small intestine) and a urostomy is an artificial outlet for the ureters. While different types of stoma and stoma systems require different care, such care usually involves firstly keeping the skin around the stoma clean (shower, shallow bath, deep bath), and secondly changing the pouches (stoma bags).

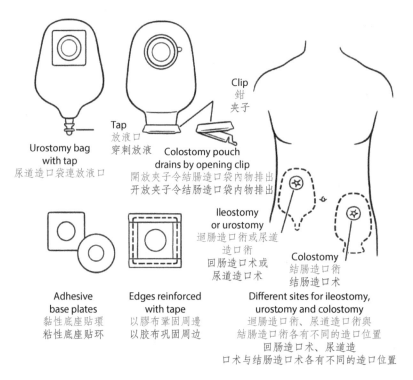

Figure 26.5 Stoma pouches and stoma sites
造口袋與造口位置
造口袋与造口位置

9. English-Chinese glossary

英漢詞彙表

English	Hong Kong & Taiwan	Mainland China
anal fissure	肛裂	肛裂
anal fistula	肛瘻	肛 (门) 瘻
antacid	制酸劑	抗酸剂
antiemetic	止吐劑; 止嘔藥	止吐药
anti-tumor necrosis factor (anti-TNF) drugs	抗腫瘤壞死因數藥物	抗肿瘤坏死因数抑制剂
antispasmodic	抗痙攣藥物; 解痙藥	镇痉剂
appendectomy	盲腸切除術; 闌尾切除術	阑尾切除术
appendicitis	盲腸炎; 闌尾炎	阑尾炎
ascites	腹水	腹水
bile	膽汁	胆汁
cholecystectomy	膽囊切除術	胆囊切除术
cholescintigraphy; HIDA scan	膽管閃爍顯像; 放射性核子膽道掃描	胆管造影
colonoscopy	結腸內窺鏡檢查	结肠镜检查
colposcopy	陰道窺鏡檢查	阴道镜检查
contrast X-ray	造影劑 X 光檢查	造影剂 X 光检查
crown	牙冠; 齒冠	(牙) 冠
CT scan; computerized tomography	電腦斷層掃描; 電腦斷層攝影; 電腦掃描	CT 掃描
digestives	消化劑	消化剂
diverticula	憩室	憩室
diverticulitis	憩室炎	憩室炎
duodenal ulcer	十二指腸潰瘍	十二指肠溃疡
emetic	催吐藥	催吐药
endoscopic retrograde cholangiopancreatography (ERCP)	內窺鏡逆行性膽胰管造影	内 (窥) 镜逆行胰胆管造影术
endoscopy	內窺鏡檢查; 內視鏡檢查	内窥镜检查; 内腔镜检查
extracorporeal shockwave lithotripsy (ESWL)	體外震 (衝擊) 波碎石術	体外震波粉碎 (肾) 结石术; 体外冲击波碎石术
filling	補牙	补牙
gallstone	膽石	胆石
gastroenterologist	腸胃科醫生	肠胃科医生

(Continued)

English	Hong Kong & Taiwan	Mainland China
gastroscopy	胃內窺鏡檢查; 胃鏡檢查	胃 (窺) 鏡檢查
Helicobacter pylori	幽門螺旋 (桿) 菌	幽门螺旋 (杆) 菌
hemorrhoid/haemorrhoid; piles	痔瘡	痔 (疮)
hepatitis	肝炎	肝炎
ileostomy	迴腸造口術	回肠造口术
ileus	腸閉塞	肠梗阻
immunomodulators	免疫調節劑	免疫调节剂
inflammatory bowel disease; Chrohn's/Crohn's disease; ulcerative colitis	發炎性腸道疾病; 腸炎; 克隆氏症; 潰瘍性結腸炎	炎 (症) 性肠病; 肠炎; 克隆 (氏) 病; 节段性回肠炎; 溃疡性结肠炎
intestinal resection	腸切除術	肠切除术
irritable bowel syndrome	過敏性腸道綜合症	过敏性 (结) 肠综合症; 肠应激综合症
lactose intolerance	乳糖不耐症	乳糖不耐 (受) 性
laparoscopy	腹腔 (內窺) 鏡檢查	腹腔镜检查
laxative	通便劑; 輕瀉劑; 瀉藥	轻泻药
magnetic resonance cholangiopancreatography (MRCP)	磁力共振膽胰管造影術	磁共振胰胆管成像
nasogastric feeding tube	鼻胃喂飼管 (俗稱「胃喉」)	鼻 (胃) 饲管
non steroidal anti inflammatory drug (NSAID)	非類固醇類消炎止痛藥	非类固醇抗炎药
pancreatitis	胰腺炎	胰腺炎
percutaneous endoscopic gastrostomy (PEG) tube	經皮內窺鏡胃造口管	经皮内镜下胃造瘘管
percutaneous transhepatic cholangiography (PTC)	經皮透肝膽管造影術	经皮肝胆管造影术
perianal abscess; anorectal abscess	肛周膿腫; 肛門直腸膿腫	肛周脓肿; 肛门直肠脓肿
peritoneal cavity	腹膜腔	腹膜腔
peritoneum	腹膜	腹膜
proctocolectomy	直腸結腸切除術	直肠结肠切除术
root canal treatment	牙髓治療; 根管治療 (俗稱「杜牙根」)	(牙) 根管疗法
sigmoidoscopy	乙狀結腸內窺鏡檢查	乙状结肠镜检查
spider naevi/angioma	蜘蛛痣; 蜘蛛形血管瘤	蛛状痣; 蜘蛛状血管瘤
stoma	造口	造口

(Continued)

English	Hong Kong & Taiwan	Mainland China
stoma pouch	造口袋	造口袋
total parenteral nutrition (TPN)	腸胃道外營養療法; 全靜脈注射營養	全肠外营养; 全静脉营养
ultrasound	超音波; 超聲波	超声波

Summary of main points

This chapter has given a brief overview of the digestive system, including:

- anatomy of the organs involved
- terms with Latin and Greek roots
- health professionals involved
- some commonly encountered conditions relating to the digestive system, together with common diagnostic tests and treatments

Chapter 27

Urology and nephrology

The urinary system

The renal and urinary systems help the body get rid of certain surplus products, including wastes.

1. Terms with Latin and Greek roots

anuria	no urine production
cyst	bladder (literally a sac filled with fluid)
cystitis	inflammation of the bladder
cystoscopy	examination of the bladder through a scope passed into the urethra
dia	through
enuresis	bedwetting
glomerulonephritis	inflammation of the glomeruli and the nephrons
glomerulus	network of capillaries where unwanted material is pushed out into the urine smallest element of the kidney (like very small filter)
hemodialysis	dialysis – rinsing out of the blood
hemofiltration	filtering the blood
-itis	inflammation of
lysis	loosening; dissolving
nephritis	inflammation of the kidneys
nephron	smallest functional unit in the kidney
oliguria	passing very little urine
peritoneum	lining of the abdomen
peritoneal dialysis	dialysis through the peritoneum
polyuria	passing a lot of urine
renal	to do with the kidneys
tract	route; canal
uremia	(high levels of) urea in the blood (urea is a breakdown product of protein which makes skin dark and itchy)

2. Anatomy of the urinary system

In a healthy person the urinary system is made up of:

- two kidneys
- the urinary tract, which consists of two ureters, the bladder and the urethra

3. The kidneys

Kidneys are the filtering and cleaning organs of the urinary system and are vital in maintaining the body's internal balance by regulating a person's state of hydration. If a person is dehydrated (dry), the kidneys will act to conserve water, so that normal body functions are maintained (i.e. blood pressure; concentration of blood nutrients; healthy acid base balance and hormonal functions). Any urine passed will be dark in color (as it is quite concentrated) and passed in smaller amounts.

In a well-hydrated person, the kidneys do not need to conserve water to maintain normal body functions. This means that a healthy person cannot become overloaded with fluid. Urine passed will be light in color and passed in larger volumes. When the kidney(s) become diseased, they cannot carry out some or all of these functions.

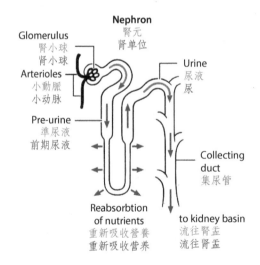

Figure 27.1 Nephron and glomerulus in the kidney
肾内的肾元及肾小球
肾内的肾单位及肾小球

4.   The urinary tract

The urinary tract provides the drainage system for the body's waste water and starts with the ureters (the two tubes leading down from the kidneys). Filtered urine drains via the renal pelvis (the central urine-collecting area of each kidney) into the ureters, flowing down into the bladder (a small reservoir that collects urine from the two kidneys). As the bladder fills, it sends signals to the brain about the amount of stretch in the bladder wall, and the person will realize that they need to empty their bladder. The emptying of the bladder can be controlled at will and the urine will then flow out through the urethra (a drainage tube leading from the bladder to outside the body).

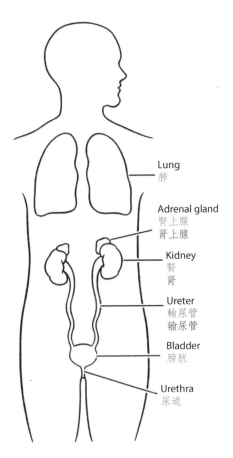

Lung
肺

Adrenal gland
腎上腺
肾上腺

Kidney
腎
肾

Ureter
輸尿管
输尿管

Bladder
膀胱

Urethra
尿道

Figure 27.2 Position of kidneys in the body
腎臟在體內的位置
肾脏在体内的位置

5.   Function of the urinary system

The kidneys:

1.   regulate the fluid environment within the body by
     –   maintaining the circulating blood volume
     –   maintaining concentration of blood constituents at a physiologically safe level
     –   maintaining acidity within safe limits on a long term basis (*Please note:* The respiratory system also regulates acidity in the body but does this on a moment-by-moment basis)
2.   remove waste products from the blood through filtering
3.   selectively reabsorb body constituents that need to be regulated according to the body's needs at the time
4.   provide a barrier against loss of large molecules such as proteins (e.g. blood cells and plasma proteins) that should not be passed out in the urine
5.   produce important hormones:
     –   The kidneys produce a hormone that is important in the production of red blood cells in the body (erythropoietin).
     –   The adrenal glands produce corticosteroids in response to the body's needs.
6.   have an integral role in the regulation of calcium and phosphate balance, which is essential for the maintenance of healthy bones (amongst other things)

6.   Health professionals

Nephrologist – Doctor who specializes in disorders of the kidneys and the urinary system.
Urologist – Doctor who specializes in disorders of the urinary system in both males and females, plus disorders of the male reproductive system.

7.   Disorders of the urinary system

1.   *Kidney failure (or renal failure)* – Occurs when kidney function is less than 15% of normal. Kidney failure is very common and relates very closely to kidney function.
     There are two forms of kidney failure. The first, acute kidney failure, is a life-threatening event that happens as a consequence to a major illness or trauma to the body, such as severe burns (which cause a large loss of fluid), or multiple major organ failure due to overwhelming infection (sepsis). The second, chronic kidney failure, involves a slow deterioration (worsening) of kidney function due to ongoing disease, which becomes so severe that the person requires dialysis or a kidney transplant to stay alive.

Causes: Diabetes; high blood pressure (hypertension); nephritis (an infective or non-infective inflammation of the kidney); blockage or obstruction of the urinary tract; genetically-linked problems such as *polycystic kidney disease.*

Symptoms: May include uremia, which relates to an excess of urea (a waste-product of protein breakdown) in the blood.

Diagnostic tests: Creatinine clearance rate (CCR); glomerular filtration rate (GFR) to check how well the kidneys are working; urine albumen test; blood urea nitrogen (BUN)

Treatment: There are three main modes of treatment for kidney failure:
- Hemodialysis – cleaning/filtering of the blood by means of a dialysis machine. The dialysis involves blood being separated from dialysis fluid by a semi-permeable membrane, which has very fine pores in it. The blood is pumped from the artery, through the tubes which lead to the dialysis machine. The blood passes to one side of the semi-permeable membrane (the filter), and extra fluid and toxins pass from the blood, through the filter into the dialyzing solution on the other side. Blood is then returned to the body and the process is repeated for another 3–4 hours. Blood that passes through the artificial kidney is treated with an anticoagulant, to stop it from forming clots while dialysis is in progress.
- Hemofiltration – a short-term treatment, similar to hemodialysis, used in Intensive Care settings to treat acute kidney failure. Also called Continuous Veno-Venous Hemofiltration (CVVH).
- Continuous ambulatory peritoneal dialysis (CAPD) – a method of dialysis done by patients themselves, in whicha permanent tube is implanted in the patient's abdominal wall and four to five times a day the patient lets the dialysis fluid run into the peritoneal cavity, where it 'dwells' for some time before being drained out again, taking with it the waste that is usually filtered by the kidney.
- Kidney transplantation – the kidney of another person is placed inside the body of a person with kidney failure. Kidney transplantation will involve taking antirejection medication (immunosuppressants) for the rest of the person's life.

2. *Acute and chronic glomerulonephritis*: – Glomeruli become inflamed, swollen, full of blood.

Causes: May be caused by bacteria, but may be due to an autoimmune reaction (e.g. in IgA nephropathy).

Symptoms: Blood and protein in urine; low blood protein; edema.

Acute glomerulonephritis: Symptoms only last 2 to 3 weeks. *Chronic glomerulonephritis*: permanent damage to nephrons which may lead to edema, coma, death.

Diagnostic tests: Blood and urine tests.

Treatment: Depending on cause: antibiotics or immunosuppressants.

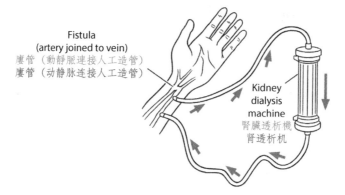

Figure 27.3 Hemodialysis
血液透析 (俗稱「洗腎」及「洗血」)

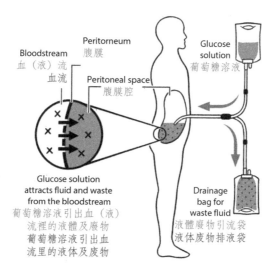

Figure 27.4 CAPD
持續流動式腹膜透析
持续流动式腹膜透析

3. *Kidney Stones* – Chemicals in urine can crystallize into stones (e.g. calcium, oxalate, phosphate).

Causes: Suspected genetic predisposition in some people; high protein/high salt diet.

Symptoms: Extreme cramping pain; blood or pus in urine.

Diagnostic tests: Imaging; urine tests.

Treatment: Lithotripsy for smaller stones (stone is crushed by high-frequency sound waves); larger stones may need to be surgically removed.

4. *Gout* – Pain and inflammation in joints (usually the big toe) caused by high levels of uric acid (hyperuricemia).

Causes: Hereditary factors; high intake of alcohol, meat, seafood; joint injury; some medications.

Symptoms: Acute joint pain.

Diagnostic tests: Blood tests.

Treatment: Anti-inflammatory medications.

5. *Pyelonephritis* – inflammation of the kidney pelvis; may be acute pyelonephritis (sudden onset) or chronic pyelonephritis (slow onset).

Causes: Bacteria comes up from the bladder, resulting in the ureters becoming blocked (e.g. a kidney stone), so the urine cannot drain out and bacteria start to multiply.

Symptoms: Fever; chills; pain in the lower back; painful urination; nausea.

Diagnostic tests: Urine tests.

Treatment: Antibiotics; treating cause of blockage.

6. *Cystitis* or *urinary tract infection* (UTI)) – Bacterial infection of the bladder lining.

Causes: Bacterial infection (often E. coli); risk factors include sexual intercourse ('alarm bells' in young children, warranting investigation into potential sexual abuse) and female anatomy.

Symptoms: Sharp, burning sensation when passing urine; frequent urge to pass urine.

Diagnostic tests: Urine tests.

Treatment: Antibiotics; alkalinizer sachets.

7. *Nephrotic syndrome* – A set of symptoms which can be due to illness or can be a disorder in itself (primary nephrotic syndrome).

Causes: Underlying illnesses may include: other forms of kidney disease (e.g. glomerulonephrosis), cancer, diabetes, systemic lupus erythematosus (SLE), immune disorders.

Symptoms: Protein in the urine, low levels of protein in the blood; edema around eyes, mouth, ankles.

Diagnostic tests: Biopsy; blood and urine tests; imaging.

Treatment: Depending on underlying cause, treatment may include corticosteroids; albumen; ACE inhibitors (see Chapter 18).

8.   *Polycystic disease* – Cysts form in the kidneys which gradually squeeze out normal kidney tissue leading to kidney failure.

Causes: Inherited.

Symptoms: High blood pressure; pain in lower back.

Diagnostic tests: Blood tests; urine tests; imaging.

Treatment: Anti-hypertensive medications; dialysis.

8.   Some common medications

diuretics	stimulate the flow of urine; used to manage heart failure or hypertension or edema (swelling)
immunosuppressants	used to suppress the body's rejection of a kidney implant
erythropoietin	helps production of red blood cells
potassium chloride (*KCl*)	used to compensate for loss of potassium as a result of the use of diuretics

9.   English-Chinese glossary

英漢 詞彙表

English	Hong Kong & Taiwan	Mainland China
blood urea nitrogen (BUN) test	血液尿素氮試驗	血液尿素氮试验; 血脲氮试验
continuous ambulant peritoneal dialysis (CAPD)	連續性流動式腹膜透析 (俗稱「洗肚」)	持续流动式腹膜透析
creatinine clearance rate (CCR)	肌酸酐廓清率	肌酐清除率; 肌酐廓清率
cystitis; urinary tract infection (UTI)	膀胱炎; 泌尿道感染	膀胱炎; 泌尿道感染
dialysis machine	透析機	透析机
dialyzing solution	透析 (溶) 液	透析 (溶) 液
diuretic	利尿劑	利尿剂
edema/oedema	水腫	水肿
erythropoietin	紅血球生成素	(促) 红细胞生成素

(Continued)

English	Hong Kong & Taiwan	Mainland China
extracorporeal shockwave lithotripsy (ESWL)	體外衝擊波碎石術	体外震波粉碎(肾)结石术; 体外冲击波碎石术
glomerular filtration rate (GFR)	腎小球過濾率	肾小球滤过率
glomeruli	腎小球	肾小球
glomerulonephritis	腎小球腎炎	肾小球肾炎
gout	痛風症	痛风症
hemodialysis/haemodialysis	血液透析(俗稱「洗腎」)	血液透析
hyperuricemia	高尿酸血症; 血(內)尿酸過多	高尿酸血(症)
IgA nephropathy	甲型球蛋白腎病變	IgA肾炎; IgA肾病; A型免疫球蛋白肾病
immunosuppressant drug	免疫抑制劑	免疫抑制剂
kidney failure; renal failure	腎衰竭	肾功能衰竭(肾衰)
kidney stone	腎石	肾(结)石
nephritis	腎炎	肾炎
Nephrologist	腎臟科醫生	肾病家
nephrotic syndrome	腎病綜合症	肾病综合症
polycystic kidney disease	多囊腎病	多囊性肾病
pyelonephritis	腎盂腎炎	肾盂肾炎
systemic lupus erythematosus (SLE)	系統性紅斑狼瘡	全身性红斑狼疮; 系统性红斑狼疮
urinary tract	(泌)尿道	尿路; 泌尿道
urine albumin test	尿蛋白試驗	尿蛋白试验
Urologist	泌尿科醫生	泌尿科医生

Summary of main points

This chapter has given a brief overview of the urological system, including:

- anatomy of the kidneys and their important role
- terms with Latin and Greek roots
- health professionals involved
- some commonly encountered conditions relating to the kidneys and urinary tract, together with common diagnostic tests and treatment methods

Chapter 28

Urology and gynecology

The reproductive systems

This chapter is divided into two sections. Section 2 covers disorders of the male and female reproductive systems, fertility and infertility, while Section 3 looks at complications of pregnancy.

1. Terms with Latin and Greek roots

benign	good (not cancerous)
brachytherapy	treatment delivered from a short distance: inserting radioactive material inside a tumor
HDR	high dose radiation
hyperplasia	overgrowth
in vitro	'in glass" i.e. in the laboratory in a test tube or specimen dish
LDR	low dose radiation
malignant	literally: bad (cancerous)
vas deferens	literally: a vessel leading out (carrying the sperm)

2. Male and female reproductive systems

2.1 Anatomy of the male reproductive system

The male reproductive system consists of:

- **two testes (testicles)** – male sperm-producing glands, in the scrotum, hanging from the spermatic cord
- **epididymis** – one of two long, tightly coiled ducts which store sperm and take it from the testes to the vas deferens
- **vas deferens** – the canal that connects the testes with the urethra and takes the sperm away from the epididymis
- **prostate gland** – gland situated directly below the bladder; the prostate gland produces a fluid that helps sperm survive

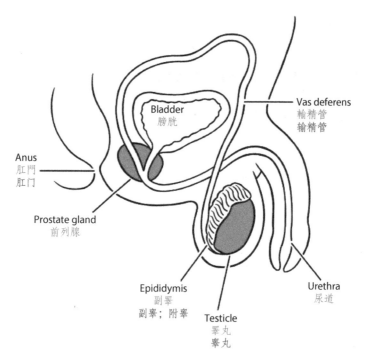

Figure 28.1 Male reproductive system
男性生殖系統

2.2 Disorders of the male reproductive system

1.   *Prostatic hypertrophy,* also referred to as *benign prostatic hyperplasia* (*BPH*) or *enlarged prostate* – occurs when the prostate gland is enlarged and presses on the urethra.

Cause: The prostate gland keeps growing very gradually from around age 40 onwards.

Symptoms: Problems with urination (dribbling, leaking, frequency) and urine retention. Can lead to bladder stones and damage to bladder and kidneys.

Diagnostic tests: Rectal examination; prostate specific antigen (PSA) blood test to check for inflammation or cancer; imaging.

Treatment: Watchful waiting; medication; avoiding coffee, alcohol, certain medications.

2.   *Prostate cancer*
See Chapter 16, page 190.

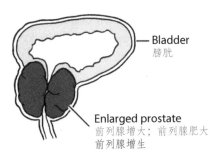

Bladder
膀胱

Enlarged prostate
前列腺增大；前列腺肥大
前列腺增生

Figure 28.2 Enlarged prostate
前列腺增大；前列腺肥大
前列腺增生

3. *Prostatitis* – Inflammation of the prostate. Can be acute or chronic.

Causes: These include bacterial infection; autoimmune response; injury and many others.

Symptoms: Acute prostatitis: Fever; chills; painful urination; swollen, tender prostate. Chronic prostatitis can occur with or without symptoms.

Diagnostic tests: Urine tests; imaging.

Treatment: Rest; increased fluid intake; antibiotics.

4. *Sexual function problems*

4a. *Infertility/Sterility* – Please see fertility/infertility, page 350ff.

4b. *Impotence (also called erectile dysfunction)* – An inability to hold an erection long enough for normal intercourse.

Causes: Circulation (vascular) disorders (diabetes and smoking may be factors); neurological disorders; psychological factors; drug side-effects; hormonal problems.

Symptoms: Inability to hold erection long enough.

Diagnostic tests: History; blood and urine tests.

Treatment: Medication; self-injection.

5. *Testicular cancer* (see Chapter 16).

6. *Undescended testes* (also referred to as *cryptorchidism*) – Either one or both testes have not come down into the scrotum.

Causes: Congenital condition.

Symptoms: Testes need to be in the scrotum because they need to be slightly below body temperature; undescended testes carry an increased risk of infertility and of testicular cancer.

Diagnostic tests: Physical examination

Treatment: Orchidopexy or orchiopexy (operation to bring testes into the scrotum).

2.3   Health professionals

Fertility specialist – Doctor specializing in managing male and female infertility problems.
Urologist – see Chapter 27

2.4   Anatomy of the female reproductive system

The female reproductive system consists of:

– two ovaries, one on either side of the womb. The ovaries are the female equivalent of the testes.
– two Fallopian tubes, one on either side of the womb
– womb or uterus
– cervix (the neck of the womb)
– vagina
– external genitals: vulva (containing the labia); the clitoris and its foreskin, and the openings of the vagina and the urethra (urine duct)

A woman's eggs mature in her ovaries. The pituitary gland in the brain produces two hormones, called follicle stimulating hormone (FSH) and luteinizing hormone (LH). The egg develops in a follicle on the surface of the ovary under the influence of FSH and LH. Once a month, ovulation takes place and an egg is pushed away from the ovary and into the Fallopian tube, where it starts travelling towards the womb. If the egg meets sperm on its way to the womb, it may be fertilized and travel on to the womb where it may imbed itself into the lining. At this stage, it is called an embryo, while in later stages of its development, it is referred to as a fetus. The lining starts producing a hormone called human chorionic gonadotropin (HCG), also referred to as pregnancy hormone, and a pregnancy test comes up as positive (positive test for HCG in the urine or in the blood).

If the egg does not meet up with any sperm, the lining of the womb which had been prepared for a possible pregnancy is shed and the woman has her menstrual period, usually approximately 14 days after the day on which she ovulated.

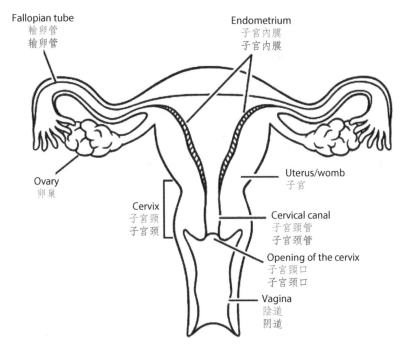

Figure 28.3 Female reproductive system
女性生殖系統

The ovarian follicle produces estrogen and progesterone, two hormones which regulate the woman's menstrual periods. When a woman goes through menopause, her ovaries stop functioning and producing these hormones. When this happens some women choose hormone replacement therapy (HRT) in which estrogen and/or progesterone (in either their bio-identical, i.e. identical to body's natural hormones, or synthetic form) are taken in order to combat menopausal symptoms such as hot flashes, irritability and fatigue. Hormone replacement therapy may also be prescribed to prevent osteoporosis and cardiovascular disease, both of which may affect women after menopause.

2.5 Health professionals

Fertility specialist – Doctor specializing in managing male and female infertility problems.
Gynecologist – see Chapter 12.

2.6   Disorders of the female reproductive system

1.   *Cervical cancer* (refer Chapter 16)

2.   *Endometrial cancer* – Cancer of the endometrium or inner lining of the womb, also referred to as *uterine cancer*. See Chapter 16.

3.   *Endometriosis* – Endometrial tissue (i.e. cells from the inner lining of the womb), is found outside of the womb, where it swells up and bleeds during every menstrual cycle. Common in women from puberty to menopause.

Cause: There are various theories, including that of retrograde (backwards) menstruation, where bits of tissue from the womb travel up into the Fallopian tubes during a period. Other theories involve certain immune system abnormalities, cells on the outside of the ovaries changing into endometrial cells, or endometrial cells travelling through the lymph system, as endometrial tissue has also been found further away from the womb.

Symptoms: Painful periods; pain during intercourse; ovulation pain; back pain; fatigue. Can lead to complications including scar tissue and adhesions (fibrous bands of scar tissue in the lower abdomen, causing organs to stick together) and infertility.

Diagnostic tests: Laparoscopy.

Treatment: Removal of endometrial tissue (e.g. by laparoscopy); hormonal treatment.

4.   *Ovarian cancer* (refer Chapter 16)

5.   *Ovarian cyst* – A sac filled with fluid or with half-solid material develops in or on the ovary. Different types of cysts exist, depending on their origins. A *follicular* cyst is the most common. It is benign and usually disappears by itself. A *dermoid* cyst is formed from cells which produce eggs and can contain bone, teeth or hair. *Corpus luteum* cysts consist of yellowish tissue which grows on the ovary after ovulation and produces progesterone. Normally these "waste away" after the period.

Causes: Ovarian cysts can be normal and may disappear by themselves; some can be malignant.

Symptoms: Constipation; frequent urination; irregular periods; abdominal pain; pain during intercourse.

Diagnostic tests: Ultrasound scan; laparoscopy; CA-125 blood test.

Treatment: Oral contraceptives (for follicular cysts); surgical removal.

6.   *Pelvic Inflammatory Disease (PID)* – An infection which starts in the neck of the womb and then moves to the tube(s) or spreads further into the abdomen.

Cause: Usually a bacterial infection, typically a sexually transmitted disease (STD) such as chlamydia or gonorrhea.

Symptoms: Foul-smelling discharge; pain in lower belly; abnormal bleeding or spotting between periods; pain during intercourse; burning sensation when passing urine. Can lead to abscess, septicemia and infertility (due to scarring of the Fallopian tubes).

Diagnostic tests: Endocervical swabs (samples taken from inside the cervix).

Treatment: Painkillers; antibiotics; tracing of (sexual) contacts.

7.   *Polycystic ovaries* – Lots of small cysts develop on the ovary which may cause the affected ovary to double in size.

Cause: Hormonal imbalance: high levels of testosterone, LH and estrogen; low levels of FSH; may be caused by problems with the adrenal glands or the pituitary gland; sometimes associated with insulin resistance.

Symptoms: No ovulation; no menstrual periods; infertility; masculine-type hair growth; low voice; weight gain.

Diagnostic tests: Blood tests; imaging.

Treatment: Often hormonal treatment; sometimes removal of part of one or both ovaries; oral diabetes medication; losing weight.

3.   Fertility and infertility

3.1   Infertility

Infertility is the inability for a couple to conceive (have a baby) and affects approximately 10% of all couples. Treatment is based on the cause of the infertility, and both partners must be investigated. The American Congress of Obstetricians and Gynecologists (ACOG) and the American Society for Reproductive Medicine (ASRM) both recommend that women under age 30 try to conceive for 12 months before seeking treatment, and that women over age 30 try for six months before seeking help from a fertility specialist. However, more recent studies suggest that couples should wait no more than 6 months of trying to conceive before seeking help.

Many conditions may lower a couple's chance of conceiving. These can include:

- decrease in the number and motility of sperm
- disorder of the vaginal mucus
- problems with the transport of sperm/eggs
- disorders of ovulation

- older parents, especially over 40 years
- sexual dysfunction
- psychological disorder
- other medical conditions
- endocrine disorders
- genetic factors
- infections (such as pelvic inflammatory disease)
- trauma to the genitals
- radiation which may have destroyed eggs or sperm
- certain drugs may interfere with ovulation
- immunological incompatibility – antibodies to sperm

Treatment: Identifying the problem; outlining the options. Treatment may include emotional counseling; coital timing (timing of sexual intercourse); donor insemination (in case of semen problems); induced ovulation and/or surgery or in vitro fertilization (IVF) in the case of tubal disease.

3.2   Men

In most cases male infertility is due to a low sperm count or poor sperm function.

Causes: Degenerative changes of the testicles through, for instance, X-rays, infection, malnutrition; sperm unable to get through due to a blockage; no or not enough viable (able to live) spermatozoa.

Symptoms: No physical symptoms.

Diagnostic tests: Semen analysis is the main test, whereby three semen samples are analyzed over the course of several weeks to check sperm count, sperm motility (sperm movement 4 hours after ejaculation) and sperm normality (counting percentage of abnormal sperm, must be < 20%). The second is a post-coital test, whereby a vaginal mucus specimen from the man's partner is examined (within 6 hours of inter-course). This test is done to analyze the penetration of mucus by the sperm and the quality of the mucus.

Treatment: Combine the few healthy sperm with the egg via IVF; donor insemination (placement of donor sperm within the cervix or uterus at ovulation).

3.3   Women

Causes: Failure to ovulate; blocked Fallopian tubes; fibroids or polyps in the womb inhibiting the egg imbedding itself in the lining of the womb; congenital abnormalities of the genital tract; unfavorable secretions; cervical or vaginal problems which make it difficult for sperm to get through. Tubal pelvic inflammatory disease is a major cause of tubal disease. Tubal damage may also follow peritonitis and pelvic adhesions after surgery. Endometriosis (uterine tissue growing outside of uterus) may also cause pelvic damage similar to tubal disease. In a number of cases no cause can be found for the infertility.

Symptoms: Failure to conceive after repeated attempts.

Diagnostic tests: Analysis of cervical mucus (should be clear and abundant, and it should be "stretchy" at ovulation time); a urine test (an ovulation predictor kit which reveals whether the woman is ovulating or not); ultrasound (detects a ripening egg); hormonal blood tests (done throughout the cycle to show variations in different hormone levels); laparoscopy to check whether the tubes are still open as well as look for any adhesions, pelvic inflammatory disease or endometriosis. Patency testing the patency of the Fallopian tubes to see whether egg and embryo can pass through, involves a colored dye being injected into the tubes.

Treatment: Ovulation failure is treated with hormonal medication. Donor eggs are used if women suffer premature ovarian failure. Tubal damage treatment involves surgery to remove adhesions, and/or IVF. If a woman is infertile due to endometriosis, IVF may be the only option.

3.4   Artificial reproduction

Artificial reproduction means that artificial means are used in order to achieve a pregnancy. This may include the following:

1.   *Artificial Insemination by Husband (AIH)*

Situations in which this may be done: Problems with the cervix; mechanical problems, such as a spinal (back) injury or a physical disability; a very low sperm count; semen stored (frozen) before chemotherapy or radiation therapy. This is also referred to as simply intra-uterine insemination (IUI).

Method: Intrauterine insemination whereby sperm is put inside the uterus through the cervix using a very fine catheter (narrow tube).

2.   *Artificial insemination by donor (AID/DI)*

Situations in which this may be done: No sperm count or a very low sperm count; abnormal sperm; risk of hereditary diseases being passed on; woman has no male partner.

Method: A speculum and syringe are used to bathe the cervix in semen. Success rates are the same as for normal conception.

3. *In vitro fertilization (IVF)*

Situations in which this may be done: Damaged tubes; low sperm count; poor move-ment of sperm; presence of anti-sperm antibodies; problems with the cervix; endome-triosis; unexplained infertility.

Method: The woman takes drugs which stimulate multiple ovulations. The eggs are removed from the woman's body using ultrasound. Eggs and sperm are treated sepa-rately then brought together outside of the body (*in vitro*). Two to three days after fer-tilization, a maximum of three embryos are placed inside the uterus. Any additional healthy embryos are frozen in case further attempts at fertilization are necessary in the future.

4. *Gamete intrafallopian transfer (GIFT)*

Situations in which this may be done: May be done if there is a "cervical barrier" to conception (problem with the cervix).

Method: The eggs are collected as for IVF and are placed into a catheter (fine tube) with fresh sperm; they are then placed in the Fallopian tube, allowing fertilization to take place.

5. *Ovum donation*

Situations in which this may be done: When the woman does not ovulate (i.e. does not produce any eggs).

Method: Eggs are donated by women (usually women who are undergoing IVF them-selves). The eggs are fertilized outside of the womb (*in vitro*) using sperm from the woman's partner. The embryos which result are then placed inside her womb.

6. *Intrauterine insemination (IUI)*

Situations in which this may be done: Unexplained fertility; ovulation problems; male partner experiences premature ejaculation or impotence; woman wants to use donor sperm.

Method: Sperm is washed to remove the fast-moving sperm, which is then placed inside the womb close to the time the woman is due to ovulate.

3.5   Contraception

Different types of contraception (methods for preventing pregnancy, sometimes referred to as family planning) exist, including the following:

1. *Natural family planning*
This involves abstinence from intercourse during the time of the month when the woman is fertile. Under ideal circumstances, this may be almost as effective as the pill,

or condoms and diaphragms, if the woman has a regular menstrual period. However, determining the fertile period may be very difficult.

2. *Condoms*
Thin, strong sheaths of rubber or similar material worn by the man, to stop the sperm from entering the vagina. Condoms may fail if they tear or if they slip off after climax. If the condom is used consistently and correctly, it is as effective as the diaphragm.

3. *Diaphragm*
A flexible rubber dome used with spermicidal cream or jelly. It is inserted into the vagina to cover the cervix and stops the sperm from getting past. The diaphragm must be left in place for at least 6 hours after intercourse and may be left in place as long as 24 hours. The diaphragm must be fitted by a specialist and must be refitted every two years or after each pregnancy. The diaphragm offers a high level of protection (failure rate is 2–3 pregnancies per 100 women). Failure may be caused by incorrect insertion or by the diaphragm being moved out of place during sexual intercourse.

4. *Intrauterine contraceptive device (IUCD).*
A small object shaped like a loop, spiral or ring, made of plastic or stainless steel. It has to be placed inside the womb by a specialist and may be left there indefinitely. Some women cannot use an IUCD, because the womb expels it, or because they have bleeding or discomfort. The IUCD is not recommended for women who have not had a child, as the womb is too small and the cervical canal too narrow. Sometimes, insertion of the IUCD may lead to inflammation of the pelvic organs.

5. *Spermicidals*
Sperm-killing chemicals inserted into the vagina to cover the surface of the vagina and the opening of the cervix. Quite effective on their own, but thought to be more effective when used together with either a diaphragm or a condom.

6. *Hormonal contraceptives* (taken by women)
Contraceptives may be taken orally (sometimes known as "the pill") or be delivered through a ring, intrauterine device, implant or injection. Hormonal contraceptives are the most effective method of contraception (apart from total abstinence or surgical sterilization). They may have some side-effects, including nausea, light bleeding (spotting) between periods, breast tenderness or enlargement, fluid retention, and weight gain. They should not be used by women who are prone to developing thrombosis.

7. *Vasectomy*
Procedure involving the cutting of the "vas," the tube which carries the sperm. Some doctors carry out "no scalpel" vasectomies, using a clamp rather than a scalpel to get through the skin.

8.   *Tubal ligation*

Abdominal surgery to tie the tubes so that eggs can no longer travel from the ovary to the womb.

4.   Pregnancy

This section will look at some of the complications which may occur in the course of a pregnancy, including gestational diabetes and pre-eclampsia. Please refer to Chapter 12 for general information on pregnancy and prenatal checkups.

A 40-week pregnancy is divided into three 3-monthly periods called *trimesters* of 13–14 weeks each. In the first trimester (conception to 13 weeks) there is rapid growth. All major organs of the fetus develop. The mother experiences major changes which affect her hormone levels, circulation, metabolism, and emotions. Mothers need folic acid to prevent neural tube defects.

In the second trimester all organs of the baby are working independently. The baby continues to grow. If born just after 24 weeks, there is a slim chance of survival but possibly impaired quality of life.

In the third trimester the baby is fully developed and preparing for birth. It is laying down fat, iron and immunity reserves. Mothers commonly experience anemia and need good nutrition, rest and relaxation.

4.1   Terms with Latin and Greek roots

Prenatal	before birth
cardiotocography (CTG)	cardio: heart; toco: contraction; graphy: recording
cervix	neck (of womb) (adjective: cervical)
ectopic	out of place
extrauterine	outside the womb
fetus	developing baby in the womb (adjective: fetal)
gestation	pregnancy (literally growing and developing)
gravid	pregnant (heavy with child)
gravidarum	belonging to pregnant women
hyster	womb (Greek)
hysterectomy	removal of the womb
intrauterine	inside the womb
menses/menstrual periods	monthly bleeding
natal	related to birth
partum	child birth
postnatal	after birth
prenatal	before birth

term	between 37 and 42 weeks gestation (i.e. ready to be born)
uterus	womb (Latin)
ovary	gland producing female hormones; eggs develop in the ovary
ovulation	egg "jumps" out of the ovary, into the Fallopian tube
ovum	egg (compare: ovaries)

4.2   Health professionals

Obstetrician-Gynecologist (Ob-Gyn) – See Chapter 12.

Midwife – Health professional specialized in the care of women during pregnancy and childbirth, as well as immediately after childbirth.

4.3   Complications of pregnancy

Minor

Nausea and vomiting – The so-called morning sickness (which can in fact last all day), usually lasts between 4–16 weeks.

Heartburn – Pain caused by gastric juices coming up into the esophagus, caused by hormone changes to the cardiac sphincter (cardia is top of the stomach). Worse from weeks 30 to 40.

Breast changes – Tingling, discomfort, feeling of fullness.

Constipation – Due to hormonal relaxation and slowing of gut.

Frequently passing urine – Due to pressure from enlarging uterus plus increased blood flow to the bladder.

Cramp and backache

Leukorrhea – White, non-irritant vaginal discharge.

Fainting – May happen more often due to vasodilation (widening of blood vessels) of extremities (arms and legs).

Varicose veins – Due to hormonal relaxing of blood vessel walls in lower legs and vulva.

Skin changes:

Linea nigra – Pigmentation line from umbilicus to top of pubic hair line.

Chloasma – Mask of pregnancy: pigmentation of face, which will fade after childbirth.

Itching of skin (urticaria): Mostly over abdomen and breasts, buttocks and upper thighs – due to liver response to pregnancy

Carpal tunnel syndrome – Numbness with pins and needles in woman's hands and fingers, due to fluid retention in the wrist, leading to pressure on the nerve in the wrist. This may require physical therapy and splints.

Insomnia – Not being able to sleep – may be caused by anxiety.

More serious

Every checkup will involve a urine test for sugar, ketones and protein. Protein in the urine may indicate pre-eclampsia, while the presence of sugar may indicate gestational diabetes. The practitioner will take the woman's blood pressure and weight to check for pre-eclampsia and will check the baby's heart tones and movements to make sure it is developing normally. The height of the fundus (top) of the uterus is checked to see if pregnancy and baby are developing normally.

1. *Abdominal pain in pregnancy*

Causes: In early weeks this may be caused by a miscarriage or an ectopic pregnancy (pregnancy within the Fallopian tube)

> *Fibroids* – benign mass in uterus
>
> *Placental abruption* – see number 12 (page 361)
>
> *Stretching of round ligaments* – not serious

Symptoms: Pain in abdomen. *Diagnostic tests*: Ultrasound scan.

Treatments: Depending on cause.

2. *Abortion* – May be spontaneous or induced. Please note the lay use of the word abortion refers to what physicians would refer to as a termination of pregnancy. Spontaneous abortion is known as a miscarriage. A missed abortion occurs when the baby has died inside the womb, but the woman continues to feel pregnant. This is also known as intrauterine fetal demise or IUFD.

Causes (*spontaneous abortion*): Often: blighted fetus (something wrong with the fetus, incompatible with life); occasionally: accidental use of teratogenic drugs (drugs which may harm or kill the fetus).

Symptoms: Usually vaginal blood loss; no fetal heartbeat.

Diagnostic tests: Ultrasound scan.

Treatment: Observation; occasionally a spontaneous abortion may not proceed and the pregnancy may continue; if miscarriage is in progress, medical staff will need to do a dila(ta)tion and curettage (D&C – see page 91) to ensure there are no products of conception left inside the womb, as this may lead to infection, bleeding or to the growth of a rare tumor.
Please note: An induced abortion is also referred to as a termination of pregnancy.

3. *Antepartum hemorrhage (APH)* (see vaginal bleeding during pregnancy).

4. *Ectopic pregnancy or extrauterine pregnancy* – This is a medical emergency and occurs when the fertilized egg implants itself outside of the womb, mostly in the Fallopian tube. As the embryo grows bigger, the tube cannot stretch to contain the egg and ruptures, causing life-threatening intra-abdominal bleeding.

Causes: Pelvic inflammatory disease (PID); damage to the tube (e.g. tubal ligation); smoking.

Symptoms: Blood loss; cramping; pain; vaginal bleeding; uterus enlarged; early breast changes; sometimes symptoms of shock.

Diagnostic tests: Ultrasound scan; blood tests.

Treatment: Methotrexate® if diagnosed early; removal of pregnancy (salpingostomy) or removal of tube (salpingectomy).

5. *Fetal alcohol syndrome* – see page 153.

6. *Gestational diabetes* (also referred to as *pregnancy diabetes*) – Diabetes is a medical condition which can seriously complicate pregnancy. The mother may have diabetes prior to pregnancy or develop it during pregnancy (*gestational diabetes mellitus*).

Causes: In gestational diabetes, the body's demand for insulin can be three times higher than normal, while the pancreas may not produce enough insulin or the body may not respond to it (insulin resistance – see Chapter 25), while the body's need for insulin may be up to three times greater than normal. Risk factors include being overweight, having a family history of diabetes or having had gestational diabetes previously. High GI food should be avoided and it is important to remember that jasmine rice has a GI that is much higher than that of sugar!

Symptoms: Excessive thirst; large volume of urine passed; weight loss; thrush; urinary tract infections.

Diagnostic tests: Sugary drink test (usually between 24 and 28 weeks of pregnancy) to see if body can process the sugar (take it out of the bloodstream).

Treatment
During pregnancy
Good control of sugar levels; delivery of baby at a hospital with a neonatal intensive care unit (NICU) available. Oral anti-diabetes medication is not used in pregnancy, as it is considered teratogenic (can lead to fetal death). Good fetal monitoring is important, including a kick chart (chart on which mother records baby's movements) and CTG; ultrasound scans and placental function tests.

During labor
IV fluids with glucose and insulin and ongoing blood glucose monitoring.

Postnatal period
Monitoring blood sugar levels for both mother and baby for 48 hours. Glucose tolerance test (GTT) for mother 6 weeks after birth.

Maternal complications of diabetes
Higher incidence of pre-eclampsia, urinary tract infections, thrush, polyhydramnion (too much amniotic fluid); long-term diabetes after pregnancy; reduced fertility; increased risk of miscarriage.

Fetal complications
Large baby, leading to difficult birth; intra-uterine death; fetal abnormalities; respiratory distress at birth; rebound hypoglycemia (baby has low blood sugar levels after birth); birth trauma due to increased risk of operative delivery; premature labor.

7.   *Hyperemesis gravidarum* – Severe and almost continuous vomiting.

Causes: These may include high levels of HCG and estrogen; many other risk factors have been studied.

Symptoms: Severe vomiting; severe dehydration and ketosis (body using protein stores instead of fat stores).

Diagnostic tests: Fluid balance chart.

Treatment: Intravenous (IV) rehydration; sometimes TPN or nasogastric feeding.

8.   *Intraturerine growth retardation (IUGR)* – A slowing down of fetal growth leading to a baby who is small for gestational age. IUGR may lead to low-birth-weight babies.
    There are two types of IUGR. Asymmetrical growth retardation is due to malnutrition in the womb, with normal growth until the third trimester, head circumference within normal limits, but low birth weight. There is a lack of body fat and the baby's head appears large when compared to the wasted appearance of body and limbs. Symmetrical (global) growth retardation is growth retardation which has occurred since early pregnancy. Head circumference is in proportion to overall size and weight; outlook not so good; may involve neurological damage.

Causes: Anything that leads to placenta not functioning well including smoking, essential hypertension; multiple pregnancy, mother weighing less than 100 pounds/45kgs; poor nutrition (e.g. dieting or junk food); problems with umbilical cord; severe anemia, pre-eclampsia; threatened abortion; prolonged pregnancy; APH; certain medications (including corticosteroids, anticonvulsants); opiates; chromosome abnormality; fetal alcohol syndrome.

Symptoms: Growth delay on scan.

Diagnostic tests: Imaging

Treatment: Bed rest; aspirin (up to 20 weeks); fetal monitoring.

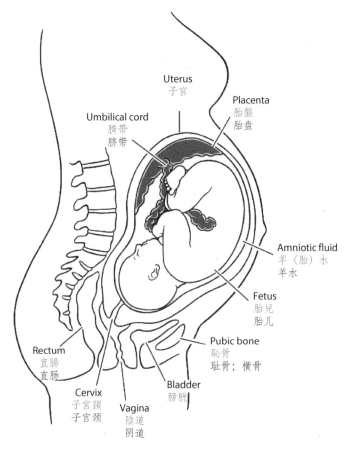

Figure 28.4 Pregnant woman at 40 weeks (baby in head down position)
懷孕40周的孕婦 (胎兒處於頭位產式位置)
怀孕40周的孕妇 (胎儿处于头位产式位置)

9.   *Malpresentation* – Any presentation other than the vertex (back of baby's head). In all malpresentations the part of the baby that presents (is ready to come out) does not fit the opening of the birth canal well. Types include breech (complete, incomplete); face; shoulder; brow. Breech is where the baby's buttocks lie lowermost in the uterus. A complete breech is when the baby is sitting cross-legged with its feet next to its bottom. A frank breech is when the baby's bottom is down, and legs are extended up, with feet next to baby's ears). Early in pregnancy babies may lie in breech position, but most turn by 34 weeks, so in preterm labor, it is quite common for baby to be breech. Other malpresentations include transverse presentation or shoulder presentation in which the baby lies sideways, or when the shoulder is the presenting part.

Cause: Often associated with early rupture of membranes (uneven pressure on bag of waters) and increased risk of prolapsed cord (when the umbilical cord falls out and is in danger of being squashed, depriving baby of oxygen). A breech may involve a uterus of abnormal shape; not enough water around baby; a mass in the uterus (e.g. a fibroid); fetal abnormality such as hydrocephalus; twins; many previous pregnancies leading to muscles around the womb being very lax; polyhydramnion (too much fluid), allowing baby to move freely.

Symptoms: Baby's heart rate may be too fast or too slow. Labor may be prolonged and can be dangerous and risky for the baby due to a lack of oxygen to the baby (both inside and outside of the womb); intracranial hemorrhage (bleed into baby's brain); bone breaks and bone dislocations; rupture of abdominal organs.

Diagnostic tests: Imaging; physical examination.

Treatment: Turning the baby inside the womb; Cesarean section.

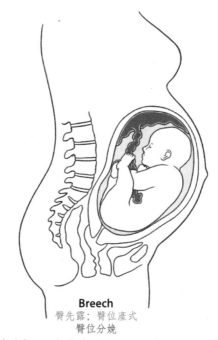

Breech
臀先露；臀位產式
臀位分娩
Baby's buttocks lie lower-most in the uterus
胎兒臀部置於子宮最底部
胎儿臀部置于子宫最底部

Figure 28.5 Pregnant woman at 40 weeks (baby in breech birth position)
懷孕40周的孕婦 (胎兒處於臀位產式位置)
怀孕40周的孕妇 (胎儿处于臀位产式位置)

10. *Miscarriage* – Products of conception (baby and placenta) come away from the womb before 24 weeks. Spontaneous abortion most often occurs between 9 and 11 weeks.

Causes: Fetal chromosomal abnormalities are involved in 60% of spontaneous abortions.

Can also be due to the mother acquiring diseases i.e. rubella; severe fever; drug overdoses; industrial chemicals; ABO (blood group) incompatibilities; thalassemia (see Chapter 20), retroverted uterus (womb is tipped backwards); bicornate uterus (abnormally shaped womb with two *horns*); cervical incompetence (cervix will not stay closed due to placental abruption or placenta previa).

11. *Multiple Pregnancy* – The development of more than one fetus in the uterus. Twins may be monozygotic (one egg and one sperm; two amniotic sacs; one placenta; connection of circulation; same sex) or dizygotic (two eggs and two sperm; two amniotic sacs; two placentas; no connected circulation, may be different sex).

Causes: Unknown; sometimes the result of fertility treatment.

Symptoms: All minor disorders of pregnancy, i.e. nausea, heartburn, may be worse; anemia due to greater demands on iron and folic acid; hypertension more common; polyhydramnion (more amniotic fluid than usual) is common, especially with monozygotic twins; more pressure symptoms caused by the increased weight and size of the uterus. Pressure symptoms include varicose veins and swelling of legs, backache; breathlessness and indigestion. Can lead to further complications such as polyhydramnion; premature rupture of membranes; fetal abnormality; prolapse of cord; malpresentations; prolonged labor; post-partum hemorrhage; delay in birth of second twin. Labor is often early due to overstretching of uterus.

Diagnostic tests: Ultrasound; uterus feels larger than expected for gestation; size of baby is small, which means there may be more than one baby.

Treatment: Careful monitoring of both babies is important, if there are any signs of fetal distress (baby/babies in trouble) doctors need to do an emergency Caesarean section.

12. *Placental abruption* – Placenta comes away from the womb after 28 weeks. Occurs in approximately 2% of pregnancies. Abruption can be mild, moderate or severe.

Causes: No cause found (very common); sometimes due to eclampsia, diffuse intravascular coagulation (DIC); essential hypertension; fall, blow, accident; polyhydramnion with ruptured membranes.

Symptoms: Pain and visible bleeding may occur.

Diagnostic tests: Ultrasound scan (if there is time).

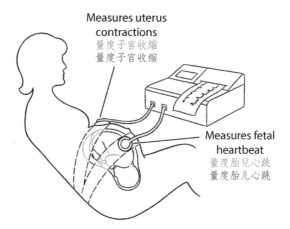

Measures uterus
contractions
量度子宮收縮
量度子宫收缩

Measures fetal
heartbeat
量度胎兒心跳
量度胎儿心跳

Figure 28.6 Cardiotocography
胎心宮縮圖
胎心宫缩图

Treatment: Depends on severity. If mild, then hospitalization: observation, monitoring baby's condition. If moderate, cases will include an assessment of the baby's condition; if not good, mother must be induced (induction of labor) or an emergency Caesarean section must be done if fetus is still alive; blood transfusions for mother.

13.   *Placenta previa* – Painless bleeding from separation of an abnormally situated placenta. The placenta lies partly or wholly in the lower uterine segment.

There are 4 grades of severity. With grades 1 and 2, the placenta partly covers the neck of the womb (*os*); vaginal delivery may be tried. In grades 3 and 4, the placenta covers the neck of the womb in front of the baby: Caesarean section is required.

Symptoms: Often first sign of placenta previa is bleeding (if not detected by ultra-sound).

Bleeding may occur at rest and may vary from very light to extremely heavy, causing a serious threat to baby and mother.

Diagnostic tests: Ultrasound scan

Treatment: Regular scans to check the position of placenta; hospitalization for check-ups and rest; plan of delivery; monitoring baby's movement. No vaginal examinations.

14.   *Pre-eclampsia (also known as pregnancy induced hypertension (PIH) or toxemia or gestational proteinuria hypertension (GPH)*

Cause: Not fully known, but may involve problem with blood vessels in the placenta, so blood pressure rises to ensure the developing child receives enough blood (oxygen and nutrients). Other factors may include family history of diabetes; high blood pressure;

kidney problems; autoimmune disorders; diet; first pregnancy; multiple pregnancy; age (over 35) and obesity.

Mainly occurs after 20 weeks and disappears after delivery. Between 6–7% of all pregnancies are complicated by hypertension (Fleming et al. 2005) and in 80% of these cases pre-eclampsia occurs.

Symptoms: Hypertension; swelling in hands, neck, face; protein in the urine (kidneys leaking protein into urine); sudden weight gain (>2 pounds or >1 kg a week). Can lead to eclampsia, a very serious state in which convulsions occur and in which the placenta may come away from the womb, leading to the child's death; bleeding inside blood vessels; drop in platelets; major organs damaged (lungs, kidneys, liver); capillaries in eye may be damaged, resulting in blindness.

Diagnostic tests: Women rarely have any symptoms until the condition has already become advanced. Therefore prenatal checkups should always include blood pressure, weight and urine checks.

Practitioners look for a change in blood pressure of 15–20 mm Hg above the normal reading (e.g. if blood pressure is normally 120/70, it may now be 135/85 or 140/90); proteinuria (protein in the urine) without any signs of a urinary infection; swelling and rapid weight gain, which may mean the body is retaining fluid.

Treatment: Careful monitoring of fetus and symptoms; may need hospitalization, careful monitoring and bed rest; lying on left side. Sometimes it is necessary to deliver the baby prematurely if symptoms worsen. Mother may be given corticosteroids to help baby's lungs develop more quickly (see Chapter 12.1).

15. *Rhesus disease* (See Chapter 28) – Health professionals are worried about mothers who are Rhesus negative (Rh-ve), because if the baby is Rhesus positive (Rh+ve) and there is any mixing of blood between mother and baby, the mother can form antibodies against the Rhesus D-antigen on her baby's red blood cells. During further pregnancies, antibodies in the mother's bloodstream may cross the placenta and destroy the baby's red blood cells.

The first pregnancy is usually not affected, because at that stage the mother has not yet formed antibodies (unless the mother has had a blood transfusion with Rhesus positive blood and formed antibodies then).

Causes: The blood groups of mother and baby may mix due to hypertension; placental abruption; trauma to placenta during amniocentesis; external cephalic version (turning a breech baby); placenta previa; previous blood transfusion to mother of Rhesus positive blood.

Symptoms: Baby's blood will flow more quickly because it will be thinner, due to hemolysis and anemia (see Chapter 20).

Diagnostic tests: Doppler sound test of baby's blood circulation.

Treatment: Mother is given anti-RhD immunoglobulin (Rho(D)) to prevent her blood from making antibodies, thus preventing Rhesus disease in following pregnancies.

16. *Vaginal bleeding in pregnancy*

Any vaginal blood loss during pregnancy should always be investigated. Bleeding can be due to:

- *Abortion or miscarriage* (see above)
- *Cervical incompetence* – The cervix opens, causing a spontaneous abortion, usually between 16 and 22 weeks. Congenital condition (born with it). Factors may include damage/injury during previous termination of pregnancy; lacerations (damage) during previous childbirth. A purse string suture is put in the cervix (to keep it closed) and taken out at 38 weeks.
- *Cervical lesion* – Changes in the lining of the cervix, can be benign or cancerous.
- *Ectopic pregnancy* (see above)
- *Implantation bleeding* – Bleeding caused by embryo implanting in the lining of the womb. Usually occurs on the 7th day after fertilization; may last 3–4 days. Sometimes mistaken for a menstrual period.
- *Increased blood supply in pregnancy* – Bleeding may occur especially after intercourse; this does not affect the pregnancy.
- *Placenta previa* (see above).

4.4   Some common diagnostic tests

Please refer to Chapter 12.

5.   Sexual health

Please see pages 344 and 347 for an overview of the anatomy of the male and female reproductive systems.

Common problems include what is referred to as sexual risk-taking behavior which may result in:

- Increased prevalence of HIV infection (see Chapter 24)
- Increased prevalence of unwanted pregnancies, resulting in abortions or unwanted children
- Increased prevalence of sexually transmitted diseases (STDs), which are also referred to as sexually transmitted infections or STIs

Having repeated abortions (terminations of pregnancy) may result in problems maintaining a pregnancy once the woman has reached a stage in her life where she does wish to have children. Repeated terminations may result in scarring of the inner lining of the uterus (endometrium), making implantation of the embryo problematic.

Repeated terminations may also lead to what is sometimes referred to as an incompetent cervix or weakened cervix, where the cervix opens too soon during the later stages of pregnancy. Please note that a weakened cervix may also be due to other causes, including previous cervical surgery, damage to the cervix during a difficult birth, or to congenital malformations.

5.1   Most common STDs

1.   *Chlamydia* – one of the most common STDs in many countries

Causes: Sexually transmitted infection with the Chlamydia trachomatis bacteria.

Symptoms: Burning sensation when passing urine; discharge from penis, vagina or rectum; in females symptoms of pelvic inflammatory disease (PID), salpingitis (inflammation of the Fallopian tubes) or hepatitis (inflammation of the liver). Please note: chlamydia may lead to infertility in females, mainly due to scarring of the Fallopian tubes; up to 25% of infected males may not experience any symptoms. When someone is diagnosed with chlamydia, they should also be checked for other STDs, including gonorrhea and syphilis.

Diagnostic tests: Antibody tests or culture of samples of discharge from penis, vagina or rectum.

Treatment: Antibiotics, tetracyclines.

2.   *Genital warts* – may also be referred to as *condyloma acuminate* or *venereal warts*.

Causes: Infection by specific strains of the human papillomavirus or HPV, usually strains 6 and 11.

Please note: Other *specific* strains of HPV (e.g. strains 16, 18, 31 and 45) have been linked to cervical cancer and throat cancer.

Symptoms: Grey or flesh-colored warts, usually in genital areas. Note: if found in children, this may be suspicious for sexual abuse.

Diagnostic tests: Applying acetic acid solution; colposcopy; cervical smear test.

Treatment: Cryotherapy; laser treatment; electrodesiccation (using electric current to destroy the warts).

3. *Gonorrhea* – common STD, also referred to as "the clap" or "the drip."

Causes: Sexually transmitted infection with the Neisseria gonorrhoeae bacteria.

Symptoms: Burning sensation when passing urine; white, yellow or green discharge from penis, vagina or rectum; pain in the testicles in males; females may have symptoms of pelvic inflammatory disease (PID), salpingitis (inflammation of the Fallopian tubes); fever, rash and joint pain if the infection spreads through the bloodstream. Symptoms usually appear within 2 to 5 days after the infection, but may take up to 1 month to appear in some men.

Please note: Gonorrhea may lead to infertility in females, mainly due to scarring of the Fallopian tubes. When someone is diagnosed with gonorrhea, they should also be checked for other STDs including chlamydia, HPV and syphilis.

Diagnostic tests: Cultures of samples of the discharge (fluid) or blood culture.

Treatment: Antibiotics; if relevant: vaccinations against hepatitis B and HPV; the person's sexual contacts should be traced and also checked for the infection.

4. *Syphilis* (see Chapter 17).

6. English-Chinese glossary

英漢詞彙表

English	Hong Kong & Taiwan	Mainland China
abortion	流產; 小產; 墮胎	流产; 小产
amniotic sac	羊膜囊	羊膜囊
antepartum hemorrhage/ haemorrhage (APH)	產前出血	产前出血
artificial insemination by donor (AID/DI)	以捐精者精子作人工授精	他精人工授精
artificial insemination by husband (AIH)	以夫精人工授精	夫精人工授精
bag of waters	羊水囊; 羊膜囊	羊水囊; 羊膜囊
bicornate uterus	雙角子宮	双角子宫
blighted fetus/foetus	胎兒萎縮	胎儿萎缩
breech	臀先露; 臀位產式	臀先露; 臀位分娩
carpal tunnel syndrome	腕管綜合症	腕管综合症
cervical cancer	(子) 宮頸癌	子宫颈癌

(*Continued*)

English	Hong Kong & Taiwan	Mainland China
cervix	(子) 宮頸	(子) 宮颈
Cesarean section	剖腹生產	剖腹产 (术); 剖宫产 (术)
chlamydia	衣原體; 披衣菌屬	衣菌体; 衣原体 (属)
chloasma	黃褐斑	褐黄斑
chromosome abnormality	染色體異常	染色体异常
contraception	避孕	避孕; 节育
contraceptive	避孕藥	避孕药
cord prolapsed	臍帶脫垂	脐带脱垂
cryotherapy	冷凍療法	冷冻疗法
dermoid cyst	皮樣囊腫	皮样囊肿
dizygotic twins	雙卵雙胎	双卵双胎; 双卵孪生; 二卵双生 (儿)
diaphragm	橫膈膜	膈膜
diffuse intravascular coagulation (DIC)	彌漫性血管內凝血; 散播性血管內凝血	弥散性血管内凝血; 播散性血管内凝血
ectopic pregnancy; extra-uterine pregnancy	宮外孕	异位妊娠; (子) 宫外孕
electrodesiccation	電乾燥治療法	电干燥治疗法
endocervical swab	內宮頸拭子	子宫颈内拭子
endometrial cancer	子宮內膜癌	子宫内膜癌
endometriosis	子宮內膜異位	子宫内膜异位
erectile disfunction	勃起障礙; 陽痿	勃起障碍
fertility specialist	生殖醫學專科醫生	生育专家
fetal/foetal alcohol syndrome	胎兒酒精綜合症	胎儿酒精综合症
fetal/foetal distress	胎兒窘迫	胎儿窘迫
fibroids	纖維瘤	纤维瘤
follicle stimulating hormone (FSH)	濾泡刺激素	(促) 卵胞 (刺) 激素; 促卵胞成熟激素
follicular cyst	毛囊囊腫; (卵巢) 濾泡性囊腫	毛囊囊肿; 滤泡囊肿; 卵泡囊肿
frank breech	單臀先露; 臀先露	臀先露
gamete intra-fallopian transfer (GIFT)	輸卵管內配子移植	配子输卵管内移植; 输卵管内受精; 输卵管内配偶子移植
genital warts	生殖器肉贅; 生殖器疣 (俗稱「椰菜花」)	生殖器疣
gestational diabetes	妊娠期糖尿病	妊娠 (期) 糖尿病
glucose tolerance test (GTT)	葡萄糖耐量試驗	葡萄糖耐量试验

(*Continued*)

English	Hong Kong & Taiwan	Mainland China
gonorrhea/gonorrhoea	淋病	淋病
Gynecologist	婦科醫生	妇科医生
heartburn	胃灼熱; 燒心; 胸口爍痛	胃灼热; 懊侬; 烧心
hormone replacement therapy (HRT)	荷爾蒙補充治療	激素替补疗法
human chorionic gonadotropin (HCG)	人體絨毛膜促性腺素; 絨促性素; 生殖素	人 (类) 绒毛膜促性腺 (激) 素
human papilloma virus (HPV)	人類乳突病毒; 人類乳頭狀瘤病毒	人类乳突病毒; 人乳头状瘤病毒
hydrocephalus	腦積水	脑积水
hyperemesis gravidarum	妊娠劇吐	妊娠剧吐
immunological incompatibility	免疫不相容性	免疫不相容性
implantation bleeding	(卵) 植入期出血	孕卵植入期出血
in vitro fertilization (IVF)	體外受孕	体外受精; 试管内受精
induction of labor	引產	引产
infertility	不孕; 不育	不孕; 不育
intrauterine contraceptive device (IUCD)	子宮內避孕器; 子宮環	宫内节育器; 宫内避孕器
intrauterine fetal/foetal demise (IUFD)	胎死宮中	胎死腹中; 胎死宫内
itrauterine growth retardation (IUGR)	胎兒宮內發育遲緩	胎儿宫内生长迟缓; 子宫内生长迟滞
IUI – Intrauterine insemination (also referred to as Artificial Insemination by Husband (AIH)	宮腔內人工授精 (亦稱以夫精人工授精)	宫腔内人工授精 (亦称夫精人工授精)
labia	陰唇	阴唇
labor/labour	分娩	分娩
laparoscopy	腹腔 (內窥) 鏡檢查	腹腔镜检查
leukorrhea	白帶	白带
linea nigra	妊娠線	妊娠线
luteinizing hormone (LH)	黃體生成素	促黄体 (生成) 激素; 黄体化激素
malpresentation	先露異常; 胎位不正	先露异常 (胎儿产式异常)
membranes	(胎) 膜	(胎) 膜
Midwife	助產士	助产师; 助产士
miscarriage; spontaneous abortion	流產; 小產; 自然流產	流产; 小产; 自然流产
missed abortion	過期流產	稽留流产; 过期流产

(Continued)

English	Hong Kong & Taiwan	Mainland China
monozygotic twins	單卵雙胎	同卵双生; 单卵双胎
multiple pregnancy	多胎妊娠	多胎妊娠
oral contraceptive	口服避孕藥	口服避孕药
orchidopexy; orchiopexy	睪丸固定術	睾丸固定术
ovarian cancer	卵巢癌	卵巢癌
ovarian cyst	卵巢囊腫	卵巢囊肿
ovum donation	卵子捐贈; 捐卵	捐卵
pelvic inflammatory disease (PID)	盆腔炎	盆腔炎
placenta previa/praevia	胎盤前置	前置胎盘
placental abruption	胎盤過早剝離; 胎盤早離	胎盘早期剥离; 胎盘早离
polycystic ovaries	多囊卵巢	多囊卵巢
Polyhydramnion/ Polyhydramnios	羊 (胎) 水過多	羊水过多
polyps	息肉	息肉
preeclampsia; pregnancy induced hypertension (PIH); gestational proteinuria hypertension (GPH); toxemia	子癇前期; 妊娠高血壓綜合症; 妊娠性蛋白尿高血壓; (妊娠) 毒血症	子痫前期;妊娠诱发高血压; 妊娠性高血压; 妊高症; 妊娠蛋白尿高血压; 毒血症
prostate cancer	前列腺癌	前列腺癌
prostate specific antigen (PSA)	前列線特異抗原	前列腺特异 (性) 抗原
prostatic hypertrophy; benign prostatic hyperplasia (BPH); enlarged prostate	前列腺肥大; 良性前列腺增生; 前列腺增大	前列腺肥大; 良性前列腺增生; 前列腺增生
prostatitis	前列腺炎	前列腺炎
rebound hypoglycemia	反彈性低血糖 (症)	反弹性低血糖 (症)
Rhesus disease	溶血性疾病	猕猴 (溶血) 病
salpingectomy	輸卵管切除術	输卵管切除术
salpingitis	輸卵管炎	输卵管炎
salpingostomy	輸卵管造口術	输卵管造口术
sexually transmitted disease (STD)	性接觸傳染病	性 (行为) 传播疾病; 性传染病; 性传播病
spermicidals	殺精劑	杀精 (子) 剂
syphilis	梅毒	梅毒
teratogenic drug	致畸胎藥	致畸胎药
termination of pregnancy; induced abortion	終止懷孕; 終止妊娠; 人工流產	终止怀孕; 终止妊娠; 人工流产
testicular cancer	睪丸癌	睾丸癌

(Continued)

English	Hong Kong & Taiwan	Mainland China
tubal ligation	輸卵管結紮術	输卵管结扎
undescended testes; cryptorchidism	睪丸未降 (隱睪症)	睾丸未降; 隐睾
Urologist	泌尿科醫生	泌尿科医生
uterine cancer	子宮癌	子宫癌
vasectomy	輸精管切除術	输精管切除术
vertex	頂先露	头顶先露

Summary of main points

This chapter has covered disorders of the male and female reproductive systems including:

- a brief overview of anatomy of the organs involved
- terms with Latin and Greek roots
- health professionals involved
- fertility and infertility
- complications of pregnancy
- sexual health, some common consequences of sexual risk-taking behaviors

Appendix

Some common diagnostic tests

Blood tests:

Blood culture	Page 145
Blood gases	Page 145
Blood grouping	Page 255
Chromosome study	Page 145
Cholesterol	Page 256
Clotting time	Page 255
CRP	C-Reactive protein, Page 270–271
Electrolytes	Page 145
ESR	Erythrocyte Sedimentation Rate, Page 269, 291.
Full blood count	Also: Complete Blood Count, Page 145
Genetic study	Page 145
Glucose	Pages 145
Group and Coombs test	Page 145
PKU (phenylketonuria)	Page 145
PSA	Pages 184
SBR	Serum Bilirubin, Page 145
Thyroid function tests	Page 145
Urea, Creatinine	Page 145
Enzymes	Elevated liver enzymes may be found in blood in case of a liver condition; elevated cardiac enzymes may be found in the blood after a heart attack
INR	regular test to monitor patient on blood-thinning medication (such as warfarin)

Biopsies	**some living cells taken for testing (e.g. for cancer)**
Bone marrow aspiration	biopsy of bone marrow
hook wire biopsy	deep biopsy of breast tissue
fine needle biopsy	biopsy using fine hollow needle and local anesthetic
smear test	checking cervical cells for abnormal cells
liver biopsy	checking for liver disease, liver cancer or liver secondaries

Imaging
Radiological tests

Abdominal X-Ray	Page 145
Chest X-Ray	Pages 145

Contrast X-rays:

Angiogram/angiography	Page 227
Barium meal/barium swallow	Page 191
Barium enema	Page 187
Cholangiogram	contrast X-Ray of gall-ducts
IVP	contrast X-Ray of kidneys and ureters
Myelogram	contrast X-Ray of space around the spinal cord

Ultrasonography: examinations by sound waves

Cranial ultrasound	Page 145
Echo or echocardiogram	Page 145
Renal ultrasound	Page 145

Urine tests

culture microscopy and sensitivity	Checking if bacteria grow on urine sample in the lab, and what antibiotics they are sensitive to
Early Morning Urine (EMU)	

Respiratory studies

Acid Fast Bacilli Tests	Page 244
Bronchoscopy	Page 184
Lung function test	Page 244
Mantoux test	Page 244
Oxygen saturation	Page 244
Peak flow meter	Page 244
Pulse oximetry	Pages 244
Spirometry	lung function test, Page 244
Sputum specimen	Page 244
Transbronchial biopsies	Page 244
Ziehl-Neelsen (Zn) stain test	Page 244

Endoscopies: looking inside an organ through a (flexible) fiber-optic tube

Arthroscopy	(looking inside a joint, e.g. knee joint)
Bronchoscopy	Page 184
Cystoscopy looking inside the bladder	Pages 184
Gastroscopy (Stomach)	looking inside the stomach, Page 185

Hysteroscopy	looking inside the uterus, Page 185
Laparoscopy (Abdomen)	looking inside the abdomen, Page 185
Esophagoscopy	looking inside the gullet, Page 184 (also esophagoscopy)
Colposcopy	viewing cervix and vagina, Page 184

Scanning

CT scan	*Computerized tomography,* Pages 210
Cardiac CT	Page 228
MRI scan	Magnetic Resonance Imaging, Page 210
PET scan	Positron Emission Tomography – scan using radioactive material to monitor areas of high activity (high cell turnover) in the body
Radionuclide (Nuclear) Scan	imaging using small amounts of radioactive material
VQ scan	ventilation perfusion scan of the lungs

Electrical tests

EEG	ElectroEncephaloGram (testing brain activity), Page 210
EMG	ElectroMyoGram (testing muscle activity), Page 274
EKG	ElectroCardioGram (testing heart activity), Page 227

Other diagnostic tests

Audiometry	hearing test
Bleeding time	Page 254
CTG (CardioTocoGraphy)	Pages 128
D & C (Dilatation and Curettage)	Page 92, 356
Doppler scanning	ultrasound scanning of a moving structure, such as blood flowing through an area
Endotracheal aspirate Culture	keeping a specimen taken from an endotracheal tube in the lab to see if it grows any bacteria
Exercise Tolerance Test	EKG while patient is on the treadmill, Page 228
Fertility Tests	Pages 349–351
Gastric aspirate	Page 146
Heart Catheterization	catheter (narrow tube) inserted in artery in arm or groin and guided through to the heart; contrast dye injected into coronary
Holter monitor	monitoring EKG for a longer time, using a portable tape, recorder, while patient carries on normal everyday activities

Lumbar puncture	Page 210
PTCA	see Heart Catheterization, Page 227
Radio-Active	
Iodine Uptake Test	patient swallows radio-active iodine tablet/liquid; 6–24 hours later radio-active activity in the thyroid is measured.
Spinal Tap	Page 146, 210 (see lumbar puncture)
Telemetry	Monitoring EKG from a distance, using a portable transmitter
TORCH study	Page 146
Viral study	Page 146
Visual Acuity	Eyesight test, Page 242, 243

References

Adams, F. M. & Osgood, C. E. (1973). A cross-cultural study of the affective meanings of color. *Journal of Cross-Cultural Psychology, 4*(2), 135–156. doi: 10.1177/002202217300400201

Andonova, A. & Taylor, H. A. (2012). Nodding in dis/agreement: A tale of two cultures. *Cognitive Process, 13*(Suppl 1): S79–S82. doi: 10.1007/s10339-012-0472-x

Angelelli, C. (2008). The role of the interpreter in the healthcare setting: A plea for a dialogue between research and practice. In C. Valero Garcés & A. Martin (Eds.), *Building bridges: The controversial role of the community interpreter*, pp. 139–152. Amsterdam: John Benjamins. doi: 10.1075/btl.76.08ang

Angelelli, C. (2004). *Medical interpreting and cross-cultural communication.* Cambridge, England: Cambridge University Press. doi: 10.1017/cbo9780511486616

Battle, D. (Ed.) (2002). *Communication disorders in multicultural populations* (3rd ed.). London, England: Butterworth.

Bolden, G. (2000). Toward understanding practices of medical interpreting: Interpreters' involvement in history taking. *Discourse Studies, 2*, 387–419. doi: 10.1177/1461445600002004001

Bontempo, K. (2013a). The chicken and egg dilemma: Academizing interpreter education. In E. Winston & C. Monikowski (Eds.), *Evolving paradigms in interpreter education*, pp. 33–41. Washington, DC: Gallaudet University Press.

Bontempo, K. (2013b). Interpreting by design: A study of aptitude, ability and achievement in Australian Sign Language interpreters. *New Voices in Translation Studies*, (10).

Bontempo, K. & Napier, J. (2011). Evaluating emotional stability as a predictor of interpreter competence and aptitude for interpreting. *Interpreting, 13*(1), 85–105. doi: 10.1075/intp.13.1.06bon

Bontempo, K., Goswell, D., Levitzke-Gray, P., Napier, J. & Warby, L. (in press). Towards the professionalization of Deaf interpreters in Australia: Testing times. In R. Adam, C. Stone, S. Collins, & M. Metzger (Eds.), *Deaf interpreters at work: International insights*. Washington, DC: Gallaudet University Press.

Bot, H. (2007). Gespreksvoering met behulp van een tolk. *De Psycholoog, 42*, 362–367.

Bot, H. (2005). Dialogue interpreting as a specific case of reported speech. *Interpreting, 7*(2), 237–261. doi: 10.1075/intp.7.2.06bot

Bowe, H. & Martin, K. (2007). *Communication across cultures. Mutual understanding in a global world.* Melbourne, Australia: Cambridge University Press. doi: 10.1017/cbo9780511803925

California Healthcare Interpreters Association. (n.d.). *California standards for healthcare interpreters: Ethical principles, protocols, and guidance on roles and intervention.* Los Angeles, CA: California Healthcare Interpreters Association. doi: 10.1075/btl.70.19ang

Canadian Healthcare. (2007). *Canadian health care: Canada health act.* Retrieved 25 December 2015 from: http://www.canadian-healthcare.org/page2.html

Cambridge, J. (1999). Information loss in bilingual medical interviews through untrained interpreters. *The Translator, 5*(2), 201–219. doi: 10.1080/13556509.1999.10799041

Camplin-Welch, V. (2007). Cross-cultural resource for health practitioners working with CulturAlly and Linguistically Diverse (CALD) clients. Auckland, New Zealand: Waitemata District Health Board and Refugees As Survivors New Zealand Trust.

Candlin, C. & Gotti, M. (Eds.) (2004a). *Intercultural aspects of specialized communication.* Bern, Switzerland: Peter Lang.

Candlin, C. & Candlin, S. (2003). Health care communication: A problematic site for applied linguistics research. *Annual Review of Applied Linguistics, 23*, 134–154. doi:10.1017/S0267190503000230

Candlin, C. & Gotti, M. (Eds.) (2004b). *Intercultural discourse in domain-specific English.* Special issue of *Textus* 17/1, Genoa, Italy: Tilgher.

Chabner, D.E. (2011). *The language of medicine* (9th ed.). Philadelphia, PA: Elsevier/Saunders.

Chen, A. (2003). *In the right words: Addressing language and culture in providing health care,* Asian and Pacific Islander American health forum, remarks at Grantmakers in Health Issue Dialogue. San Francisco, CA.

Chen, T. W. 陳子瑋. (2011). Community interpreting – A New Horizon in interpreting research in Taiwan [社區口譯—臺灣口譯研究新領域]. *Compilation and Translation Review, 4*(2), 207–214.

Chesher, T. (1997). Rhetoric and reality: Two decades of community interpreting and translating in Australia. In S. E. Carr, R. Roberts, A. Dufour & D. Steyn (Eds.), *The critical link: Interpreters in the community,* pp. 277–289. Amsterdam: John Benjamins. doi:10.1075/btl.19.29che

Clifford, A. (2005). Healthcare interpreting and informed consent: What is the interpreter's role in treatment decision-making. *TTR: Traduction, Terminologie, Redaction, 18*(2), 225–247. doi:10.7202/015772ar

Coney, S. (1988). *The unfortunate experiment. The full story behind the inquiry into cervical cancer treatment.* Auckland, New Zealand: Penguin Books.

Crezee, I. (2015). Semi-authentic practices for student health interpreters. *Translation & Interpreting, 7*(3), 50–62.

Crezee, I. (2009a). The development of the interpreting profession. In D. Clark & C. McGrath (Eds.), *Interpreting in New Zealand: The pathway forward,* pp. 75–80. Wellington: Crown.

Crezee, I. (2009b). Interpreting and the New Zealand healthcare system. In D. Clark & C. McGrath (Eds.), *Interpreting in New Zealand: The pathway forward,* pp. 102–107. Wellington: Crown.

Crezee, I. (2003). Health interpreting: The cultural divide. In L. Brunette, G. Bastin, I. Hemlin & H. Clarke (Eds.), *The Critical Link 3. Interpreters in the community,* pp. 249–259. Amsterdam: John Benjamins. doi:10.7202/016741ar

Crezee I., Atkinson, D., Pask, R., Au, P., & Wong S. (2015). When interpreting leaves interprets negatively affected: Teaching interprets about self-care. *International Journal of Interpreter Education, 7*(3).

Crezee I. & Grant, L. (in press). Thrown in the deep end. Challenges of interpreting informal paramedic language. *Translation and Interpreting.*

Crezee, I. & Grant, L. (2013). Missing the plot? Idiomatic language in interpreter education. *International Journal of Interpreter Education, 5*(1), 17–34.

Crezee, I., Mikkelson, H. & Monzon-Storey, L. (2015*). Introduction to healthcare for Spanish-speaking interpreters and translators.* Amsterdam: John Benjamins. doi:10.1075/z.193

Crezee, I. & Sachtleben, A. (2012) Teaching health interpreting in multilingual and multicultural classrooms: Towards developing special pedagogies. Paper delivered at the *AUSIT Jubilation Conference,* Sydney, Australia, 1–3 December 2012.

Crezee, I., Jülich, S. & Hayward, M. (2013). Issues for interpreters and professionals working in refugee settings. *Journal of Applied Linguistics and Professional Practice, 8*(3), 254–273. doi:10.1558/japl.v8i3.253

Department of Health. (2007). *Departmental Report 2007.* London, England: Department of Health. doi:10.1037/e558652010-001

Dijk, T. van. (1977). *Text and context. Explorations in the semantics and pragmatics of discourse.* London, England: Longman. doi:10.1017/s002222670000640x

Dysart-Gale, D. (2007). Clinicians and medical interpreters: Negotiating culturally appropriate care for patients with limited English ability. *Family & Community Health, 30*(3), 237–246. doi:10.1097/01.fch.0000277766.62408.96

Eggleston, K. (2012). Health care for 1.3 billion: An overview of China's health system. Working paper series on health and demographic change in the Asia-Pacific: Stanford University. Walter H. Shorenstein Asia-Pacific Research Center Asia Health Policy Program. Retrieved from http://iis-db.stanford.edu/pubs/23668/AHPPwp_28.pdf

Faden, R. & Beauchamp, T. (1986). *A history and theory of informed consent.* New York, NY: Oxford University Press.

Ferner, S. & Liu, H. (2009). Comprehensive strategy towards delivering better communications and better health care to non-English speaking New Zealanders? *Journal of the New Zealand Medical Association, 122*(1304), 123–125.

Fischbach, H. (Ed.) (1998). *Translation and medicine.* American Translators Association Scholarly Monograph Series. Volume X 1998. Philadelphia, PA: John Benjamins. doi:10.1075/ata.x

Flores G. (2006). Language barriers to health care in the United States. *New England Journal of Medicine, 355*(3), 229–231. doi:10.1056/nejmp058316

Flores, G. (2005). The impact of medical interpreter services on the quality of health care: A systematic review. *Medical Care Research and Review, 62*(3), 255–299. doi:10.1177/1077558705275416

Flores, G., Barton Laws, M. & Mayo, S. (2003). Errors in medical interpretation and their potential clinical consequences in paediatric encounters. *Pediatrics, 111*(1), 6–14. doi:10.1542/peds.111.1.6

Gentile, A., Ozolins, U. & Vasilakakos, M. (1996). *Liaison interpreting: A handbook.* Melbourne, Australia: Melbourne University Press. doi:10.7202/001984ar

Gile, D. (1995). *Basic concepts and models for interpreter and translator training.* Amsterdam: John Benjamins. doi:10.7202/002162ar

Gill, P. S., Shankar, A., Quirke, T. & Fremantle, N. (2009). Access to interpreting services in England: secondary analysis of national data. *BMC Public Health, 9*(1), 12. doi:10.1186/1471-2458-9-12

Ginori, L. & Scimone, E. (1995). *Introduction to interpreting.* Sydney, Australia: Lantern Press.

Gonzalez Davies, M. (2004). *Multiple voices in the translation classroom: Activities, tasks and projects.* Amsterdam: John Benjamins. doi:10.1075/btl.54

Gonzalez Davies, M. (1998). Student assessment by medical specialists. In H. Fischbach (Ed.), *Translation and medicine.* American Translators' Association Scholarly Monograph Series. Volume X 1998, pp. 93–102. Amsterdam: John Benjamins. doi:10.1075/ata.x.11gon

Gray, B., Hilders, J. & Stubbe, M. (2012). How to use interpreters in general practice: The development of a New Zealand toolkit. *Journal of Primary Health Care, 4*(1), 52–61.

Grice, P. (1975). Logic and conversation. In P. Cole & J. Morgan (Eds.), *Syntax and semantics, 3: Speech acts,* pp. 41–58. New York, NY: Academic Press. doi:10.1017/s0022226700005296

Hale, S. (2014). Interpreting culture. Dealing with cross-cultural issues in court interpreting. *Perspectives: Studies in Translatology, 22*(3), 321–331. doi:10.1080/0907676X.2013.827226

Hale, S. (2012). Are we there yet? Taking stock of where we are up to and where we are heading. Jill Blewett Memorial Lecture delivered at the *AUSIT Jubilation Conference,* Sydney, Australia, 1–2 December 2012.

Hale, S. (2008). Controversies over the role of the court interpreter. In C. Valero-Garcés & A. Martin (Eds.), *Crossing borders in community interpreting. Definitions and dilemmas,* pp. 99–122. Amsterdam: John Benjamins. doi:10.1075/btl.76.06hal

Hale, S. (2007). *Community interpreting. Research and practice in Applied Linguistics.* Basingstoke, England: Palgrave Macmillan.

Hale, S. (2005). The interpreter's identity crisis. In J. House, J. R. Martín Ruano & N. Baumgarten (Eds.), *Translation and the construction of identity. IATIS Yearbook 2005,* pp. 14–29. Manchester/Northampton, MA: St Jerome.

Hale, S. (2004). *The discourse of court interpreting: Discourse practices of the law, the witness and the interpreter.* Amsterdam: John Benjamins. doi:10.1075/btl.52

Hale, S. (1996). Pragmatic considerations in court interpreting. *The Australian Review of Applied Linguistics, 19*(1), 61–72.

Hale, S. & Napier, J. (2013). *Research methods in interpreting: A practical resource.* London, England: Bloomsbury.

Hall, E. T. & Hall, M. R. (1990). *Understanding cultural differences.* Yarmouth, ME: Intercultural Press.

Hammell, K. W. (2009). Self-care, productivity, and leisure, or dimensions of occupational experience? Rethinking occupational "categories". *Canadian Journal of Occupational Therapy, 76*(2), 107–114. doi:10.1177/000841740907600208

Health Media. (1988). *Counselling with interpreters sexual Assault interviews.* Sydney, Australia: Department of Health NSW. (Video resource).

Helman, C. (1991). *Culture, health and illness 2.* Oxford, England: Butterworth-Heinemann. doi:10.1046/j.1365–2923.2002.01059.x

Hermann, A. (2002). Interpreting in antiquity. (Translated by Ruth Morris). In F. Pöchhacker & M. Shlesinger (Eds.), *The interpreting studies reader,* pp. 15–22. London, England: Routledge.

HIN (Healthcare Interpretation Network). (2007). *National standard guide for community interpreting services.* Toronto: Healthcare Interpretation Network.

Hofstede, G. H. (2001). *Culture's consequences: Comparing values, behaviors, institutions, and organizations across nations.* Thousand Oaks, CA: Sage Publications.

Hofstede, G. (2003). *Culture's consequences, comparing values, behaviors, institutions, and organizations.* London, England: Sage Publications. doi:10.2307/3556622

Hofstede, G. (1980). *Culture's consequences: International differences in work-related values (cross cultural research and methodology).* London, England: Sage Publications. doi:10.1177/017084068300400409

Holmes, S. (2013). *Fresh fruit, broken bodies. Migrant workers in the United States.* Berkely, CA: University of California Press. doi:10.5250/resilience.1.2.013

Holt, R., Crezee, I. & Rasalingam, N. (2003). *The communication gap: Immigrant healthcare in Aotearoa New Zealand.* Auckland, New Zealand: Auckland University of Technology School of Languages and the New Zealand Federation of Ethnic Councils.

Hunt, L. M. & Voogd, K. B. (2007). Are good intentions good enough? Informed consent without trained interpreters. *Journal of General Internal Medicine, 22*(5), 598–605. doi:10.1007/s11606-007-0136-1

IMIA/MMIA (International Medical Interpreters Association/Massachusetts Medical Interpreters Association) and Education Development Center. (1996). *Medical interpreting standards of practice.* Boston: IMIA/MMIA.

Jackson, K. (2006). *Fate, spirits and curses: Mental health and traditional beliefs in some refugee communities.* Auckland, New Zealand: Rampart.

Johnston, T. & Napier, J. (2010). Medical Signbank – bringing deaf people and linguists together in the process of language development. *Sign Language Studies, 10*(2), 258–275. doi:10.1353/sls.0.0042

Kaufert, J. & Putsch, R. (1997). Communication through interpreters in healthcare: Ethical dilemmasarising from differences in class, culture, language, and power. *Journal of Clinical Ethics, 8*(1), 71–87.

Keesing, R. (1981). *Cultural anthropology: A contemporary perspective.* New York, NY: Holt, Rinehart and Winston. doi:10.1017/s0047404500006023

Ko, W. M. (2013). HK healthcare is a dual-track system. Remarks by Secretary for Food & Health Dr Ko Wing-man at the Asian ministers panel discussion session of the World Health Summit Regional Meeting – Asia in Singapore on April 9. Retrieved from: http://www.news.gov.hk/en/record/html/2013/04/20130409_190409.shtml

Kübler-Ross, E. & Kessler, D. (2008). *On grief and grieving: Finding the meaning of grief through the five stages of loss.* New York, NY: Simon and Schuster.

Kübler-Ross, E. (1969). *On death and dying.* New York, NY: Macmillan. doi:10.1177/004057367002700112

Lai, M., Heydon, G. & Mulayim, S. (2015). Vicarious trauma among interpreters. *International Journal of Interpreter Education, 7*(1), 3–22.

Langdon, H. (2002). *Interpreters and translators in communication disorders; A practitioner's handbook.* Eau Clair, WI: Thinking Publications.

Langdon, H. & Chen, L. L. (2002). *Collaborating with interpreters and translators.* Eau Clair, WI: Thinking Publications.

Lave, J. (1996). Teaching, as learning, in practice. *Mind, Culture, and Activity, 3*(3), 149–164. doi:10.1207/s15327884mca0303_2

Lave, J. (1991). Situated Learning in Communities of Practice. In L. B. Resnick, J. M. Levine & S. D. Teasley (Eds.), *Perspectives on socially shared cognition*, pp. 64–82. Pittsburgh, PA: Learning Research and Development Center, University of Pits-burgh/American Psychological Association.

Lave, J. (1990). Views of the classroom: Implications for math and science learning research. In J. W. Stigler, R. A. Schweder & G. Herdt (Eds.), *Cultural psychology: Essays on comparative human development*, pp. 309–327. Cambridge, England: Cambridge University Press. doi:10.1017/CBO9781139173728.010

Lave, J. & Wenger, E. (1991). *Situated learning: Legitimate peripheral participation.* Cambridge, England: Cambridge University Press. doi:10.1017/cbo9780511815355

Lee, T. Y. & Ballard, E. Y. (2011). Assessing Mandarin speaking clients: cultural and linguistic considerations. *ACQuiring Knowledge in Speech, Language and Hearing, 13*(3), 132–136.

Lee, T., Lansbury, G. & Sullivan, G. (2005). Health care interpreters: A physical therapy perspective. *Australian Journal of Physical therapy, 51,* 161–165. doi:10.1016/s0004-9514(05)70022-2

Lim, S., Mortensen, A., Feng, K., Ryu, G. & Cui, C. (2012). Waitemata DHB cultural responsiveness to its Asian, migrant and refugee populations – cultural competence concepts and initiatives. Paper presented to the *Growing Pacific Solutions Conference*, Auckland, New Zealand, April 2012.

Low, P. K. C. & Ang, S. L. (2010). The foundation of traditional Chinese medicine. *Journal of Chinese Medicine, Scientific Research, 1,* 84–90. Available at SSRN: http://ssrn.com/abstract=1760869. doi:10.4236/cm2010.13016

Mairs, R. (2011). Translator traditor: The interpreter as traitor in classical tradition. *Greece & Rome, 58,* 1. doi:10.1017/s0017383510000537

Major, G., Napier, J., Ferrara, L. & Johnston, T. (2012). Exploring lexical gaps in Australian Sign Language for the purposes of health communication. *Communication & Medicine, 9*(1), 7–47.

Mason, I. (2004). Conduits, mediators, spokespersons: Investigating translator/interpreter. In C. Schäffner (Ed.), *Translation research and interpreting research. Traditions, gaps and synergies*, pp. 88–87. Clevedon, Oh.: Multilingual Matters.

Meador, H. E. & Zazove, P. (2005). Health care interactions with deaf culture. *The Journal of the American Board of Family Practice, 18*(3), 218–222. doi:10.3122/jabfm.18.3.218

Merlini, R. & Favaron, R. (2005). Examining the "voice of interpreting" in speech pathology. *Interpreting, 7*(2), 263–302. doi:10.1075/intp.7.2.07mer

Meyer, B. (2000). *Medizinische Aufklärungsgespräche: Struktur und Zwecksetzung aus diskursanalytischer Sicht.* University of Hamburg, Germany: Sonderforschungsbereich 538 (Mehrsprachigkeit – Working Papers on Multilingualism).

Meyer, B. (2001). How untrained interpreters handle medical terms. In I. Mason (Ed.), *Triadic exchanges: Studies in dialogue interpreting,* pp. 87–106. Manchester/Northampton, MA: St. Jerome.

Meyer, B., Apfelbaum, B., Pöchhacker, F. & Bischoff, A. (2003). Analysing interpreted doctor-patient communication from the perspectives of linguistics, interpreting studies and health sciences. In L. Brunette, G. Bastin, I. Hemlin & H. Clarke (Eds.), *The Critical Link 3. Interpreters in the community,* pp. 67–80. Amsterdam: John Benjamins. doi:10.1075/btl.46.11mey

Morris, R. (1999). The gum syndrome: Predicaments in court interpreting. *Forensic Linguistics, 6*(1), 6–29. doi:10.1558/sll.1999.6.1.6

Napier, J. (2010). An historical overview of signed language interpreting research: Featuring highlights of personal research. *Cadernos de Tradução, 2*(26), 63–97. doi:10.5007/2175-7968.2010v2n26p63

Napier, J. (2011). If a tree falls in a forest and no one is there to hear it, does it make a noise? *Advances in Interpreting Research: Inquiry in Action, 99,* 121. doi:10.1075/btl.99.09nap

Napier, J., Major, G. & Ferrara, L. (2011). Medical Signbank: A cure-all for the aches and pains of medical sign language interpreting? In L. Leeson, S. Wurm & M. Vermeerbergen (Eds.), *Signed language interpreting: Preparation, practice and performance,* pp. 110–137. Manchester, England: St Jerome.

National Center for State Courts (NCSC). (2011). *Guide to translation of legal materials.* Retrieved from http://www.ncsc.org/Topics/Access-and-Fairness/Language-Access/Resource-Guide.aspx.

NCIHC (National Council on Interpreting in Healthcare). (2004). *A national code of ethics for interpreters in health care.* Washington, DC: NCIHC.

National Council on Interpreting in Health Care. (2005). *National standards of practice for interpreters in health care.* San Francisco, CA: NCICH.

National Immigration. (2015). 2015 Outline of the ministry of the interior. Retrieved from: http://www.moi.gov.tw/outline/en-11.html.

O'Neill, M. (1998). Who makes a better medical translator: The medically knowledgeable linguist or the linguistically knowledgeable medical professional? A physician's perspective. In H. Fischbach (Ed.), *American translators association series: Translation and medicine,* pp. 69–80. Amsterdam: John Benjamins. doi:10.1075/ata.x.09one

Ozolins, U. & Hale, S. (2009). Introduction: Quality in interpreting – A shared responsibility. In S. Hale, U. Ozolins & L. Stern (Eds.), *The Critical Link 5: Quality in interpreting – a shared responsibility,* pp. 1–10. Amsterdam: John Benjamins. doi:10.1075/btl.87.01ozo

Pan American Health Organization. (September 2005). Regional declaration on the new orientations of primary health care. Retrieved from http://new.paho.org

Phelan, M. (2001). *The interpreter's resource.* Clevedon, Oh.: Multilingual Matters.

Pöchhacker, F. (2004). *Introducing interpreting studies.* London, England: Routledge. doi:10.1075/intp.6.2.14gar

Pöchhacker, F. & Shlesinger, M. (2007). *Healthcare interpreting: Discourse and interaction.* Amsterdam: John Benjamins. doi:10.1075/bct.9

Pöchhacker, F. & Shlesinger, M. (Eds.) (2002). *The interpreting studies reader.* London, England: Routledge. doi:10.1075/intp.6.1.11ilg

Pritzker, S., Hui, K. & Zhang, H. (2014). *Considerations in the translation of Chinese medicine.* Retrieved 28 January 2016 from: http://cewm.med.ucla.edu/wp-content/uploads/CM-Considerations-4.10.14-FINAL.pdf

Pym, A., Shlesinger, M. & Jettmarová, Z. (2006). *Sociocultural aspects of translating and interpreting.* Amsterdam: John Benjamins. doi:10.1075/btl.67

Risse, G.B. (1999). *Mending bodies, saving souls: A history of hospitals.* Oxford, England and New York, NY: Oxford University Press. doi:10.1056/nejm199911043411921

Roat C. (2000). Healthcare interpreting: An emerging discipline. *ATA Chronicle, 29*(3), 18–21.

Roat C. (1999a). Certifying medical interpreters: Some lessons from Washington State. *ATA Chronicle, 28*(5), 23–26.

Roat, C. (1999b). *Bridging the gap: A basic training for medical interpreters.* Seattle, WA: The Cross Cultural Health Care Program, 1995, 1999.

Roat, C. E., & Crezee, I. (2015). Healthcare interpreting. In H. Mikkelson & R. Jourdenais (Eds.), *Handbook of interpreting*, pp. 236–253. London, England: Routledge.

Roberts-Smith, L., Frey, R. & Bessell-Browne, S. (1990). *Working with interpreters in law, health & social work.* Sydney, Australia: National Accreditation Authority for Translators and Interpreters.

Roy, C. (2002). The problem with definitions, descriptions and the role metaphors of interpreters. In F. Pöchhacker & M. Shlesinger (Eds.), *The interpreting studies reader*, pp. 344–353. London, England: Routledge.

Roy, C. (2000). *Interpreting as a discourse process.* New York, NY: Oxford University Press. doi:10.1017/s0047404501322054

Rudvin, M. (2007). Professionalism and ethics in community interpreting: The impact of individualist versus collective group identity. *Interpreting, 9*(1), 47–69. doi:10.1075/intp.9.1.04rud

Rudvin, M. (2004). Professionalism and contradictions in the interpreter's role. Paper delivered at the Critical Link 4 Conference in Stockholm, 20–23 May 2004.

Samovar, L. A., Porter, R. E., McDaniel, E. R. & Roy, C. S. (2013). *Communication between cultures.* Boston, MA: Cengage Learning.

Sarangi, S. (2004). Towards a communicative mentality in medical and healthcare practice. *Communication & Medicine, 1*(1), 1–11. doi:10.1515/come.2004.002

Scollon, R. & Scollon, S. (2001). *Intercultural communication: A discourse approach.* Malden, MA: Blackwell Publishing. doi:10.1017/s0047404503255056

Searle, J. (1969). *Speech acts.* Cambridge, England: Cambridge University Press. doi:10.1017/s0012217300029073

Searle, J. (1975). Indirect speech acts. In P. Cole & J. Morgan (Eds.), *Syntax and semantics, 3: Speech acts*, pp. 59–82. New York, NY: Academic Press. doi:10.1017/s0022226700005296

Simon, C. M., Zyzanski, S. J. & Durand, E. (2006). Interpreter accuracy and informed consent among Spanish-speaking families with cancer. *Journal of Health Communication, 11*(5), 509–522. doi:10.1080/10810730600752043

Slatyer, H. (2014). Unpublished Ph.D. dissertation. *Multilingual interpreter education. Curriculum design and evaluation.* Macquarie University, Sydney, Australia.

Stewart, M. A. (1995). Effective physician-patient communication and health outcomes: A review. *CMAJ: Canadian Medical Association Journal, 152*(9), 1423–1433.

Strengthening Access to Primary Healthcare (SAPHC). (2006). Literature review: Examining Spanish-speaking patients' satisfaction with interpersonal aspects of care. *Medical Care Research and Review, 62*(3), 255–299.

Sultz, H. A. & Young, K. M. (2006). *Health care USA: Understanding its organization and delivery.* Sudbury, MA: Jones and Bartlett.

Swabey, L. & Nicodemus, B. (2011). Bimodal bilingual interpreting in the US healthcare system. *Advances in Interpreting Research: Inquiry in Action, 99*, 241–260. doi:10.1075/btl.99.14swa

Tate, G. & Turner, G. H. (2002). The code and the culture. Sign language interpreting – in search of the new breed's ethics. In F. Pöchhacker & M. Shlesinger (Eds.), *The interpreting studies reader,* pp. 372–383. London, England: Routledge.

Tebble, H. (2004). Discourse analysis and its relevance to ethical performance in medical interpreting. In C. Wadensjö, B. Dimitrova & A. L. Nilsson (Eds.), *Critical Link 4: Professionalisation of interpreting in the community: 4th International Conference on Interpreting in Legal, Health and Social Service Settings,* p. 57. Amsterdam: John Benjamins. doi:10.1075/intp.10.1.12mik

Tebble. H. (2003). Training doctors to work effectively with interpreters. In L. Brunette, G. Bastin, I. Hemlin & H. Clarke (Eds.), *The Critical Link 3. Interpreters in the community. Selected papers in legal, health and social service settings,* pp. 81–98. Amsterdam: John Benjamins. doi:10.1075/btl.46.12teb

Tebble, H. (1998). *Medical interpreting: Improving communication with your patients.* Canberra and Geelong, Australia: Deakin University.

Tellechea Sánchez, M. T. (2005). El intérprete como obstáculo: Fortalecimiento y emancipación del usuario y para superarlo. In C. Valero Garcés (Ed.), *Traducción como mediación entre lenguas culturas,* pp. 114–122. Alcalá de Henares, Spain: Universidad de Alcalá de Henares.

Tylor, E. G. (1871). *Primitive culture.* New York, NY: J.P. Putnam's Sons.

US Census Bureau. (2011). State and county quick facts. Retrieved from: http://quickfacts.census.gov/qfd/states/00000.html

Valero-Garcés, C. & Martin, A. (Eds.) (2008). *Crossing borders in community interpreting: Definitions and dilemmas.* Amsterdam: John Benjamins. doi:10.1075/btl.76

van Dijk, T. (1977). *Discourse as social interaction. Discourse studies: A multidisciplinary introduction,* Vol. 2. London, England: Sage. doi:10.1177/096394709800700206

Vazquez, C. & Javier, R. (1991). The problem with interpreters: Communications with Spanishspeaking patients. *Hospital and Community Psychiatry, 42,* 163–165.

Venuti, L. (Ed.) (2000). *The translation studies reader.* London, England: Routledge. doi:10.4324/9780203446621

Wadensjö, C. (2002). The double role of a dialogue interpreter. In F. Pöchhacker & M. Shlesinger (Eds.), *The interpreting studies reader,* pp. 354–370. London, England: Routledge.

Wadensjö, C. (1998). *Interpreting as interaction.* London, England & New York, NY: Longman. Waitemata District Health Board (WDHB), Asian Health Support Services (AHSS). (2012). *CALD 9: Working with Asian clients in mental health.* Auckland: Waitemata DHB. Retrieved from http://www.caldresources.org.nz/info/Home.php

Walker, P. F., & Barnett, E. D. (2007). *Immigrant medicine.* Philadelphia, PA: WB Saunders.

Wall, B. M. (n.d.). History of hospitals. Retrieved from http://www.nursing.upenn.edu/nhhc/Welcome%20Page%20Content/History%20of%20Hospitals.pdf

Wiseman, N. A. R. (2000). *Translation of Chinese medical terms: A source-oriented approach.* University of Exeter, England: Unpublished doctoral thesis. Retrieved 28 January 2016 from: http://www.paradigm-pubs.com/sites/www.paradigm-pubs.com/files/files/ex.pdf

Woodward, B. (2006). *State of Denial.* New York, NY: Simon & Schuster.

Wu, T. Y. (2010). An overview of the healthcare system in Taiwan. *London Journal of Primary Care, 2010*(3), 115–119. Retrieved from http://www.kleykampintaiwan.com/files/Social_Issues/TaiwanHealthCareSystem2010.pdf. doi:10.1080/17571472.2010.11493315

Yang, J. M., Ye, N. Y., & Sha, X. H. 楊金滿、葉念雲、沙信輝. (2010). *A study of the execution of the database platform for translation and interpretation professionals. An internal study by the national immigration agency of the ministry of the interior* [通譯人才資料庫使用平台執行情形之研究。內政部入出國及移民署自行研究報告].

Suggested further readings for Parts II and III

Aberg, J. A., Kaplan, J. E., Libman, H., Emmanuel, P., Anderson, J. R., Stone, V. E., Oleske, J. M., Currier, J. S. & Gallant, J. E. (2009). Primary care guidelines for the management of persons infected with human immunodeficiency virus: 2009 update by the HIV medicine Association of the Infectious Diseases Society of America. *Clinical Infectious Diseases, 49*(5), 651–681. doi:10.1086/605292

Abraham, D., Cabral, N. & Tancredi, A. (Eds.) (2004). *A handbook for trainers: language interpreting in the healthcare sector.* Toronto, Canada: Healthcare Interpretation Network.

Alberti, K. G. M. M. & Gries, F. A. (2009). Management of non-insulin-dependent diabetes mellitus in Europe: A concensus view. *Diabetic Medicine, 5*(3), 275–281. doi:10.1111/j.1464–5491.1988.tb00984.x

Albers, J. R., Hull, S. K. & Wesley, R. M. (2004). Abnormal uterine bleeding. *American Family Physician, 69*(8), 1915–1934.

Allman, K. & Wilson, I. (Eds.) (2011). *Oxford handbook of anaesthesia.* Oxford, England: Oxford University Press. doi:10.1093/med/9780199584048.001.0001

American Nurses Association. (2006). *Nursing facts: Today's Registered Nurse – Numbers and demographics.* Washington, DC: American Nurses Association.

American Psychiatric Association. (2013). *Diagnostic and statistical manual of mental disorders* (5th ed.). Arlington, VA: American Psychiatric Publishing. doi:10.1007/s11019-013-9529-6

Anandan, C., Nurmatov, U., van Schayck, O. & Sheikh, A. (2010). Is the prevalence of asthma declining? Systematic review of epidemiological studies. *Allergy, 65*(2), 152–167. doi:10.1111/j.1398–9995.2009.02244.x

Anatomical Chart Company. *The world's best anatomical charts* (3rd ed.). Philadelphia, PA: Lippincott Williams & Wilkins.

Apgar, V. (1953). A proposal for a new method of evaluation of the newborn infant. *Current Research in Anesthesia and Analgesia, 32*(4), 260–267. doi:10.1213/00000539-195301000-00041

Atkinson, F., Foster-Powell, K. & Brand-Miller, J. (2008). International tables of Glycemic Index and Glycemic Load values. *Diabetes Care, 31*(12), 2281–2283. doi:10.2337/dc08-1239

Bancroft, M. (2013). The voice of love. http://www.volinterpreting.org

Beers, M. & Berkow, R. (Eds.) (2000). *The Merck manual of geriatrics* (3rd ed.). New York, NY: John Wiley & Sons.

Bhattacharya, V. (2011). *Postgraduate vascular surgery the candidate's guide to the FRCS.* Leiden, the Netherlands: Cambridge University Press. doi:10.1017/cbo9780511997297

Biggs, W., Bieck, A., Pugno, P. & Crosley, P. (2011). Results of the 2011 national resident matching program: Family medicine. *Family Medicine, 43*(9), 619–624.

Bisno, A. & Stevens, D. (2009). *Streptococcus pyogenes.* In G. Mandell, J. Bennett & R. Dolin (Eds.), *Principles and practice of infectious diseases* (7th ed.). Philadelphia, PA: Elsevier Churchill Livingstone. doi:10.1086/655696

Braddom, R. L. (2011). *Physical medicine and rehabilitation* (4th ed.). Philadelphia, PA: Elsevier/Saunders.

Burgers, J. S., Fervers, B., Haugh, M., Brouwers, M., Browman, G., Philip, T. & Cluzeau, F. A. (2004). International assessment of the quality of clinical practice guidelines in oncology using the appraisal of guidelines and research and evaluation instrument. *Journal of Clinical Oncology*, *22*(10), 2000–2007. doi:10.1200/jco.2004.06.157

Camargo, C. A., Rachelefsky, G. & Schatz, M. (2009). Managing Asthma exacerbations in the emergency department summary of the national Asthma education and prevention program expert panel report 3 guidelines for the management of asthma exacerbations. *Proceedings of the American Thoracic Society*, *6*(4), 357–366. doi:10.1513/pats.p09st2

Camm, A. J., Kirchhof, P., Lip, G. Y., Schotten, U., Savelieva, I., Ernst, S., ... & Folliguet, T. (2010). Guidelines for the management of atrial fibrillation The Task Force for the Management of Atrial Fibrillation of the European Society of Cardiology (ESC). *Europace*, *12*(10), 1360–1420. doi:10.1093/europace/euq350

Chabner, D. E. (2011). *The language of medicine* (9th ed.). Philadelphia, PA: Elsevier/Saunders.

Christian, S., Kraas, J. & Conway, W. (2007). Musculoskeletal infections. *Seminars in Roentgenology* *42*, 92–101. doi:10.1053/j.ro.2006.08.011

Chung, J. H., Phibbs, C. S., Boscardin, W. J., Kominski, G. F., Ortega, A. N. & Needleman, J. (2010). The effect of neonatal intensive care level and hospital volume on mortality of very low birth weight infants. *Medical care*, *48*(7), 635–644. doi:10.1097/mlr.0b013e3181dbe887

Cieza, A. & Stucki, G. (2005). Understanding functioning, disability, and health in rheumatoid arthritis: the basis for rehabilitation care. *Current opinion in rheumatology*, *17*(2), 183–189. doi:10.1097/01.bor.0000151405.56769.e4

Cloherty, J. P., Eichenwald, E. C., Hansen, A. R. & Stark, A. R. (2012). *Manual of neonatal care*. Philadelphia, PA: Lippincott Williams & Wilkins.

Colledge, N., Walker, B. & Ralston, S. (Eds.) (2010). *Davidson's principles and practice of medicine* (21st ed). Edinburg, Scotland: Churchill Livingstone. doi:10.12968/hmed.2011.72.2.117

Craig, D.I. (2008). Medial tibial stress syndrome: Evidence-based prevention. *Journal of Athletic Training*, *43*(3), 316–318. doi:10.4085/1062-6050-43.3.316

Crezee, J., Van Haaren, P., Westendorp, H., De Greef, M., Kok, H., Wiersma, J., Van Stam, G., Sijbrands, J., Zum Vörde Sive Vörding, P., Van Dijk, J., Hulshof, M. & Bel, A. (2009). Improving locoregional hyperthermia delivery using the 3-D controlled AMC-8 phased array hyperthermia system: A preclinical study. *International Journal of Hyperthermia*, *25*(7), 581–592. doi:10.3109/02656730903213374

Davidson, J. E., Powers, K., Hedayat, K. M., Tieszen, M., Kon, A. A., Shepard, E., Spuhler, V., Todres, I. D., Levy, M., Barr, J., Ghandi, R., Hirsch, G. & Armstrong, D. (2007). Clinical practice guidelines for support of the family in the patient-centered intensive care unit: American College of Critical Care Medicine Task Force 2004–2005. *Critical Care Medicine*, *35*(2), 605–622. doi:10.1097/01.ccm.0000254067.14607.eb

Dolk, H., Loane, M. & Garne, E. (2011). Congenital heart defects in Europe: Prevalence and perinatal mortality, 2000 to 2005. *Circulation*, *123*(8), 841–849. doi:10.1161/circulationaha.110.958405

Drake, R. L., Vogl, A. W. & Mitchell, A. W. M. (2010). *Gray's Anatomy for students*. Philadelphia, PA: Churchill Livingstone. doi:10.1016/b978-0-443-06952-9.00003-5

Eddleston, M. & Pierini, S. (2000). *Oxford handbook of tropical medicine* (Vol. 158). New York, NY: Oxford University Press.

Eng, D. (2006). Management guidelines for motor neuron disease patients on non-invasive ventilation at home. *Palliative Medicine*, *20*, 69–79. doi:10.1191/0269216306pm1113oa

Engstrom, P. F., Benson 3rd, A. B., Chen, Y. J., Choti, M. A., Dilawari, R. A., Enke, C. A., Fakih, M. G., Fuchs, C., Kiel, K., Knol, J. A., Leong, L. A., Ludwig, K. A., Martin, E. W. Jr., Rao, S., Saif, M. W., Saltz, L., Skibber, J. M., Venook, A. P. & Yeatman, T. J. (2005). Colon cancer clinical practice guidelines in oncology. *Journal of the National Comprehensive Cancer Network: JNCCN, 3*(4), 468–491.

Faucy, A. (2006). *Harrison's rheumatology.* New York, NY: McGraw-Hill.

Finster, M. & Wood, M. (April 2005). The Apgar score has survived the test of time. *Anesthesiology, 102*(4), 855–857. doi:10.1097/00000542-200504000-00022

Fleisher, G. R. & Ludwig, S. (Eds.) (2010). *Textbook of pediatric emergency medicine.* Philadelphia, PA: Lippincott Williams & Wilkins.

Fleming, S. M., O'Gorman, T., Finn, J., Grimes, H., Daly, K. & Morrison, J. J. (2005). Cardiac troponin I in pre-eclampsia and gestational hypertension. *BJOG: An International Journal of Obstetrics & Gynaecology, 107*(11), 1417–1420. doi:10.1111/j.1471-0528.2000.tb11658.x

Fox, G. F., Hoque, N. & Watts, T. (2010). *Oxford handbook of neonatology.* Oxford, England: Oxford University Press. doi:10.1093/med/9780199228843.003.04

Friedman-Rhodes, E. & Hale, S. (2010). Teaching medical students to work with interpreters. *JoTrans, 14.*

Gallagher, P. F., Barry, P. J., Ryan, C., Hartigan, I. & O'Mahony, D. (2008). Inappropriate prescribing in an acutely ill population of elderly patients as determined by Beers' Criteria. *Age and Ageing, 37*(1), 96–101. doi:10.1093/ageing/afm116

Gérvas, J., Starfield, B. & Heath, I. (2008). Is clinical prevention better than cure? *Lancet, 372,* 1997–99. doi:10.1016/s0140-6736(08)61843-7

Gore, R. M., Levine, M. S. & Laufer, I. (2008). *Textbook of gastrointestinal radiology* (Vol. 1). Philadelphia, PA: Saunders/Elsevier.

Gregory, K. D., Niebyl, J. R. & Johnson, T. R. (2012). Preconception and prenatal care: Part of the continuum. *Obstetrics: Normal and Problem Pregnancies,* 101–124. doi:10.1016/b978-0-443-06930-7.50007-4

Griffiths, J., Austin, L., & Luker, K. (2004). Interdisciplinary teamwork in the community rehabilitation of older adults: an example of flexible working in primary care. *Primary Health Care Research and Development, 5,* 228–239. doi:10.1191/1463423604pc202oa

Hall, B. & Chantigian, R. (2003). *Anesthesia. A comprehensive review.* Philadelphia, PA: Mosby. doi:10.1016/b978-0-323-06857-4.10024-6

Hammer, C., Detwiler, J. S., Detwiler, J., Blood, G. & Dean Qualls, C. (2004). Speech-Language Pathologists' training and confidence in serving Spanish-English Bilingual children. *Journal of Communication Disorders, 37*(2), 91–108. doi:10.1016/j.jcomdis.2003.07.002

Hampton, J. R., Harrison, M. J., Mitchell, J. R., Prichard, J. S., & Seymour, C. (1975). Relative contributions of history-taking, physical examination, and laboratory investigation to diagnosis and management of medical outpatients. *British Medical Journal, 2*(5969), 486–489. doi:10.1136/bmj.2.5969.486

Harris, B., Lovett, L., Newcombe, R., Read, G., Walker, R. & Riad-Fahmy, D. (1994). Maternity blues and major endocrine changes: Cardiff puerperal mood and hormone study II. *British Medical Journal, 308,* 949–953. doi:10.1136/bmj.308.6934.949

Hart, I., Sathasivam, S. & Sharshar, T. (2007). Immunosuppressive agents for myasthenia gravis. *Cochrane Database of Systematic Reviews, 4,* cd005224. doi:10.1002/14651858.cd005224

Heaney, R. & Rafferty, K. (2001). Carbonated beverages and urinary calcium excretion. *American Journal of Clinical Nutrition, 74*(3), 343–347.

Hedrick, J. (2003). Acute bacterial skin infections in pediatric medicine: Current issues in presentation and treatment. *Pediatric Drugs, 5*(Supplement 1), 35–46.

Hwa-Froelich, D. & Westby, C. (2003). Considerations when working with interpreters. *Communication Disorders Quarterly, 24*(2), 78–85. doi:10.1177/15257401030240020401

Isaac, K. (2002). *Speech pathology in cultural and linguistic diversity.* London, England: Whurr. International Classification of Primary Care (ICPC). Retrieved from http://www.globalfamilydoctor.com/wicc/icpcstory.html

Jang, I., Gold, H., Ziskind, A., Fallon, J., Holt, R., Leinbach, R., May, J. & Collen, D. (1989). Differential sensitivity of erythrocyte-rich and platelet-rich arterial thrombitolysis with recombinant tissue-type plasminogen activator. A possible explanation for resistance to coronary thrombolysis. *Circulation, 79*(4), 920–928. doi:10.1161/01.cir.79.4.920

Jenkins, D., Kendall, C., McKeown-Eyssen, G., Josse, R., Silverberg, J. & Booth, G. (2008). Effect of a low–glycemic index or a high–cereal fiber diet on Type 2 Diabetes. *Journal of the American Medical Association, 300*(23), 2742–2753. doi:10.1001/jama.2008.808

Jenkins, D., Wolever, T., Taylor, R., Barker, H., Fielden, H. Baldwin, J., Bowling, A, Newman, H., Jenkins, A. & Goff, D. (1981). Glycemic index of foods: A physiological basis for carbohydrate exchange. *American Journal of Clinical Nutrition, 34,* 362–366.

Johnston, M. (2011). Encephalopathies. In R. Kliegman, R. Behrman, H. Jenson & B. Stanton (Eds.), *Nelson textbook of pediatrics* (19th ed.). Philadelphia, PA: Saunders Elsevier.

Jones, R., Hunt, C., Stevens, R., Dalrymple, J., Driscoll, R., Sleet, S., & Smith, J. B. (2009). Management of common gastrointestinal disorders: quality criteria based on patients' views and practice guidelines. *The British Journal of General Practice, 59*(563), e199. doi:10.3399/bjgp09x420761

Kaemmerer, H., Meisner, H., Hess, J. & Perloff, J. (2004). Surgical treatment of patent ductus arteriosus: a new historical perspective. *American Journal Of Cardiology, 94*(9), 1153–1154. doi:10.1016/j.amjcard.2004.07.082

Kambanaros, M. & van Steenbrugge, W. (2004). Interpreters and language assessment: Confrontation naming and interpreting. *Advances in Speech-Language Pathology, 6*(4), 247–252. doi:10.1080/14417040400010009

Kauffman, T. J. & Barr, M. M. (Eds.) (2007). *Geriatric rehabilitation manual* (2nd ed.). Edinburgh, Scotland & New York, NJ: Churchill Livingstone Elsevier.

Kemp, C. & Rasbridge, L. (2004). *Refugee and immigrant health: A handbook for health professionals.* Cambridge, England: Cambridge University Press.

Kingsnorth, A. (2011). *Fundamentals of surgical practice: A preparation guide for the Intercollegiate MRCS Examination.* Leiden, the Netherlands: Cambridge University Press. doi:10.1017/cbo9780511984785

Kitzmiller, J. L., Wallerstein, R., Correa, A., & Kwan, S. (2010). Preconception care for women with diabetes and prevention of major congenital malformations. *Birth Defects Research Part A: Clinical and Molecular Teratology, 88*(10), 791–803. doi:10.1002/bdra.20734

Kussmaul, W. G. (2012). Guidelines on diagnosis and treatment of stable Ischemic Heart Disease: Keeping up with a constantly evolving evidence base. *Annals of Internal Medicine, 157*(10), 749–751. doi:10.7326/0003-4819-157-10-201211200-00015

Langdon, H. & Quintanar-Sarellana, R. (2003). Roles and responsibilities of the interpreter in interactions with Speech-Language Pathologists, parents, and students. *Seminars in Speech and Language, 24*(3), 235–244. doi:10.1055/s-2003-42826

Leeseberg Stamler, L. & Yiu, L. (2005). *Community health nursing: A Canadian perspective.* Upper Saddle River, NJ: Prentice Hall.

Longmore, M., Wilkinson, I., Davidson, E., Foulkes, A. & Mafi, A. (2010). *Oxford handbook of clinical medicine*. Oxford, England: Oxford University Press. doi:10.1093/med/9780199232178.001.0001

Longo, D. (2012). *Harrisons online: Principles of internal medicine*. New York, NY: McGraw-Hill. Mancia, G., Laurent, S., Agabiti-Rosei, E., Ambrosioni, E., Burnier, M., Caulfield, M.J., Cifkova, R., Clément, D., Coca, A., Dominiczak, A., Erdine, S., Fagard, R., Farsang, C., Grassi, G., Haller, H., Heagerty, A., Kjeldsen, S.E., Kiowski, W., Mallion, J.M., Manolis, A., Narkiewicz, K., Nilsson, P., Olsen, M.H., Rahn, K.H., Redon, J., Rodicio, J., Ruilope, L., Schmieder, R.E., Struijker-Boudier, H.AJ., van Zwieten, P.A., Viigimaa, M. & Zanchetti, A. (2009). Reappraisal of European guidelines on hypertension management: a European Society of Hypertension Task Force document. *Journal of Hypertension, 27*(11), 2121–2158. doi:10.1097/hjh.0b013e328333146d

Martinez, G. (2008). Language-in-healthcare policy, interaction patterns, and unequal care on the U.S.-Mexico border. *Language Policy, 7*, 345–363. doi:10.1007/s10993-008-9110-y

Marx, J., Hockberger, R. & Walls, R. (2009). *Rosen's emergency medicine-concepts and clinical practice* (7th ed.). Maryland Heights, MI: Mosby/Elsevier. doi:10.1016/b978-0-323-05472-0.00205-x

Mayo Clinic. (2012). Cholesterol levels. Retrieved 28 June 2012 from http://www.mayoclinic.com/health/cholesterol-levels/CL00001.

McLatchie, G., Borley, N. & Chikwe, J. (2007). *Oxford handbook of clinical surgery*. Oxford, England: Oxford University Press. doi:10.1093/med/9780198568254.003.0011

McVary K., Roehrborn C., Avins A.L., et al. (2011). Update on AUA guideline on the management of benign prostatic hyperplasia. *Journal of Urology, 185*(5), 1793–1803. Epub 2011 Mar 21. doi:10.1016/j.juro.2011.01.074

Melman, A. & Newnham, R. (2011). *A what-comes-next guide to a safe and informed recovery*. New York, NY: Oxford University Press.

Miller, D. & Leary, S. (2007). Primary-progressive multiple sclerosis. *Lancet Neurology, 6*, 903–912. doi:10.1016/s1474-4422(07)70243-0

Miller, B. (2010). *General surgical lists and reminders*. Brisbane, Australia: University of Queensland Press.

Nicodemus, B. (2009). *Prosodic markers and utterance boundaries in American Sign Language interpretation*. Washington, DC: Gallaudet University Press. doi:10.1075/sll.16.1.04dac

Nicolaides, K. H., Syngelaki, A., Ashoor, G., Birdir, C. & Touzet, G. (2012). Noninvasive prenatal testing for fetal trisomies in a routinely screened first-trimester population. *American Journal of Obstetrics and Gynecology, 206*(2012), 322.e1–322.e15. doi:10.1016/j.ajog.2012.08.033

Nursing and Midwifery Council. (2010). *Changes to pre-registration nursing programmes: FAQs*. Nursing and Midwifery Council. Retrieved from http://nmc-uk.org

Qaseem, A., Fihn, S. D., Williams, S., Dallas, P., Owens, D. K. & Shekelle, P. (2012). Diagnosis of stable Ischemic Heart Disease: Summary of a clinical practice guideline from the American College of Physicians/American College of Cardiology Foundation/American Heart Association/American Association for Thoracic Surgery/Preventive Cardiovascular Nurses Association/Society of Thoracic Surgeons. *Annals of Internal Medicine, 157*(10), 729–734. doi:10.7326/0003-4819-157-10-201211200-00010

Qureshi, A. (2011). *Textbook of interventional neurology*. Leiden, the Netherlands: Cambridge University Press. doi:10.1017/CBO9780511975844

Ramos, G. A., Chopra, I. J. & Bales, S. R. (2012). Endocrine disorders in pregnancy. *Women's health review: A clinical update in Obstetrics-Gynecology (Expert Consult-Online)*, 226–234.

Ramsay, N. A., Kenny, M. W., Davies, G. & Patel, J. P. (2005). Complimentary and alternative medicine use among patients starting warfarin. *British Journal of Haematology, 130*(5), 777–780. doi:10.1111/j.1365-2141.2005.05689.x

Reiss, U., Zucker, M. & Hanley, J. (2002). *Natural hormone balance for women*. New York, NY: Atria Books.

Robertson, A. (1998). *Preparing for birth: Background notes for pre-natal classes* (3rd ed). Glebe, Australia: Ace Graphics.

Roehrborn, C. (2011). Male lower urinary tract symptoms (LUTS) and benign prostatic hyperplasia (BPH). *Medical Clinics of North America, 95*(1), 87–100. doi:10.1016/j.mcna.2010.08.013

Roseberry-McKibbin, C. (2002). *Multicultural students with special language needs* (2nd ed.). Oceanside, CA: Academic Associates.

Schenker, Y., Wang, F., Selig, S. J., Ng, R. & Fernandez, A. (2007). The impact of language barriers on documentation of informed consent at a hospital with on-site interpreter services. *Journal of General Internal Medicine, 22*(Suppl 2), 294–299. doi:10.1007/s11606-007-0359-1

Sinclair, A. & Dickinson, E. (1998). *Effective practice in rehabilitation: The evidence of systematic reviews*. King's Fund.

Singh, J., Christensen, R., Wells, G., Suarez-Almazor, M., Buchbinder, R., Lopez-Olivo, M., Tanjong Ghogomu, E. & Tugwell, P. (2012). Update of the 2008 ACR recommendations for use of DMARDs and biologics in the treatment of Rheumatoid Arthritis. *Arthritis Care & Research*, 625–639. doi:10.1002/14651858.cd007848.pub2

Smyth, R. & Openshaw, P. (2006). Bronchiolitis. *Lancet, 368*(9532), 312–322. doi:10.1016/s0140-6736(06)69077-6

Sobin, L., Gospodarowicz, M. & Wittekind C. (Eds.) (2009). *TNM Classification of Malignant Tumors* (7th ed.). Oxford, England: Wiley-Blackwell.

Soper, N. & Kaufman, D. (2011). *Northwestern handbook of surgical procedures*. Evanston, Ill.: Northwestern University.

Sperry, L. (2006). *Cognitive behavior therapy of DSM-IV-TR personality disorders 2*. New York, NY: Routledge. doi:10.4324/9780203961582

Tanner, J. M., Whitehouse, R. H. & Hughes, P. C. R. (1976). Relative importance of growth hormone and sex steroids for the growth at puberty of trunk length, limb length, and muscle width in growth hormone-deficient children. *The Journal of pediatrics, 89*(6), 1000–1008. doi:10.1016/s0022-3476(76)80620-8

Tarrant, A., Ryan, M., Hamilton, P. & Bejaminov, O. (2008). A pictorial review of hypovolaemic shock in adults. *British Journal of Radiology, 81*, 252–257. doi:10.1259/bjr/40962054

Tasker, R. C., McClure, R. J. & Acerini, C. L. (2013). *Oxford handbook of paediatrics*. Oxford, England: Oxford University Press. doi:10.1093/med/9780199608300.001.0001

Tesio, L. U. I. G. I. (2007). Functional assessment in rehabilitative medicine: Principles and methods. *Europa Medicophysica, 43*(4), 515–523.

Turner, S., Paton, J., Higgins, B. & Douglas, G. (2011). British guidelines on the management of asthma: What's new for 2011? *Thorax, 66*(12), 1104–1105. doi:10.1136/thoraxjnl-2011-200213

University of Virginia. (2013). *Refusal of treatment of minors*. Retrieved from: http://www.med-ed. virginia.edu/courses/rad/consent/4/refusal_of_treatment.html

Van Tulder, M., Malmivaara, A. & Koes, B. (2007). Repetitive strain injury. *Lancet, 369*(9575), 1815–1822. doi:10.1016/s0140-6736(07)60820-4

Varney, H., Kriebs, J. M. & Gegor, C. L. (2004). *Varney's Midwifery* (4th ed.). Burlington, MA: Jones & Bartlett Learning. doi:10.1016/j.jmwh.2003.10.021

Walker, P. F. & Barnett, E. D. (2007). *Immigrant medicine*. Philadelphia, PA: WB Saunders.

Weng, Y. H., Chiu, Y. W. & Cheng, S. W. (2012). Breast milk jaundice and maternal diet with Chinese herbal medicines. *Evidence-Based Complimentary and Alternative Medicine*, 1–6. doi:10.1155/2012/150120

Wiemels, J. (2012). Perspectives on childhood leukemia. *Chemico-biological Interactions* 2012 Apr 5; *196*(3), 59–67. doi:10.1016/j.cbi.2012.01.007. Epub 2012 Feb 2

Wiesel, S. W. & Delahay, J. N. (Eds.) (2010). *Essentials of orthopedic surgery.* New York, NY: Springer.
Wyatt, J. P., Illingworth, R. N., Graham, C. A. & Hogg, K. (2012). *Oxford handbook of emergency medicine.* Oxford, England: Oxford University Press. doi:10.1093/med/9780199589562.001.0001

Xiong, L. (2009). Complete lung whiteout. *Nursing Critical Care*, July 1, 2009. doi:10.1097/01.ccn.0000357490.54310.68

Useful websites

Websites which are managed by bona fide professional bodies are an extremely useful source of information, as information tends to be continually updated and reviewed by the relevant (medical) professionals. Some recommended websites are:

American Association for Thoracic Surgery (AATS): http://www.aats.org/ American College of Cardiology: http://www.cardiosource.org/acc American College of Emergency Physicians: http://www.acep.org/ American College of Gastroenterology: http://gi.org/

American College of Radiology: http://www.acr.org/

American College of Rheumatology: http://www.rheumatology.org/ American College of Surgeons: http://www.facs.org/

American Congress of Obstetricians and Gynecologists (ACOG): http://www.acog.org/ American Heart Association (AHA): http://www.heart.org/HEARTORG/

American Pregnancy Association: http://www.americanpregnancy.org/ American Society for Reproductive Medicine (ASRM): http://www.asrm.org/

Canadian Medical Association: http://www.cma.ca

Cancer Topics. National Cancer Institute: http://www.cancer.gov/cancertopics/ Clinical Nutrition Certification Board: http://www.cncb.org/

Graduate Medical School Admissions Test: http://www.gamsatuk.org/

Harrison's Online on Access Medicine: http://www.accessmedicine.com/public/learnmore_hol.aspx Health Resources and Services Administration. Maternal and Child health: http://mchb.hrsa.gov/

International Council of Nurses (ICN). http:// www.icn.ch/ National Cancer Institute at the National Institutes of Health.

National Council on Interpreting in Health Care. http://www.ncihc.org/

National Digestive Diseases Information Clearinghouse (NDDIC): http://digestive.niddk.nih.gov/ National Eye Institute: http://www.nei.nih.gov/

National Kidney Disease Education Program (NKEDEP): http://www.nkdep.nih.gov

Useful websites re healthcare insurance:

Glossary of Health Coverage and Medical Terms. (2014). http://www.dol.gov/ebsa/pdf/SBCUniform Glossary.pdf Accessed May 30, 2014.

Health Information Privacy. (2014) http://www.hhs.gov/ocr/privacy/ Accessed May 29, 2014.

Health Pocket: Top 10 Healthcare Services Excluded Under Obamacare. (2014). http://www.health pocket.com/healthcare-research/infostat/top-10-excluded-services-obamacare#.U5pUPm wLCc Accessed September 18, 2014.

Medicaid.gov: Keeping America Healthy. (2014). http://www.medicaid.gov/ Accessed May 30, 2014

Medicare.gov: The Official U.S. Government Website for Medicare. (2014). https://www.medicare.gov/ Accessed May 30, 2014.

Veterans Health Administration. (2014). http://www.va.gov/health/aboutVHA.asp Accessed September 18, 2014.

Useful websites professional organizations

American Translators Association (ATA): http://ata.net.org Auslan Medical Signbank: http://www.auslan.org.au/medical/ http://www.avlic.ca/ethics-and-guidelines

HIN – Healthcare Interpreter Network www.hcin.org

Healthcare Interpretation Network healthcareinterpretationnetwork.ca/ NCIHC – National Council on Interpreting in Health Care www.ncihc.org IMIA – International Medical Interpreters Association www.imiaweb.org

ILCA – International Lactation Consultant Association. http://www.ilca.org/i4a/pages/index.cfm?pageid=1

Interpreting in health care settings: http://healthcareinterpreting.org/new/ Medical Interpreting: www.medicalinterpreting.org

Useful websites for health information (continually updated)

North American Registry of Midwives: http://www.narm.org

MedlinePlus: Health information from the National Library of Medicine http://www.nlm.nih.gov/ medlineplus/

PubMed MEDLINEV: http://www.ncbi.nlm.nih.gov/pubmed/

Society for Cardiovascular Angiography and Interventions (SCAI) http://www.scai.org/Default. aspx   The American Board of Family Medicine: https://www.theabfm.org/

The Mayo Clinic: http://www.mayoclinic.com/

The Merck Manual Illustrated:. http://www.merckmanuals.com

U.S. Department of Health and Human Services, Centers for Medicare & Medicaid Services:

U.S. National Library of Medicine. National Institutes of Health. http://www.nlm.nih.gov/

US Centers for Disease Control and Prevention: http://www.cdc.gov/ US National Library of Medicine http://www.nlm.nih.gov.

World Health Organization (WHO): http://www.who.int

National Heart, Lung and Blood Institute. http://www.nhlbi.nih.gov/health/

Index